Psychonephrology

Ana Hategan • James A. Bourgeois
Azim S. Gangji • Tricia K.W. Woo
Editors

Psychonephrology

A Guide to Principles and Practice

Springer

Editors
Ana Hategan
Department of Psychiatry and Behavioral Neurosciences
McMaster University
Hamilton, ON, Canada

James A. Bourgeois
Department of Psychiatry
Baylor Scott and White Health
Central Texas Division
Temple, TX, USA

Azim S. Gangji
Department of Medicine
McMaster University
Hamilton, ON, Canada

Tricia K.W. Woo
Department of Medicine
McMaster University
Hamilton, ON, Canada

ISBN 978-3-030-84739-5 ISBN 978-3-030-84740-1 (eBook)
https://doi.org/10.1007/978-3-030-84740-1

This Springer imprint is published by the registered company Springer Nature Switzerland AG
The registered company address is: Gewerbestrasse 11, 6330 Cham, Switzerland

Foreword

I was thrilled by Dr. Ana Hategan and her colleagues' decision to use the word "psychonephrology" in the title of this impressive textbook, and when they extended an invitation to me to provide a brief history of the term.

When the formidable internist, Dr. Eli Friedman, decided to institute one of the first dialysis units in the United States at SUNY Downstate Medical Center, in Brooklyn, New York, he approached two of my consultation-liaison psychiatry mentors, Drs. Franz Reichsman and Norman Levy.

"I have a problem," he announced. "Help me decide who is going to live, and who is going to die."

In the early 1960s, Dr. Belding Scribner, a nephrologist at the University of Washington Medical School, had developed the first shunt, allowing patients to receive continuous dialysis of their blood. Insertion of the simple plastic tube was nothing less than a medical miracle for people with end-stage renal disease (ESRD).

A *Life Magazine* article[1] about the artificial kidney caught the public's attention when it described the "ugly" ESRD death that John Myers, 37, had been facing: "his heart was pounding violently. He could not stop coughing. Blood was running from his nose. He had an indescribable headache, a horrible taste in his mouth, dreadful nausea. His face and lips were grossly swollen."

But instead of dying, Seattle's experimental outpatient dialysis program—2 nights/week of 10 to 12 hours of treatment—allowed Myers to resume working and to continue being a loving presence in the lives of his wife and three children.

By the summer of 1961, the medical team in Washington State had established a novel double-screening process for potential patients that selected Myers for treatment. The seven lay members of the "Life or Death Committee" consisted of a lawyer, minister, banker, homemaker, official of state government, labor leader, and surgeon. Their task was to identify patients for the handful of available dialysis slots. A medical evaluation board first screened out children, adults over 45, and physically and psychiatrically unsuitable patients. The committee then performed their Solomonic undertaking by examining the patient's age and sex, marital status,

[1]Alexander S. They decide who lives, who dies: Medical miracle puts a moral burden on a small committee. Life Magazine. 1962; November 9: 102-125. https://www.originallifemagazines.com/product/life-magazine-november-9-1962/.

and number of dependents, income, net worth, emotional stability with regard to the capacity to accept treatment, educational background, and occupation.

Journalists dubbed the committee the "God squad," and they were amazed at the humility and compassion evidenced by its members as they went about their unique assignment. However, critics also surfaced who were displeased that the choice of candidates was based to some degree on "good citizenship," which led, for example, to the selection of married churchgoers with children, while immediately excluding single men with criminal records.

Politicians paid attention to both the good and bad publicity, and in 1972, Congress agreed that *all* US patients with ESRD would qualify for Medicare. The availability of government funding promptly led to a rapid growth of dialysis programs throughout the country. Within a couple of years, the unavailability of dialysis facilities had become a historical footnote, as was the "God squad"—although the latter became the model for today's bioethics consultation services.

The infusion of Federal funds impacted Dr. Friedman's research and clinical goals, and his request to Drs. Reichsman and Levy changed accordingly. Instead of trying to get them to duplicate Seattle's double tiered system, they were asked to limit the screening process to identifying patients who did not have psychoses and could reasonably comply with the treatment's basic requirements.

As dialysis programs sprung up around the world, Dr. Levy and others recognized that they would benefit from a multidisciplinary team approach involving nephrologists, renal nurses, and social workers supplemented by input from psychiatrists and psychologists. Dr. Levy decided that a forum to discuss psychosocial issues would be valuable, and he came up with the term "psychonephrology." A series of international conferences were initiated bearing that name.

The first of these was held in 1978 in the largest available room at Downstate—the gymnasium—and featured a psychiatric colleague from Hadassah Medical Center. During subsequent conferences, the subjects included: psychological aspects related to dependence on a machine, depression, suicide and noncompliance, delirium, anxiety and panic, sexual disorders, and disruptive behavior.

Dr. Levy—now 89 years old—is sufficiently proud of the word psychonephrology, which he legally registered as a trademark. He recently told me with a delightful chuckle how pleased he is to allow the textbook's editors to make use of it!

The 11th International Conference of Psychonephrology was the final meeting coordinated by Dr. Levy, and it convened in 2000 in Yokohama, Japan. I was fortunate to attend and presented on a prospective study of dialysis discontinuation and my team's efforts to integrate palliative care.

In the two decades since, it has been thrilling to see how the field continues to evolve. The topics covered in this textbook represent a magnificent expansion of psychonephrology, and they should be a source of pride for everyone connected with this ambitious project. Like the original series of conferences, this book will be a treasured resource for its readers.

Northampton, MA, USA Lew Cohen

Preface

Patients with chronic kidney disease, including end-stage kidney disease, face various comorbid psychiatric illnesses, in addition to personal and social burdens, during the time leading up to dialysis and/or renal transplantation[1]. These patients may experience high levels of distress due to their chronic complex health issues, including a high risk for comorbid depressive disorder, delirium, and vascular major neurocognitive disorder (formerly vascular dementia). They also frequently suffer from medication side effects, from both systemic and central nervous system-active medications.

In renal transplant patients, specific stressors commonly include situational anxiety associated with placement on the transplant wait list, ongoing health complications and hospitalizations, worry of eventual organ rejection and subsequent graft failure, plus a significant risk of psychiatric side effects of the required post-transplant immunomodulators. It is the duty of all nephrology clinicians to be aware of these problems and to inquire about them, so that the appropriate involvement of psychiatric consultants and other mental health clinicians can be coordinated for optimally collaborative multispecialty and multidisciplinary care.

Moreover, dialysis patients have high rates of comorbid depressive disorder, anxiety disorder, delirium, and other neurocognitive disorders. As a result, they have three times higher risk of hospitalization, compared to those with other chronic systemic illnesses, resulting in significantly higher overall mortality rates[2]. However, even acknowledging this likely *still underestimate*s the burden of comorbid psychiatric illness in this population. Patients with end-stage kidney disease have a high central nervous system symptom comorbidity burden. These patients experience multiple psychiatric symptoms, which significantly impact their quality of life, health outcomes, and overall daily function.

"Psychonephrology" is a term encompassing concepts from the specialties of nephrology and psychiatry, mainly based on the concept of consultation-liaison psychiatry within the biopsychosocial model of mind-body unity. Norman B. Levy, a leading authority on the psychological aspects of kidney transplantation and

[1] Simões E Silva AC, Miranda AS, Rocha NP, Teixeira AL. Neuropsychiatric disorders in chronic kidney disease. Front Pharmacol. 2019;10:932.

[2] Kimmel PL, Fwu CW, Abbott KC, et al. Psychiatric illness and mortality in hospitalized ESKD dialysis patients. Clin J Am Soc Nephrol. 2019;14:1363–1371.

dialysis treatment, is considered the "father of psychonephrology."[3] The editors and chapter authors owe Dr. Levy a debt of gratitude for the original conceptualization and nomenclature describing psychonephrology[3]. In the decades since the term was introduced, it has become evident that psychiatry and nephrology have significant clinical intersection far beyond the original focus on psychological factors and psychiatric illness in the context of chronic kidney disease and dialysis. There has been a great deal of advancement in the availability of kidney transplant, making it available to a broader range of patients, including those with chronic psychiatric illness antedating their kidney disease. The specific nephrotoxic effects of the important psychotropic medication lithium are commonly seen and appreciated clinically. The numerous psychiatric side effects of immunomodulators are now well understood in the post-op kidney transplant patient. Several psychotropic medications are either avoided or dosed more conservatively in renal disease patients. The editors of this book, therefore, take a modern, expansive, and inclusive stance on psychonephrology to reflect the current clinical literature and practice. Ultimately, it is their hope that this book will lead to more regular conceptual focus on the term and the field, beyond the clinical pragmatism which also is emphasized.

Written and edited by academic psychiatrists, nephrologists, geriatricians, family physicians, psychologists, and medical educators, ***Psychonephrology: A Guide to Principles and Practice*** covers three main domains: (i) psychiatric pharmacotherapy for treatment of patients with "primary" psychiatric disorders and interventions adversely affecting the kidneys and medication adjustments due to comorbid kidney disease; (ii) interventions for complex and often multiple psychiatric comorbidity of chronic kidney disease and transplant patients; and (iii) mental health care for clinicians *themselves* involved in the care of patients with end-stage kidney disease, dialysis, and transplantation.

In this book, the term "gender" is used to reflect socially constructed distinctions among male and female, as well as other genders, while the term "sex" is used to reflect primarily biological/anatomic/hormonal constructs. The editors appreciate that there is much progress in both the biological sciences and social sciences in these areas and the accompanying language continues to evolve accordingly. While gender and sex are not the main foci of the book, the editors seek to use the language in this way in this book. Furthermore, regarding terminology employed, "end-stage kidney disease" is also known as "end-stage renal disease," and these two terms are used interchangeably in this volume. The book's key features include content-specific guidance, easy-to-reference advice, and illustrative clinical vignettes. The vignettes are either created extemporaneously for this book and/or are composites of cases of the authors. Any similarity to real/actual cases in the clinical vignettes presented in the volume is purely coincidental.

This book focuses on pharmacological and non-pharmacological approaches of psychiatric syndromes that commonly occur in patients with kidney disease. These patients typically have multiple needs that differ among individuals based on the complexity of their illness, as well as caregiver supports and resources available to

[3] Levy NB. What is psychonephrology? J Nephrol. 2008;21 Suppl 13:S51–53.

them. The coexistence of psychiatric syndromes in kidney disease patients who require specialized medical treatments represents a challenge to nephrologists regarding diagnosis and ongoing treatment. Since few studies relating to the treatment of psychiatric disorders occurring in patients with end-stage kidney disease have been reported, general recommendations for treating these patients have been usually based upon clinical outcomes among those *without* chronic kidney disease.

Therefore, principles of psychotherapy and psychopharmacology are reviewed, with emphasis on organ impairment and drug-drug interactions specific to nephrology. For example, the book discusses the psychopharmacokinetics of medications used to treat patients with chronic kidney disease, which requires special consideration of the route of elimination, volume of distribution of the drug, hydrophilicity, and drug-protein binding; all these are factors that affect the ability to dialyze a drug.

Kidney transplant patients may experience the same psychiatric problems as many other groups of patients. However, the immunotherapy used in kidney transplant recipients may induce psychiatric adverse effects, which require independent management. Poor patient adherence to prescribed medications and other aspects of medical treatment post-transplant can adversely affect the transplant outcomes. Therefore, this book covers issues with medication nonadherence in patients with chronic kidney disease and psychiatric comorbidity, as well as the associated issues in dialysis and renal transplantation.

The medicolegal context for the practice of medicine is ever-changing. This desirable trend reflects tremendous progress in management of these illnesses, as well as a greater focus on comorbidity, appreciation of the social determinants of health, and greater integration of bioethical principles into clinical decision-making. Clinically based matters such as including bioethics committees; deliberations regarding discussion on patients' wishes to decline, discontinue, or withhold dialysis and palliative care; and issues of patient's capacity for decision-making during the time leading up to kidney transplantation and other inflection points in clinical management are often complex and strictly regulated, and are discussed in depth. The book also covers various additional topics addressing an active stance towards health promotion in chronically ill patients, including the critical role of the diet and physical activity. Such advice is often complex and changing depending on the stage of chronic kidney disease and the individual needs of the patient.

The goal of care is to have patients with kidney disease empowered and fully included in a shared-care model or collaborative care model between psychiatric and nephrology/transplant services. Implementing a collaborative care model for kidney patients with psychiatric comorbidity has important implications for nephrology practice. Such collaboration between specialties may reduce burden on dialysis and transplant centers and allows resources to be distributed more efficiently in the benefit of the patient. The shared care between specialized services in nephrology and psychiatry (either the consultation-liaison psychiatry service in the hospital setting, or the community psychiatry service in the outpatient setting) should also improve accessibility to care. A collaborative environment between these medical specialties is much needed to meet the patient's complex care needs, with a more coordinated approach to patient care.

Interspecialty and interdisciplinary collaboration among psychiatrists, nephrologists, transplant surgeons, and other clinicians to address renal patients' health problems is promoted throughout this book. It is the editors' hope that further development of the role and place of psychonephrology within medical practice will help to maintain higher quality care and quality of life of renal patients with psychosocial stressors and psychiatric comorbidity. The editors hope that this book becomes a valuable reference and teaching tool that provides an opportunity for learning across a rapidly evolving medical field.

Hamilton, ON, Canada — Ana Hategan
Temple, TX, USA — James A. Bourgeois
Hamilton, ON, Canada — Azim S. Gangji
Hamilton, ON, Canada — Tricia K. W. Woo

Contents

Contributors

Sehrish Ali Section of Nephrology, Department of Medicine, Baylor College of Medicine, Houston, TX, USA

Section of Nephrology, Michael E. DeBakey Veterans Affairs Medical Center, Houston, TX, USA

James A. Bourgeois Department of Psychiatry, Baylor Scott & White Health, Central Texas Division, Department of Medical Education, College of Medicine, Texas A&M University Health Science Center, Temple, TX, USA

Teresa M. Chan Division of Education & Innovation/Division of Emergency Medicine, Department of Medicine & Office of Continuing Development, Faculty of Health Sciences, McMaster University, Hamilton, ON, Canada

Natasha N. Dave Strive Health, Denver, CO, USA

Alan Eppel Department of Psychiatry & Behavioural Neurosciences, McMaster University, St. Joseph's Hospital, Hamilton, ON, Canada

Azim S. Gangji Division of Nephrology, Department of Medicine, McMaster University, St. Joseph's Healthcare Hamilton, Hamilton, ON, Canada

Emma Gregory Department of Psychiatry and Behavioural Neurosciences, Michael G. DeGroote School of Medicine, McMaster University, Hamilton, ON, Canada

Ana Hategan Division of Geriatric Psychiatry, Department of Psychiatry & Behavioural Neurosciences, Faculty of Health Sciences, Michael G. DeGroote School of Medicine, McMaster University, Hamilton, ON, Canada

Calvin H. Hirsch Division of General Medicine (Geriatrics), University of California Davis Medical Center, Sacramento, CA, USA

Poh Choo How Department of Psychiatry and Behavioral Sciences, University of California, Davis, Sacramento, CA, USA

Briana S. Howarth Geriatric & Consultation Liaison Psychiatry, Halton Healthcare, Oakville, ON, Canada

Department of Psychiatry & Behavioural Neurosciences, McMaster University, Hamilton, ON, Canada

Meera Joseph Division of Nephrology, Department of Medicine, McMaster University, St. Joseph's Healthcare Hamilton, Hamilton, ON, Canada

Nick Kates Department of Psychiatry and Behavioural Neurosciences, Michael G. DeGroote School of Medicine, McMaster University, Hamilton, ON, Canada

Jelena P. King Department of Psychiatry & Behavioural Neurosciences, St. Joseph's Healthcare Hamilton, Clinical Neuropsychology Services, Hamilton, ON, Canada

Julia Danielle Kulikowski Department of Psychiatry and Behavioural Neurosciences, McMaster University, Hamilton, ON, Canada

Vanessa Lentz Department of Psychiatry and Behavioural Neurosciences, Michael G. DeGroote School of Medicine, Faculty of Health Sciences, McMaster University & St. Joseph's Healthcare Hamilton, Hamilton, ON, Canada

Margaret Leung Department of Palliative Care Services, Kaiser Permanente, Roseville, CA, USA

Anika Lucas Division of Nephrology, Department of Medicine, Duke University School of Medicine, Durham, NC, USA

Shyam Maharaj Department of Medicine, McMaster University, Hamilton, ON, Canada

Lynda Marfisi Hemodialysis Program, Grand River Hospital, Kitchener, ON, Canada

Heather E. McNeely Department of Psychiatry and Behavioural Neurosciences, McMaster University, St. Joseph's Healthcare Hamilton, Clinical Neuropsychology Services, Hamilton, ON, Canada

Vishnu P. Parvathareddy Section of Nephrology, Department of Medicine, Baylor College of Medicine, Houston, TX, USA

Stanislav Pasyk Department of Psychiatry and Behavioural Neurosciences, Michael G. DeGroote School of Medicine, McMaster University, Hamilton, ON, Canada

Sarah Candace Payne Department of Psychiatry and Behavioural Neurosciences, McMaster University, Hamilton, ON, Canada

Joseph R. Pellizzari St. Joseph's Healthcare Hamilton, McMaster University, Hamilton, ON, Canada

Veronica Perez Department of Psychiatry, Baylor Scott & White Health, Central Texas Division, Temple, TX, USA

College of Medicine, Texas A&M University Health Science Center, Temple, TX, USA

Tara Riddell Department of Psychiatry and Behavioural Neurosciences, McMaster University, Hamilton, ON, Canada

Silvi Shah Division of Nephrology, Kidney CARE Program, Department of Internal Medicine, University of Cincinnati College of Medicine, Cincinnati, OH, USA

Amanjot Sidhu Division of Geriatric Medicine, Department of Medicine, Faculty of Health Sciences, McMaster University, Hamilton, ON, Canada

Natasha Snelgrove Department of Psychiatry and Behavioural Neurosciences, McMaster University, Hamilton, ON, Canada

Matthew A. Sparks Division of Nephrology, Department of Medicine, Duke University, Durham, NC, USA

Renal Section, Durham Veterans Affairs Health Care System, Durham, NC, USA

Javeed Sukhera Division of Child and Adolescent Psychiatry, Department of Psychiatry, Schulich School of Medicine, Western University, London, ON, Canada

Joel M. Topf Department of Internal Medicine, Oakland University, Detroit, MI, USA

Tyler G. Tulloch Kidney Urinary Program, St. Joseph's Healthcare Hamilton, Department of Psychiatry and Behavioural Neurosciences, McMaster University, Hamilton, ON, Canada

Heather Waters Department of Family Medicine, McMaster University, Hamilton, ON, Canada

Michele MacDonald Werstuck Nutrition Program Coordinator, Hamilton Family Health Team, Hamilton, ON, Canada

Tricia K. W. Woo Division of Geriatric Medicine, Department of Medicine, McMaster University, Hamilton, ON, Canada

Glen Xiong Department of Psychiatry and Behavioral Sciences, University of California, Davis, Sacramento, CA, USA

April Zehm Department of Medicine, Division of Geriatric and Palliative Medicine, Medical College of Wisconsin, Milwaukee, WI, USA

Part I

Fundamentals of Psychonephrology

Psychiatric Examination in Nephrology

1

Sarah Candace Payne and Vanessa Lentz

1.1 Introduction

As in all areas of medicine, the diagnostic interview remains a fundamental skill of a clinician. This skill is particularly indispensable in the specialty of psychiatry given the heterogeneous nature of psychiatric illness and often inadequate supportive objective testing to aid diagnostic clarity. The psychiatric examination and mental status examination are both key diagnostic tools in the clinician's toolbox. This chapter reviews basic concepts on how to effectively complete a psychiatric assessment in a renal patient and serves to introduce the clinician to notable aspects of the mental status examination that may be seen in patients with renal disease.

The primary aims of the psychiatric interview are to understand the patient's symptoms within a biopsychosocial framework while simultaneously building a therapeutic alliance with the patient [1]. In developing a formulation of the patient, the clinician postulates what biological, psychological, and social factors may be contributing to the patient's current presentation. Examples can include family history of neuropsychiatric illness (biological), a history of traumatic experience (psychological), or new interpersonal stressors (social). Throughout the psychiatric assessment, it is important to assess what predisposing and precipitating factors may be contributing to the patient's current presentation. This will inform both the

S. C. Payne (✉)
Department of Psychiatry and Behavioural Neurosciences,
McMaster University, Hamilton, ON, Canada
e-mail: sarah.payne@medportal.ca

V. Lentz
Department of Psychiatry and Behavioural Neurosciences, Michael G. DeGroote School of Medicine, Faculty of Health Sciences, McMaster University & St. Joseph's Healthcare Hamilton, Hamilton, ON, Canada
e-mail: vlentz@stjosham.on.ca

A. Hategan et al. (eds.), *Psychonephrology*,
https://doi.org/10.1007/978-3-030-84740-1_1

diagnostic profile and the treatment plan. The formulation allows a clinician to move beyond solely placing a diagnostic label on the patient's symptoms; rather, it allows a clinician to begin to understand the patient's experience, which is integral to the building of a positive therapeutic alliance. Ultimately, the clinician should aim for the patient to feel that their perspective has been heard [2].

While many clinicians may initially experience anxiety when first approaching a psychiatric interview, it is important to remember that many of the aspects of the psychiatric interview are similar to the diagnostic evaluations used in other areas of medicine. However, there are several key distinctions that should be highlighted (Table 1.1). Similarly, the mental status examination can be conceptualized as the psychiatric equivalent of the physical examination, and it provides essential information in forming the clinician's overall diagnostic impression [1].

The following discussion reviews the basic structure of the psychiatric assessment (as summarized in Table 1.2) and highlights key information that should be collected during the interview.

Table 1.1 Key tasks in completing a psychiatric interview

⇒ It is important to review limits of confidentiality at the start of the psychiatric assessment.
⇒ Establish chronology: It is important to construct a thorough timeline of events to understand what led up to the patient's current presentation [2].
⇒ It is also important to gather collateral history when completing a psychiatric assessment; this may include reviewing additional history from previous medical records and interviewing family members.
⇒ The use of open-ended questions is integral to obtaining a valid psychiatric assessment (e.g., "how would you describe your mood?" compared to "have you been feeling depressed?"). This will also allow the patients the opportunity to elaborate on their thoughts and experiences rather than the clinician relying on a rapid-fire approach to interviewing. Closed-ended questions can then be helpful in gathering more specific details as required.
⇒ A flexible approach to interviewing may be necessary for the psychiatric patient. For example, when a patient is presenting in crisis, it may not be possible (or appropriate) to gather all details of the history on initial approach, and one may need to re-approach over time. Some patients may also require more of a structured approach to the interview than others (e.g., overly inclusive patients), and this will often become evident early in the interview.

Table 1.2 Basic structure of a psychiatric history

The psychiatric history	Identifying data
	Chief complaint
	History of presenting illness
	Psychiatric review of systems
	Substance history
	Past psychiatric history
	Past medical history and medications
	Family history
	Personal history

1.2 The Psychiatric Interview

1.2.1 Identifying Data

Gathering of identifying data should include learning the patient's preferred name and preferred pronoun, age, sex/gender, relationship status, housing situation, and financial and occupational status. It represents a snapshot of the person before you and provides some context before delving into the interview.

Clinical Pearl

- Starting off the interview with identifying data can generally serve as a nonthreatening lead into the psychiatric assessment, allowing the patient time to settle into the interview. For the anxious patient, it may be helpful for the clinician to comment on their anxious appearance and give the patient an opportunity to share their worries (e.g., "I wonder if you are feeling anxious about what kind of questions I am going to ask you today…").
- It may also be helpful for the patient to know what to expect during the assessment, and the clinician can consider reviewing this prior to the start of the psychiatric interview.

1.2.2 The Chief Complaint

The chief complaint represents the patient's perspective on why they are seeing you and should typically be recorded in the patient's own words [1]. The patient's concerns will then be further elucidated in the history of presenting illness. In some cases, the patient's chief complaint may be different from the reason why they were referred, or the patient may not actually have any concerns about their own mental health; this is important to know upfront because it may change how the clinician approaches the interview.

1.2.3 History of Presenting Illness

The history of presenting illness provides an account of the onset and nature of the presenting complaint(s) [3]. The goal is to appreciate why this person is before you: *why here* and *why now*? It is also important to understand how the patient arrived for assessment and whether they are there of their own volition or due to the intervention of others (e.g., did a family member urge the patient to seek medical intervention or was the patient brought in by police?). An open-ended question such as, "What brings you here today?" can be a helpful starting point.

The history of presenting illness should focus on understanding onset of the presenting concern(s), precipitating and alleviating factors, severity and frequency of symptoms, and course of the symptoms [1]. Examples of common precipitating factors may include a change in relationship status, job loss, grief, medical illness, or medication changes. It can often be helpful to take a chronological approach when reviewing the evolution of the symptoms [3]. In assessing severity, evaluation should reveal how symptoms are impacting the patient's daily functioning. The suicide and violence risk assessment are standard components of the history of presenting illness and also speak to severity of illness [1]. The risk assessment will be reviewed in Sect. 1.4.

1.2.4 Review of Systems and Substance History

In addition to identifying what symptoms are *present*, it is also necessary to identify what symptoms are **absent**. The psychiatric review of systems includes assessment of any concurrent psychiatric symptoms with which the patient may be struggling. As some patients may not disclose symptoms beyond their chief complaint, the skilled clinician must be attentive to not miss any pertinent positives. The review of systems is therefore essential to the development of a thorough differential diagnosis and prognostic profile. In considering the differential diagnosis, physical symptoms should also be assessed as there are many systemic illnesses that may present with psychiatric symptoms. Figure 1.1 reviews common symptoms that should be screened for in the psychiatric review of systems. The focus of the review of symptoms will often be tailored to the patient as well as the context within which the clinician is seeing the patient.

In many medical assessments, the substance history may be reviewed as part of the social history. However, in the psychiatric assessment, it is necessary to screen for substance misuse *early* in the patient interview. This is because substance use can mimic many psychiatric syndromes or be comorbid with other psychiatric illnesses [4]. Substance use can also increase a patient's risk of suicide and violence [1]. It is therefore important to consider substance use disorders early in the assessment.

The substance use history should include details such of the type of substance(s) being used as well as the frequency, quantity, and pattern of use over time [1]. In addition to assessing the impact substance use is having on functioning, it is important to gauge the patient's level of insight into the impacts of their substance use and their motivation for change (Fig. 1.2). Using the model of Prochaska's stages of change [5] may help anchor this discussion. This review should also include an exploration of the patient's past treatments for substance use and if and how the patient feels they benefitted.

Clinical Pearl

- It can be helpful to begin the substance use history with a normalizing statement. Examples can include: "Many individuals use alcohol or other drugs at some point in their lives and we know that this can impact a person's mental health. For this reason, I want to ask you some questions about your pattern of use."

The Psychiatric Review of Systems

- Mood
  - Depressive symptoms ("SIGECAPS")
  - Hypomanic/manic symtoms ("DIGFAST")
- Sleep
  - Insomnia: Initial, middle, terminal
  - Hypersomnia
- Anxiety
  - Generalized anxiety, health anxiety, social anxiety, panic attacks, etc.
- Obsessive-compulsive symptoms
  - Intrusive thoughts and compulsive behaviors
- Trauma
  - Experience of trauma
  - Intrusive symptoms, avoidance behaviors, hyperarousal, negative cognitions/alterations in mood
- Psychosis
  - Hallucinations
  - Delusions
  - Disorganized thoughts/behavior
- Behavioral concerns (e.g. disordered eating, self-harming, gambling, impulse control behaviors, ADHD)
- Cognitive concerns
  - Features of delirium
  - Impairment in various cognitive domains (e.g., memory, learning, executive functioning, visuospatial abilities, attention,language

Fig. 1.1 Common psychiatric symptoms that are explored in the psychiatric review of systems. ***SIGECAPS***, **S**leep (insomnia or hypersomnia); **I**nterest (reduced, or loss of pleasure); **G**uilt (often unrealistic); **E**nergy (mental and physical fatigue); **C**oncentration (distractibility, indecisiveness, memory disturbance); **A**ppetite (decreased or increased); **P**sychomotor (retardation or agitation); **S**uicide (thoughts, plans, behaviors). ***DIGFAST***, **D**istractibility (poorly focused); **I**nsomnia (decreased need for sleep); **G**randiosity (inflated self-esteem); **F**light of ideas (complaints of racing thoughts); **A**ctivities (increased goal-directed activities, psychomotor agitation); **S**peech (talkativeness); **T**houghtlessness (risk-taking behaviors; e.g., sexual, financial, driving); **ADHD**, **A**ttention **D**eficit **H**yperactivity **D**isorder

1.2.5 The Past Psychiatric History

The past psychiatric history is an essential component of the assessment because many psychiatric disorders have a pattern of recurrence with high rates of psychiatric comorbidity [1]. The past psychiatric history provides an account of past episodes of mental health difficulties as well as previous contact with mental health professionals. Any history of admission to hospital and past psychiatric diagnoses should be specifically inquired into. Similarly, it is necessary to specifically assess for history of suicide attempts and/or self-harming behaviors. A thorough past psychiatric history should also explore previous treatments and treatment responses. It is important to establish the patient's functional baseline during any periods of recovery to better understand the overall prognosis.

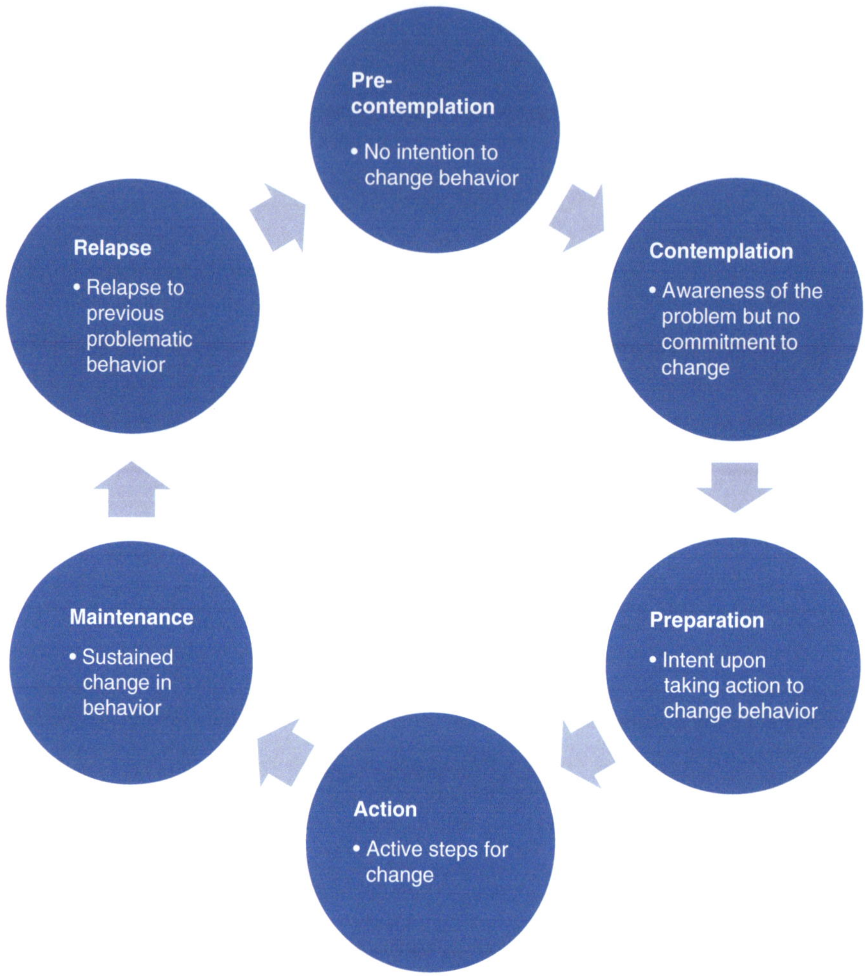
Pre-
contemplation
• No intention to change behavior
Contemplation
• Awareness of the problem but no commitment to change
Preparation
• Intent upon taking action to change behavior
Action
• Active steps for change
Maintenance
• Sustained change in behavior
Relapse
• Relapse to previous problematic behavior

Fig. 1.2 Prochaska's stages of change [5]

Clinical Pearl
- Collateral history from family members or thorough review of previous medical documentation can be helpful in fully elucidating the past psychiatric history.

1.2.6 Past Medical History and Medications

This part of the assessment aims to review what physical health problems may be contributing to the patient's presentation. Systemic medical illness can often mimic or precipitate a psychiatric illness; it can also affect treatment options available to the patient [1]. A history of head injury, seizures, and other neurological or endocrine disorders are particularly relevant in the psychiatric assessment as these conditions can impact treatment response and treatment options [1]. The patient's current medication regimen should also be documented. This includes any routine use of over-the-counter medications. Given high rates of poor medication adherence in the general population [6] – with patients with renal disease being no exception – assessment of medication adherence is also important to review.

Recommendation

- A comprehensive review of the patient's medication regimen, including over-the-counter medications, is essential due to the risks associated with drug-drug interactions. A number of psychotropic medications require dosing adjustments in patients with renal and liver dysfunction, and thus it is essential for the clinician to have access to an updated medication list and review any available investigations.

1.2.7 Family History

Many psychiatric illnesses have a genetic predisposition, and, for this reason, a review of the patient's family history is necessary. This component of the patient history focuses on the pertinent positives and pertinent negatives within the family history in terms of relevant psychiatric symptoms and/or diagnoses including substance use disorders and history of attempted or completed suicide. In addition, it is important to assess for medical illnesses that may run in the family as these may impact the patient's differential diagnosis and treatment plan (e.g., cautious use of certain second-generation antipsychotics may be necessary if there is a strong family history of metabolic syndrome).

1.2.8 Personal History

The personal history provides a narrative of the patient's life history including a review of his or her early development, educational history, and his or her current life circumstances. Significant life events (e.g., divorce, losses in the family, occupational changes) should be explored insofar as they have affected the patient's life story. It can often be helpful to approach the personal history chronologically – starting with details of the person's early life and leading up to present day [1]. In exploring the developmental history, questions can include where the person was born, who they resided with growing up, the quality of early life relationships, and their educational experience. It is also important to review the patient's current social situation including significant relationships, sources of stress, hobbies or interests, as well as the patient's main sources of financial and social support.

Religious and cultural background can also be explored as religious and cultural connections can be protective factors for many individuals.

Clinical Pearl

- Details of the personal history may come up at various points during the patient interview, and exploration of the patient's social history need not be left to the end of the interview.
- The depth to which the personal history is explored may depend on the circumstances of the clinical interview (e.g., it is not indicated to do so when interviewing an agitated patient).

1.3 The Mental Status Examination

The mental status examination (MSE) can be likened to the psychiatric version of the physical examination. The goal of the MSE is to objectively describe the patient's physical and cognitive states at the time of the assessment. It requires close observation on the part of the clinician to be able to do so effectively.

The mental status is assessed throughout the interview, and the order with which the components of the mental status examination are documented can vary. The features included within the mental status examination are summarized in Table 1.3.

1.3.1 Starting with the ABCs: Appearance, Behavior, and Cooperation

An important role of a clinician is to immediately assess if the patient before you requires urgent intervention (e.g., chemical restraint for safety, initiation of an emergency legal hold). The patient's physical *appearance*, *behavior*, and level of *cooperation* (the ABCs) provide numerous clues to help the clinician get a sense of the patient's mental status early on in the interview. With regard to appearance, features such as the patient's hygiene, and the state of his or her clothing can provide a sense

Table 1.3 Basic structure of the mental status examination

The mental status examination	The ABCs: appearance, behavior, cooperation
	Speech
	Mood and affect
	Thought process and thought content
	Perceptual disturbances
	Cognition (e.g., orientation, attention, abstraction, memory)
	Insight and judgment
	Risk assessment

of how well the patient is functioning. When assessing the patient's behavior and level of cooperation, it is necessary to look for any signs of agitation or aggression to ensure the safety of all involved.

1.3.2 Speech

This involves assessment of the rate, rhythm, volume, and pattern of the patient's speech. Certain abnormalities of speech can be associated with specific psychiatric disorders (e.g., rapid/pressured speech in mania, mutism in catatonia). Speech abnormalities such as dysarthria or aphasia can be suggestive of potential neurological disorders such as cerebrovascular events or neurodegenerative disorders [3].

1.3.3 Mood vs. Affect

Mood and affect are distinct but related components of the mental status examination. To assess a patient's mood, the clinician asks the patient directly *how he or she is feeling*. Conversely, affect is the mood state or emotional tone that the *clinician objectively observes* during the assessment [7]. Affect can be described as euphoric, dysphoric, irritable, tearful, and flat, for example. When there is no disturbance of mental state, the affect can be described to be euthymic.

The range of affect being displayed during the assessment should be considered and can be described as restricted, normal, or labile. It is important to also reflect on the degree of congruence between the described mood state and the observed affect (e.g., the patient who describes their mood to be happy but presents as tearful throughout the interview is displaying incongruency between stated mood and observed affect); such situations are common especially in psychotic and neurocognitive disorders and can provide important insight into diagnosis and what interventions may be required.

Clinical Pearl

- Discussing with a patient his or her mood state can be a natural transition into completion of the suicide risk assessment. The risk assessment will be reviewed in Sect. 1.4.

1.3.4 Thought Process

Thought process, or thought form, refers to the rate and flow of thought production and describes how appropriately a patient can connect his or her ideas. Normal thought form tends to be organized, logical, and goal-directed. There are many types of disordered thought forms, and certain thought forms can be characteristic of specific psychiatric diagnoses (e.g., tangential thought process as seen in mania or thought blocking as seen in psychosis). Table 1.4 reviews some common

Table 1.4 Common descriptors of disordered thought form

Disordered thought forms	Perseveration: Repetition of a response with an inability to switch to a different idea
	Circumstantiality: A circuitous and overinclusive pattern of speech
	Tangentiality: A response that is only partially connected to the original idea
	Loose associations: Illogical shifting between unrelated ideas such that the meaning is lost
	Flight of ideas: A response that jumps from one idea or theme to another at a rapid rate
	Thought blocking: Abrupt interruption of a thought with impaired ability to then complete the thought

descriptors of disordered thought form. In the case of patients with severe renal disease, disordered thought form should cue the clinician to the possibility of the presence of delirium. This will be further discussed in Sect. 1.6.

1.3.5 Thought Content

Thought content describes the central themes that occupy the patient's thoughts. Examples of disordered thought content can include the presence of overvalued ideas, delusions, and obsessions.

Clinical Pearl

- As defined in the *Diagnostic and Statistical Manual for Mental Disorders, fifth Edition* (DSM-5) [8], delusions are fixed false beliefs that can either be bizarre or non-bizarre in nature.
- While it is important for the clinician to not be drawn into the patient's delusional schema, it is generally not helpful to directly challenge these beliefs either.

1.3.6 Perceptual Disturbances

The most common perceptual abnormalities are hallucinations – perceptions that occur in the absence of external stimuli. Hallucinations can be auditory, visual, olfactory, or tactile in nature. In assessing for the presence of auditory hallucinations, it is necessary to inquire about command hallucinations (i.e., hallucinations that order the patient to act in a specific manner) as this can be associated with increased risk of harm to self or others [4].

1.3.7 Cognition and Orientation

An assessment of a patient's cognition is an important component of the mental status examination as it provides information about how well a patient can function. While the clinician may gain a general sense of the patient's cognitive functioning while completing the psychiatric interview, objective cognitive testing can be helpful in many instances. The Mini-Mental State Examination (MMSE®) or Montreal Cognitive Assessment (MoCA®) are commonly used standardized cognitive assessments [9, 10]. These assess areas such as visuospatial skills, attention, memory, and orientation to time, place, and person. In cases of suspected delirium and/or major neurocognitive disorder/dementia, repeat cognitive testing over time is essential.

1.3.8 Insight and Judgment

Insight describes a patient's ability to understand their symptoms and how he or she is impacted by these symptoms. The patient's understanding of treatment options and the need for treatment can also reflect his or her insight into their illness. Conversely, judgment concerns a person's ability to anticipate the consequences of his or her behavior and to make informed decisions based on this. Judgment can be assessed by exploring the patient's recent choices and decisions or by assessing their problem-solving abilities.

Clinical Pearl

In evaluating insight and judgment, questions can include:

- "Do you feel that your [psychiatric symptoms] are problematic?"
- "Do you believe that you would benefit from treatment?"
- "If you begin to smell smoke in your home, what would you do?"

Table 1.5 summarizes the various components of the mental status examination.

Table 1.5 Basic structure of the mental status examination

Appearance	Hygiene and grooming, clothing (appropriateness for the weather, style of dress), body habitus, posture, approximate age
Behavior	Abnormal movements or mannerisms (e.g., tics, posturing, tardive dyskinesia), level of motor activity (i.e., psychomotor agitation vs. psychomotor retardation), degree of eye contact
Cooperation	Attitude toward the interviewer (e.g., polite vs. hostile), openness vs. guardedness/suspiciousness
Speech	Rate, volume, prosody, dysarthria, poverty of content
Mood and affect	Range, stability, appropriateness for context, congruence (i.e., match between mood and affect)
Thought process	Flow and rate of speech production, coherence and organization of thought form
Thought content	Obsessions, delusions, overvalued ideas, ideas of reference
Perceptual disturbances	Illusions, depersonalization/derealization; auditory, visual, tactile, olfactory hallucinations
Cognition	Orientation, attention, abstraction, memory, intelligence
Insight and judgment	Areas of impairment
Risk assessment	Suicidal and homicidal ideation

1.4 The Risk Assessment

It can be argued that one of the most important components of the psychiatric examination is the risk assessment. By the end of a psychiatric assessment, the clinician should have an understanding of the patient's immediate risk in order to be able to determine the most appropriate disposition plan.

Clinical Pearl

- It is a myth that asking a patient about suicide may put the idea into their head [1, 11].

The suicide assessment involves an analysis of both static and dynamic risk factors (Table 1.6) [12, 13]. It is also necessary to assess the patient's protective factors – the characteristics that may reduce his or her risk of attempting or completing suicide (Table 1.6). While it is important to understand how these various factors may increase or decrease suicide from an epidemiological perspective, yet, there is no evidence-based algorithm that can accurately predict a patient's risk of suicide [11]. For this reason, clinical judgment is ultimately what will decide the clinical formulation of risk. Note that physical illness – including renal disease and its sequelae – serves as a static risk factor for suicide (Table 1.6).

In assessing suicidality, the clinician needs to determine the extent of the patient's suicidal ideation as well as how far they have gone in acting upon their suicidal thoughts. There are various strategies that can help the clinician to bring up the topic of suicide in a sensitive manner. Normalization is one such strategy whereby the clinician communicates to the patient that he or she is not alone in experiencing these thoughts; e.g., "Sometimes when people are going through similarly difficult experiences, they have thoughts that they would be better off dead. Have you had any thoughts like this?". In addition, first questioning around passive suicidal

Table 1.6 Summary of static and dynamic risk factors and protective factors that form part of the suicide risk assessment [12, 13]

Static risk factors	Dynamic risk factors	Protective factors
Personal history of suicide attempts Family history of suicide Male Older age Single, divorced, or widowed marital status Systemic illness/disability	Psychiatric illness (e.g., depressive, psychotic, substance use disorder) Psychosocial stress Physical illness Access to suicidal means Hopelessness	Spirituality Family supports Parental responsibilities Access to treatment/ psychosocial intervention Hope for the future

ideation can be a more delicate way of leading into questioning about active suicidal ideation. The following scenario provides such an example:

Clinician: Sometimes when people are experiencing depression like yourself, they have thoughts that life is no longer worth living. Have you had any thoughts like this?
Patient: Yes, I've been thinking that over the past few weeks.
Clinician: How often do you have these thoughts?
Patient: Oh, every day now.
Clinician: Can you give me an example of what thoughts come to mind?
Patient: I think about how my family would be better off if I wasn't around anymore and how I wouldn't have to suffer anymore.
Clinician: Do these thoughts come and go or do they stick with you?
Patient: I'm finding it harder and harder to push them away now.
Clinician: Have you ever thought about taking steps to end your life?
Patient: Yes….
Clinician: What have you considered?
Patient: It's hard for me to talk about… but I've thought about hanging myself….

It is now incumbent upon the clinician to question the patient on their plan and to evaluate the patient's level of intent on completing suicide in the immediate future. This would involve questioning the patient on when, where, and how they would act on the plan and whether or not they have taken any active steps to do so (e.g., purchasing a rope, tying a noose, visiting the planned location for the attempt). Persistence is key as knowing these details will speak to the level of suicidal intent as well as allow the clinician to determine the potential degree of lethality. Furthermore, the clinician should also question the patient about protective factors (e.g., "What has kept you from acting on these thoughts of suicide?" and "Do you have hope that things can still get better?").

It is important to note that some patients who have decided upon suicide may be less than forthcoming when the clinician broaches this line of questioning because they do not want to be stopped from acting on their plan. For this reason, the clinical formulation of risk should also include information from collateral history. There are additional factors that may also inform the risk formulation, e.g., the patient's nonverbal communication and the patient's level of engagement. For example, the patient who did not seek medical attention on their own accord and is now not making eye contact or being forthcoming in their responses could potentially have a higher degree of risk than the help-seeking, engaged individual. Additional clues that the patient may be actively suicidal can include the giving away of possessions, the preparation of a will, and writing of a suicide note. Depending on the clinician's overall impression of risk, an emergency legal hold and/or admission to hospital may be required. Depending on the clinical setting, assistance from the consultation-liaison psychiatry team or psychiatrist on call may be required.

Recommendation

- Careful documentation of the suicide risk assessment is critical. Documentation should include whether or not the patient has access to means, details of any plan(s) the patient may have divulged, degree of intent, and degree of future-orientation. Collateral information should also be documented when available.

Apart from taking active steps to end his or her life, a patient can also be at risk of harm due to his or her inability or lack of motivation to care for their own personal needs. The presence of self-neglect (e.g., due to severely depressed mood, psychosis, cognitive impairment) would also weigh into the overall assessment of risk.

Finally, the risk assessment also includes an evaluation of risk of harm to others; it is important for this to become a routine part of a clinician's psychiatric examination so that he or she becomes comfortable asking these potentially sensitive questions. Screening around risk for violence can be integrated into the psychiatric history in a manner that connects to the topic under discussion. For example, in patients endorsing persecutory delusions, the clinician can assess whether the patient has felt the need to protect themselves against the individual who the patient believes is meaning them harm as well as whether they have approached the individual or have thoughts of harming the individual. Because clinicians have a duty to warn/protect potential victims of planned violence in most jurisdictions, the clinician must also determine if there is an identifiable individual (or group of individuals) that the patient means to harm and whether or not the patient has access to this individual (or group of individuals). Like the suicide risk assessment, the clinician must understand the patient's level of intent and the immediacy of the risk of harm. In so doing, it is necessary to consider (and document) the patient's access to weapons. The patient's history of legal charges can also inform the violence risk assessment as a history of violence increases future risk of violence [1].

1.5 Concluding the Psychiatric Interview

As described throughout this chapter, the goal of the psychiatric examination is to establish the presence of a mental disorder but also to understand how the patient's symptoms are impacting his or her functioning and quality of life. Developing a treatment plan in collaboration with the patient is then the next step. It is important to provide patients with the opportunity to ask questions. While a psychiatric assessment does tend to focus on symptoms of mental illness, it is also important to highlight the patient's strengths which became clear during the interview (e.g., courage, resiliency, openness). This is the strength-based approach to psychiatric care and can play an important role in psychiatric recovery [14]. Ultimately, without providing false reassurance, it is important to leave the patient with a message of hope.

1.6 Special Considerations in the Psychiatric Examination in Nephrology

In this section, the clinician is introduced to some common aspects of the psychiatric examination in nephrology, with particular emphasis on the mental status examination. As will be reviewed in detail in this volume, the prevalence of psychiatric disorders in patients with chronic kidney disease (CKD) or end-stage renal disease (ESRD) is significant, secondary to a multitude of factors including (but not limited to) high physical burden of illness, considerable anticipatory anxiety and distress, and significant social stressors [15, 16]. In those with impending need for transplant, anxiety in relation to their position on the waiting list or concern about organ rejection may serve to further increase mood and/or anxiety burden. Patients with ESRD are 50% more likely to experience depression compared to those without [15, 16]. Patients undergoing dialysis also have high comorbidity rates of delirium and other neurocognitive disorders [16]. For these reasons, it is important to be able to recognize cues on mental status examination that may suggest the presence of a primary depressive, anxiety, or neurocognitive disorder. Early recognition may assist with treatments that can improve health outcomes (both physical and mental), as well as enhance overall quality of life indices.

1.6.1 Depression

Depression remains the most common psychiatric disorder in patients with ESRD [15, 16]. Furthermore, many of the signs and symptoms of ESRD may overlap with those of major depressive disorder, further complicating the clinician's assessment [17]. Patients experiencing the burden of frequent dialysis sessions may report symptoms such as low mood, decreased energy, fatigue, and/or a sense of hopelessness. Patients with uremia may report poor sleep, fatigue, and loss of interest and may appear depressed, with little range in their affect and/or a slowed thought process [17].

1.6.1.1 Case Vignette 1

Mr. G, a 55-year-old male with ESRD undergoing dialysis three times per week, presents on Monday morning for his regularly scheduled dialysis treatment. Normally a jovial presence on the unit, he appears withdrawn, sullen, and extremely fatigued. During his session, he sits quietly with his head down. When approached by his nurse, he appears to stare off into space and has difficulty formulating his thoughts. He reports increased stress at home recently. There is a significant family history of depression. Bloodwork is within the expected ranges for him.

1.6.1.2 Case Vignette 1 Analysis

Mr. G is first assessed by his nephrologist who suspects a possible depressive episode after the patient admits that he has been feeling depressed for a couple of weeks, worsened over the weekend after learning of the sudden death of a neighbor. His nephrologist requests the assistance of a psychiatric consultant to the dialysis clinic, who confirms the presence of a major depressive episode. Mr. G is started on an antidepressant and referred for outpatient treatment and starts noting an improvement in his symptoms in about 4 weeks. His depression is fully remitted within about 4 months, and he returns to his previous outgoing self.

1.6.2 Anxiety

Anxiety has not been studied as frequently as other psychiatric conditions in patients with chronic kidney disease [15, 17], although its burden cannot be underemphasized. Like depression, anxiety in patients with ESRD appears to be associated with increased morbidity and negative impacts to quality of life [15–17]. On mental status examination, patients with significant anxiety may present with a self-described report of "worry" or anxiety, signs of psychomotor agitation (e.g., physical restlessness, hand wringing, pacing), and clear evidence of anxious affect, including fear or episodes of crying. Repeated requests for reassurance are also common [18].

1.6.2.1 Case Vignette 2

Ms. L is a 63-year-old female with a recent diagnosis of ESRD and has started dialysis only in the last couple of weeks. At each session thus far, she appears to be very anxious, with mild hyperventilation, wringing of her hands, and scrutinizing of her fistula, and repeatedly seeks reassurance from her nurse that she is "okay." She also continually watches the clock to count down the minutes to the end of her session. She has very limited social supports and discloses that she "watched [her] mother die on the transplant list" while waiting for a lung transplant after a diagnosis of idiopathic pulmonary fibrosis. She states that she "can't bear this continuing," as she fears "dying" after each dialysis session. She experienced a headache after each previous session and wonders if she is having a "stroke." She has a long history of generalized anxiety, including separation anxiety as a child, for which she has never sought medical intervention.

1.6.2.2 Case Vignette 2 Analysis

Ms. L appears to be experiencing severe anxiety – likely generalized anxiety disorder, with possible somatization – manifested by reported statements suggesting significant worry, psychomotor agitation, hypervigilance, and probable catastrophizing, as well as reassurance seeking. Her limited social supports are likely adding to her anxiety and her previous familial experiences with transplant that have potentially reinforced in her mind that no successful outcomes are possible in the context of organ failure. Ms. L would likely benefit from a first-line antidepressant for anxiety, as well as referral for cognitive behavioral therapy (CBT).

1.6.3 Delirium

Delirium and other neurocognitive disorders are commonly seen in patients with ESRD [15–17]. Chronic kidney disease has been noted to be an independent risk factor for cognitive impairment and neurocognitive disorders, and the presence of cognitive impairment in this group is estimated at 30–60% [19, 20]. Evidently, patients missing a dialysis session are at increased risk of delirium, and although the signs and symptoms of uremia can vary significantly, central nervous symptoms may begin with mild cognitive dysfunction, fatigue, and headache, eventually progressing most commonly to hypoactive delirium; in untreated cases, coma may result [17]. In addition to such acute changes in mental status, the clinician should also be mindful that slower, more progressive changes particularly in the setting of multiple comorbidities – may occur in the patient's cognition over the course of months or years on dialysis, with a major neurocognitive disorder/dementia eventually becoming apparent.

1.6.3.1 Case Vignette 3

Mr. K is a 76-year-old male who missed his dialysis session 2 days ago after his wife fell unexpectedly ill and herself was hospitalized. His past medical history is significant for ESRD, a history of transient ischemic attacks (TIAs), chronic anemia, and type 2 diabetes mellitus. He was also given a recent diagnosis of mild neurocognitive disorder. He was brought in to the emergency department (ED) this morning by his son after Mr. K was unable to get out of bed. According to his son, other than some fatigue yesterday, Mr. K was in his usual state of health until last evening, but he is now very drowsy and appeared to be confused in the little that he was able to communicate. He also appears dazed. He mumbles to his son "just let me die." Bloodwork is significant for a small drop from his baseline hemoglobin and a significant increase in blood urea nitrogen.

1.6.3.2 Case Vignette 3 Analysis

Mr. K appears to be experiencing symptoms consistent with a hypoactive delirium, likely secondary to uremia after missing his dialysis session 2 days ago. His history of cerebrovascular disease may also be contributing. He starts a dialysis session within a couple of hours of arriving in the ED, and by evening, he is already more alert and showing some improvement in his confusion. The following morning, he is further improved and expresses utter disbelief that he made a comment that he wished to die, joking that he and his wife can't miss hosting their 50th Annual New Year's Eve party in a couple of months.

Recommendation

- It is important to distinguish between those psychiatric symptoms that may overlap with the clinical sequelae of severe renal disease.
- Careful examination in this regard can allow for early intervention in psychiatric conditions that are likely to respond to treatment and may themselves in turn decrease the morbidity and mortality frequently experienced by this patient population.

1.7 Key Takeaways

- The psychiatric examination comprises a thorough psychiatric history and mental status examination; it requires careful listening and observation on the part of the clinician.
- The gathering of information from the patient, chart, and collateral sources will allow for the clinician to arrive at the most appropriate diagnosis, which is a prerequisite for developing an effective treatment plan.
- The risk assessment is fundamental to the psychiatric examination and involves careful history taking, analysis of risk factors, and documentation.
- A strength-based approach to psychiatric care can be important to mental health recovery.
- Although the approach to the psychiatric examination is generally uniform, the clinician should be aware of the most common psychiatric signs and symptoms on examination that are frequently observed in patients with CKD or ESRD.

References

1. Houghtalen RP, Mcintyre JS. Psychiatric interview, history, and mental status examination of the adult patient. In: Sadock BJ, Sadock VA, Ruiz P, editors. Kaplan & Sadock's comprehensive textbook of psychiatry. 10th ed. Philadelphia: Lippincott Williams & Wilkins; 2017.
2. Poole R, Higgo R. Diagnosis. In: psychiatric interviewing and assessment. 2nd ed. Cambridge: Cambridge University Press; 2017.
3. Hategan A, Bourgeois JA. Psychiatric examination. In: Hategan A, Bourgeois JA, Hirsch CH, editors. On-call geriatric psychiatry: Handbook of principles and practice. Switzerland: Springer; 2016.
4. Matorin AA, Shah AA, Ruiz P. Clinical manifestations of psychiatric disorders. In: Sadock BJ, Sadock VA, Ruiz P, editors. Kaplan & Sadock's comprehensive textbook of psychiatry. 10th ed. Philadelphia: Lippincott Williams & Wilkins; 2017.
5. Prochaska J, DiClemente C. Stages and processes of self-change of smoking: toward an integrative model of change. J Consult Clin Psychol. 1983;51(3):390–5.
6. Brown MT, Bussell JK. Medication adherence: WHO cares? Mayo Clin Proc. 2011;86(4):304–14.

7. Akiskal HS. The mental status examination. In: Fatemi S, Clayton P, editors. The medical basis of psychiatry. New York: Springer; 2016.
8. American Psychiatric Association. Diagnostic and statistical manual of mental disorders (DSM-5®). American Psychiatric Pub; May 22, 2013.
9. Folstein MF, Folstein SE, McHugh PR. "mini-mental state". A practical method for grading the cognitive state of patients for the clinician. J Psychiatr Res. 1975;12(3):189–98.
10. Nasreddine ZS, Phillips NA, Bedirian V, Charbonneau S, Whitehead V, Collin I, et al. The Montreal cognitive assessment, MoCA: a brief screening tool for mild cognitive impairment. J Am Geriatr Soc. 2005;53(4):695–9.
11. Shea SC. Psychiatric interviewing: the art of understanding: a practical guide for psychiatrists, psychologists, counselors, social workers, nurses, and other mental health professionals. 3rd ed. Edinburgh: Elsevier; 2017.
12. Wasserman D. Suicide: overview and epidemiology. In: Sadock BJ, Sadock VA, Ruiz P, editors. Kaplan & Sadock's comprehensive textbook of psychiatry. 10th ed. Philadelphia: Lippincott Williams & Wilkins; 2017.
13. Bouch J, Marshall JJ. Suicide risk: structured professional judgment. Adv Psychiatr Treat 2005;11(2):84–91.
14. Xie H. Strengths-based approach for mental health recovery. Iran J Psychiatry Behav Sci. 2013;7(2):5–10.
15. Simoes e Silva AC, Miranda AS, Rocha NP, Teixeira AL. Neuropsychiatric disorders in chronic kidney disease. Front Pharmacol. 2019;10:932.
16. Kimmel PL, Fwu CW, Abbott KC, Moxey-Mims MM, Mendley S, Norton JM, et al. Psychiatric illness and mortality in hospitalized ESKD dialysis patients. Clin J Am Soc Nephrol. 2019;14(9):1363–71.
17. Cukor D, Levenson JL, Rosenthal-Asher D, Kimmel PL. Renal disease. In: Levenson JL, editor. The American Psychiatric Association publishing textbook of psychosomatic medicine and consultation-liaison medicine. 3rd ed. Washington: American Psychiatric Publishing; 2018.
18. Goh ZS, Griva K. Anxiety and depression in patients with end-stage renal disease: impact and management challenges–a narrative review. Int J Nephrol Renovasc Dis. 2018;11:93–102.
19. Madero M, Gul A, Sarnak MJ. Cognitive function in chronic kidney disease. Semin Dial. 2008;21(1):29–37.
20. Etgen T, Chonchol M, Forstl H, Sander D. Chronic kidney disease and cognitive impairment: a systematic review and meta-analysis. Am J Nephrol. 2012;35(5):474–82.

Psychometric Assessment of Neuropsychological Function in Kidney Disease

2

Heather E. McNeely, Tyler G. Tulloch, Joseph R. Pellizzari, and Jelena P. King

2.1 Introduction

Psychological stress and cognitive difficulties are common and interwoven comorbidities frequently encountered in patients with chronic kidney disease (CKD). It is well established that depressive and anxiety symptoms, suicidal ideation, and cognitive impairment, such as deficient attention, memory, and reasoning, predict poor treatment adherence and outcomes in a number of medically ill populations. The interplay between neuropsychiatric, including cognitive, symptoms and physical status is complex. Cognitive impairment can give rise to psychosocial distress which contributes to poor engagement in treatment, poor health choices or decisions, and

H. E. McNeely (✉)
Department of Psychiatry and Behavioural Neurosciences, McMaster University, St. Joseph's Healthcare Hamilton, Clinical Neuropsychology Services, Hamilton, ON, Canada
e-mail: hmcneely@stjoes.ca

T. G. Tulloch
Kidney Urinary Program, St. Joseph's Healthcare Hamilton, Department of Psychiatry and Behavioural Neurosciences, McMaster University, Hamilton, ON, Canada
e-mail: ttulloch@stjoes.ca

J. R. Pellizzari
St. Joseph's Healthcare Hamilton, McMaster University, Hamilton, ON, Canada
e-mail: jpellizz@stjosham.on.ca

J. P. King
Department of Psychiatry & Behavioural Neurosciences, St. Joseph's Healthcare Hamilton, Clinical Neuropsychology Services, Hamilton, ON, Canada
e-mail: kingj@stjosham.on.ca

A. Hategan et al. (eds.), *Psychonephrology*,
https://doi.org/10.1007/978-3-030-84740-1_2

increased morbidity and mortality in chronic medically compromised populations such as those with CKD.

As discussed elsewhere in this book, glomerular filtration rate (GFR) is the best measure of kidney function and is the number used to determine stage of renal disease. Meta-analyses have found increased severity of cognitive impairment across a number of domains of cognition as GFR decreases [1]. Physicians and other clinicians working with CKD populations should be aware of common neuropsychiatric symptoms, including cognitive presentations, appropriate screening methods/tools used for assessing presence and severity of these symptoms, and necessity of symptom monitoring, as these features may fluctuate in response to varying GFR. Clinicians should also be aware when to refer for specialized psychological assessment/treatment and formal neuropsychological assessment in order to mitigate negative outcomes, enhance or sustain patient quality of life, and enable patients and family members opportunity for advanced planning and decision-making.

This chapter will provide guidance in how to approach neuropsychological assessment in patients with CKD. Given the overlap between symptoms of uremia and those of depressive and neurocognitive disorders, special considerations must be made when assessing patients with CKD. The chapter uses case vignettes to highlight neuropsychiatric manifestations in patients with CKD and their impact on clinical status, review tools and methods used to screen for presence and severity of these symptoms, highlight clinical pearls, and identify key points to consider when making a referral for specialized psychological and/or neuropsychological services.

2.2 Psychological Assessment

Psychological assessment (also referred to as psychological or psychometric testing) is a process of testing by clinical psychologists that uses a combination of tests and other assessment tools to measure and observe a patient's behavior to help the psychiatric clinician arrive at a diagnosis and guide treatment. When and who can refer for formal psychometric testing is discussed later in the chapter.

This section will begin by reviewing common comorbid psychiatric disorders observed in renal patients. It will present some useful screening tools that can be used by frontline clinicians and mental health specialists alike and will identify when patients should be referred for more specialized psychiatric and/or psychotherapeutic services. Chapter 7 also presents an overview of psychotherapy principles for patients with CKD.

2.2.1 Common Psychiatric Presenting Concerns

Although the most common psychiatric presenting concerns are detailed elsewhere in this volume, the authors hereby review these psychiatric concerns from the perspective of presenting the components of a psychological evaluation, including tests and assessments, to aid in establishing a psychiatric diagnosis and treatment plan.

Epidemiological studies of psychiatric disorders in CKD patients are lacking; however, empirical research has focused on several commonly observed disorders, including depressive, anxiety, and sleep disorders.

2.2.1.1 Depressive Disorders

Depressive disorders are perhaps the most common psychiatric disorder observed among CKD patients, and their presence is associated with poorer clinical outcomes, including more frequent hospital admissions, lengthier hospital stays, higher rates of dialysis withdrawal, and increased risk of morbidity and mortality [2]. Not surprisingly, the estimated prevalence of depressive disorders in CKD patients varies depending on whether they are assessed via interview or questionnaire and also by stage of CKD. A meta-analysis of observational studies found that the prevalence of depressive disorder was higher when diagnosed via self- and clinician-administered questionnaires compared to clinician-administered interview, likely overestimating depression symptomology [3]. The estimated point prevalence of depressive disorder based on clinician-administered interview in this study was 21.4% among stage 1–5 CKD patients not yet on dialysis, 22.8% among stage 5 CKD patients on dialysis, and 25.7% among kidney transplant recipients. In contrast, the prevalence of depressive disorders among stage 5 CKD patients on dialysis increased to 39.3% when assessed via self- or clinician-administered questionnaire.

Despite overestimating depression symptomology, there remain many advantages to using questionnaires to screen for depression in primary care settings, including this methodology being more accessible, requiring less training, and being less costly and time-consuming to administer than a formal clinical interview. It is important to carefully interpret questionnaire results considering a given patient's CKD symptoms. This may be because there is significant overlap in symptoms of depressive disorder and uremia that, when misattributed to depression, will overestimate depression severity. These symptoms include fatigue, poor appetite, difficulty concentrating, restlessness, and sleep disturbance. When assessing a patient for depressive disorder, the clinician must judiciously decide whether shared symptoms are more likely indicative of uremia or depressive disorder. One way to accomplish this often-difficult task is to consider timing of symptoms. For example, does the patient's poor appetite coincide with periods of low mood or anhedonia, or does it fluctuate independently of these other symptoms? Of course, at least one of the hallmark symptoms of major depressive disorder, either depressed mood and/or diminished interest or pleasure in most activities, must be present most of the day nearly every day for greater than 2 weeks for a diagnosis of major depressive disorder [4]. Table 2.1 lists the comparison of depressive symptoms and select uremia symptoms [4, 41].

It should be noted that depressed mood *alone* does not necessarily indicate the presence of major depressive disorder if not accompanied by a suprathreshold number of other symptoms of major depressive disorder for at least 2 weeks. It may represent a normative reaction to significant life changes, such as starting dialysis or experiencing yet another symptom of failing kidneys. It may be part of a patient's typical daily "ups and downs," especially if there are more "downs" than "ups" when the patient attends medical appointments or dialysis treatments. Furthermore,

Table 2.1 Comparison of depressive disorder and select uremia symptoms highlighting similarities [4, 41]

Depressive disorder	Uremia
Depressed mood	Peripheral neuropathy
Anhedonia (loss of interest/pleasure)	Decreased sense of smell/taste
Feelings of worthlessness/inappropriate guilt	Itching
Thoughts of death/suicidal ideation	Cramps
Similarities between depressive disorder and uremia symptoms:	
Sleep disturbance (insomnia/hypersomnia)	Sleep disturbance
Fatigue	Fatigue
Change in appetite/weight (decrease/increase)	Poor appetite/nausea/vomiting
Difficulty concentrating/indecisiveness	Difficulty concentrating/decreased mental acuity
Psychomotor agitation/retardation	Restless legs

depressed mood could be indicative of another psychiatric disorder such as adjustment disorder or be associated with hypoactive delirium.

Clinical Pearl

- Patients may be quick to report losing interest or enjoyment in most activities.
- However, this may not be depressive disorder per se, but rather may be due to an inability to engage secondary to fatigue, pain, retinopathy, neuropathy, dyspnea, or other physical conditions.

Recommendation

- Explore if loss of interest or enjoyment exists for activities the patient is still able to engage in or if it would be present for previously enjoyed activity if the interfering symptoms went away.

2.2.1.2 Case Vignette: "An Unfortunate New Beginning"

Mr. Wilson was a 29-year-old recently divorced man with end-stage kidney disease (ESKD) who found himself in the unenviable position of having to move back into his childhood home with his parents due to financial stressors. The hospital-based dialysis center was close by, and he was settling into his new lifestyle of attending dialysis sessions three times per week. Efforts to solicit a live organ donor had come up empty, and he was now looking at a several years wait for deceased donor kidney. Circumstances found him newly unemployed, and prospects were looking grim to find employment that would reasonably accommodate his renal replacement needs. Three months later, his dialysis nurses had started to notice some recent trends: he had become less conversational in general, but particularly about his beloved Toronto Blue Jays baseball team who were enjoying a banner season. His smiles seemed more forced, he was looking thinner, and he started to call in requesting scheduling changes at the last minute. The nurses communicated these newer observations to his nephrologist prior to his next monthly follow-up. We follow this case along as the patient's psychological distress and symptoms begin to be monitored utilizing various self-report tools.

Given that most CKD patients have routine and long-term follow-up with healthcare providers after renal disease is diagnosed, typically in a multidisciplinary kidney care clinic, there is ample opportunity for depression screening at many points along the patient journey. Indeed, given the impact of untreated depressive disorder on clinical outcomes in CKD, routine screening for depression and subsequent treatment may benefit not only the patient and their loved ones but also the healthcare system in terms of reducing number of hospitalizations and length of stays. Renal programs could opt to incorporate routine screening at regular intervals (e.g., each follow-up visit, annually) or based on milestones in CKD progression (e.g., progression from one stage to another, after dialysis initiation). Screening could be done in person during clinic visits or via telemedicine for patients in rural or remote areas. When a patient screens "positive" for depression, healthcare providers would ideally have a plan in place to provide follow-up. This could include referral to an internal or external mental health specialist for diagnostic assessment and treatment. Depending on depression severity, treatment options could include active monitoring, psychoeducation, self-management programs, psychotherapy provided by a mental health specialist, and/or antidepressant medication. (See Chap. 7 for an overview of psychotherapy principles for renal patients and Chap. 10, for further information on psychiatric aspects and their treatments in the kidney patient.)

Recommendation

- Routine screening for depression should be incorporated into care for the patient with CKD.
- Consider the role of depressive disorder on adherence to medications, fluid restrictions, dietary and exercise recommendations, and dialysis attendance.

Clinical Pearl

- Unidentified and untreated depressive disorder is associated with poorer engagement in treatment and poorer clinical outcomes.

2.2.1.3 Suicidality

One important consideration in screening for depressive disorder is how to manage suicidal ideation, once identified. Suicidality in CKD patients has not been extensively researched, but there is preliminary evidence that patients on hemodialysis are at 1.25 times greater risk of completing suicide relative to age-, gender-, and geography-matched controls, with a period of further increased risk during the first 3 months after initiating hemodialysis [5]. While further research on suicidality among CKD patients is needed, this strongly supports the need for psychological intervention and routine screening of depressive disorder including suicidal ideation, especially around the time of dialysis initiation. Screening for depression using questionnaires that measure suicidal ideation, therefore, requires a plan in place for managing this once identified. Plans could include having a healthcare provider available trained in suicide risk assessment to conduct a more detailed assessment, having a consultation or referral system in place, or at the very least providing access to a local crisis outreach team.

Dialysis patients may reach a point where they begin considering the costs and benefits of remaining on dialysis versus withdrawing from care and pursuing conservative management, and this may be particularly relevant for patients who are not eligible transplant candidates. While for some patients, this may reflect underlying suicidal ideation, this is not always the case and may reflect a patient's shifting goals of care. Patients should be encouraged to discuss their wishes with loved ones and care providers to receive support and guidance with this type of decision, and suicidal ideation could be explored, but should not be assumed. Patients seeking to withdraw dialysis in this context should have their decisional capacity assessed, as comorbid neurocognitive impairment may impact decisional capacity. Training in conducting suicide risk assessment is beyond the scope of this chapter, but should typically include assessing for the presence of suicidal ideation, desire, plan/method, intent, psychiatric comorbidity, and also protective factors against suicide.

2.2.1.4 Anxiety Disorders

Anxiety disorders are common among CKD patients. According to a recent meta-analysis, 43% of patients experience anxiety symptoms, and 19% are diagnosed with at least one anxiety disorder [6]. Anxiety can be conceptualized as the anticipation of future threat and may be associated with symptoms of muscle tension, vigilance, and increased cautious and avoidant behaviors [4]. While the sensation of anxiety is a normative and often useful part of daily living, it can become excessive or persistent and lead to clinically significant distress or impairment. It is understandable that renal patients would experience anxiety symptoms, given the chronic and progressive nature of CKD and uncertainty about when new physical and neuropsychiatric symptoms will appear, how quality of life will change as the kidney disease progresses, how long the kidneys will last, what dialysis will feel like, and how effective treatment(s) will be. An important component of assessing for anxiety syndromes in renal patients, therefore, is not just identifying whether anxiety disorder is present, but to what degree it is causing clinically significant distress or impairment in daily functioning.

Anxiety disorder has been associated with adverse clinical outcomes in CKD, including reduced health-related quality of life, poorer adherence to treatment recommendations, and increased risk of mortality and progression to stage 5 CKD requiring dialysis [6]. Furthermore, while all anxiety disorders, by definition, are associated with clinically significant distress or impairment, some may have a disproportionate impact on a patient's ability to attend and tolerate life-saving treatments such as hemodialysis. Patients with blood-injection-injury (specific) phobia may have considerable difficulty coping with hemodialysis, given the need for two dialysis needles to be inserted (and remain inserted) for every dialysis treatment, typically for 4 hours, three times weekly, in an environment where blood is visibly circulating through tubing for all patients in a shared space. Agoraphobia may also make attending hemodialysis treatments challenging, given that patients are not typically provided private rooms. Patients with panic disorder may have difficulty tolerating physiological sensations associated with hemodialysis, such as changes in blood pressure, restless legs, and muscle cramping. Given the frequent medical appointments and blood work required for patients with CKD, blood-injection-injury (specific) phobia and agoraphobia may be identified long before the patient must start dialysis; however, it may be helpful, when feasible, to screen patients for the presence of treatment-interfering anxiety disorders prior to initiating hemodialysis.

Given the association between anxiety disorder and adverse clinical outcomes, early screening and treatment for anxiety disorder may help improve the patient's health-related quality of life as well as clinical outcomes. Furthermore, early identification of anxiety disorders that may specifically interfere with hemodialysis may benefit the patient in that they may be encouraged to consider peritoneal dialysis, in which needles, blood, and shared treatment settings are absent, or by providing ample opportunity to seek anxiety treatment prior to starting hemodialysis. For these reasons, it may be helpful to incorporate routine screening of anxiety symptoms and specific anxiety disorders into multidisciplinary kidney care clinics. At present, there is no consensus on the recommended frequency of screening for anxiety disorders in CKD patients. Clinicians may wish to incorporate this screening into routine clinic visits, whether in person or via telemedicine, similar to screening for depressive disorders. While there is no gold standard anxiety screening measure for CKD patients, a list of potential screening tools is further presented in this chapter.

Recommendation

- When assessing for anxiety disorder, ask the patient if there is anything they typically avoid doing or thinking about to help them feel less anxious.

Clinical Pearl

- Patients may deny feeling anxious because they have become very good at avoiding anxiety-provoking situations or thoughts.

2.2.1.5 Sleep Disorders

Sleep disorders are highly prevalent among renal patients and are associated with poorer quality of life, as well as increased risk of disease and mortality. Maung et al. present a helpful overview of the association between sleep disorders and CKD, focusing on disorders most prevalent in renal patients, including sleep apnea, insomnia, restless leg syndrome, and excessive daytime sleepiness [7]. Assessment of the two most common sleep disorders, sleep apnea and insomnia, will be discussed here.

Untreated sleep apnea is associated with excessive daytime sleepiness, cognitive impairment, hypertension, and increased risk of cardiovascular disease. It is highly prevalent among CKD patients, with estimates ranging from 70% to 80% based on polysomnographic studies [7]. Sleep apnea cannot be diagnosed through interview or questionnaire, but level of risk can be quickly calculated using questions related to snoring, tiredness during daytime, observed episodes of apnea, and high blood pressure or the STOP-BANG Questionnaire [8], described in more detail below. Patients with high scores on the STOP-BANG, or who report pauses in breathing during their sleep, should be referred for an overnight sleep study for polysomnography to diagnose sleep apnea. Given the extremely high estimated prevalence of sleep apnea among CKD patients, and the serious health impact of untreated sleep apnea, renal healthcare providers should consider routinely assessing level of risk using the STOP-BANG.

Insomnia involves difficulty falling or staying asleep or problems with early-morning awakening with inability to return to sleep [4]. Symptoms of insomnia are reported by 50% to 75% of stage 5 CKD patients on dialysis and may be associated with increased risk of cardiovascular disease and poor immune response [7]. While polysomnography is considered the gold standard for assessing many other sleep disorders, including sleep apnea, it is not recommended for the assessment of insomnia [9]. Rather, insomnia should be assessed via a patient's own self-report in the form of a 2-week prospective sleep diary such as the Consensus Sleep Diary [10]. Interpretation of sleep diary data involves some training and calculation of certain sleep parameters, such as average sleep efficiency, sleep onset latency, and wakefulness after sleep onset; therefore, it may not be a feasible assessment method in primary care settings. The Insomnia Severity Index (ISI), described below, may be a useful alternative for screening for insomnia disorder in primary care settings [11]. Insomnia disorder may also be diagnosed by clinical interview using established diagnostic criteria such as those for DSM-5 insomnia disorder [4].

2.2.2 Screening Tools

This section provides a sample of screening tools that can be used with CKD patients and is not intended to be an exhaustive inventory. These are not diagnostic tools and thus should not be used to diagnose psychiatric disorders solely on the basis of scores on scales, while the scores can support a diagnosis based on clinical interview. Rather, they provide a standardized way of screening for symptoms of psychiatric disorders in a fast and efficient format. Based on empirically derived cutoffs on these questionnaires, the clinician can then determine the appropriate course of action. Potential courses of action could include active monitoring of symptoms, providing psychoeducation, providing access to self-management programs, or referring for further clinical evaluation, diagnosis, and treatment by a psychiatrist. Many open access screening tools provide guidance to the user on what level of intervention should be offered based on symptom severity. Some, but not all of the following tools have been validated for use with CKD patients.

2.2.2.1 Depressive Disorders

There are several brief self-report measures that have been validated with renal patients for screening for depression symptomology. A recent review of depression screening tools for CKD patients suggests that more research is needed, however, to establish diagnostic accuracy of these tools in this population [12].

The Patient Health Questionnaire, 9-item version (PHQ-9), is a self-report questionnaire that screens for the presence and frequency of depressive symptoms over a 2-week period [13]. It has been validated in primary care settings and recommended clinical cutoffs of 5, 10, 15, and 20 represent mild, moderate, moderately severe, and severe depression, respectively. It has been validated in CKD patients on hemodialysis, and the suggested cutoff score indicative of a depressive disorders diagnosis in this population is 10, which is the same cutoff for the general population [14]. Given that this questionnaire assesses somatic symptoms of depression that overlap with uremic symptoms, it is wise to interpret the score judiciously. It is possible for a CKD patient to score over the cutoff while not reporting any problem with depressed mood or anhedonia. Notably, a diagnosis of depressive disorder requires depressed mood and/or anhedonia, not solely a PHQ-9 score threshold. The benefits of this questionnaire are that it is free, brief to administer, and widely used.

The Patient Health Questionnaire, 2-item version (PHQ-2), contains just the first two items of the PHQ-9 screening for the presence and frequency of low mood and anhedonia [15]. A cutoff of ≥3 is recommended for identifying patients with depression in the general population. This is a very brief and commonly used screening tool, but has not been validated specifically with CKD patients.

The Edmonton Symptom Assessment System (ESAS) was initially developed to assess symptoms relevant to palliative care patients using a visual analog scale [16]. The single items representing depression and anxiety symptoms have been validated in a hemodialysis population, using an 11-item scale ranging from 0 (no symptoms) to 10 (worst possible symptoms). This scale may also be presented in the form of a thermometer, with patients indicating their depression "temperature" on the 0 to 10 scale. A cutoff score of ≥2 was recommended for identifying patients with depression [17]. Advantages of the ESAS are that it is free to use, is simple to administer, and requires very little cognitive effort on the part of the patient. This latter feature is important, given the prevalence of cognitive impairment among CKD patients, discussed in detail below.

The Hospital Anxiety and Depression Scale (HADS) is a 14-item tool designed to assess anxiety and depression symptoms in hospitalized patients, but is now commonly used in community and primary care settings [18]. It contains two 7-item subscales to assess for depression and anxiety symptoms separately. The HADS has been validated for use with CKD patients, with recommended cutoffs of ≥7 for the depression subscale and ≥ 6 for the anxiety subscale [19]. This scale is slightly longer than the PHQ-9, but includes screening for anxiety as well as depression. Furthermore, it is free to use, and depression items relate more to mood and anhedonia rather than somatic complaints that may overlap with uremia.

Finally, the *Beck Depression Inventory, Second Edition* (BDI-II) is a 21-item screening tool to assess for depression symptom severity [20]. Out of all available depression screening tools, this has been the most widely studied for use with CKD patients [12]. There is no consensus on the optimal cutoff score for CKD patients using the BDI-II, and proposed cutoffs in the literature range from ≥10 to ≥19, with several studies recommending cutoffs between a smaller range of ≥14 and ≥ 16 [12]. Despite being widely studied, there are several disadvantages to using the BDI-II. For example, it is longer than most other depression screening tools, which may pose more of a burden to CKD patients, and is not open access, requiring a license and fee to administer.

2.2.2.2 Suicidality

The Columbia-Suicide Severity Rating Scale (C-SSRS) is a free assessment tool available to clinicians to help quantify suicide risk, including ideation and behavior [21]. It is composed of four subscales that assess different components of suicidality, including severity of ideation, intensity of ideation, past behaviors, and lethality of former attempts. Clinicians may choose a relevant time-frame (e.g., lifetime, since last contact). The C-SSRS also provides guidance on what level of intervention is recommended based on patient response to specific items. For example, patients who report thinking about *how* they might kill themselves would receive a higher level of intervention than patients who have just thought about killing themselves, but have *not* thought about how they would do it. At the time of writing this chapter, a wide selection of C-SSRS versions can be downloaded from https://cssrs.columbia.edu, each tailored to specific settings (e.g., first responders, healthcare facilities, military installations, correctional facilities, colleges/schools). Notably, although depressive disorder and suicide are linked, only about 60% of individuals who die by suicide had a history of major depressive disorder, and thus other neuropsychiatric illnesses can increase the risk for suicide (e.g., substance use disorder, borderline and narcissistic personality disorders, multiple sclerosis) [22].

2.2.2.3 Anxiety Disorders

Several brief self-report screening measures have been validated for use with CKD patients, including the HADS and ESAS which have already been described above in the context of screening for depressive disorder. Another frequently used measure, the Generalized Anxiety Disorder-7 Inventory (GAD-7) is a 7-item self-report measure of anxiety symptom severity [23]. Recommended cutoffs of 5, 10, and 15 are indicative of mild, moderate, and severe levels of anxiety. A cutoff of 10 is suggestive of generalized anxiety disorder; however, this instrument is not intended as a diagnostic tool independent of the clinical interview. The GAD-7, though widely used, has not been validated with CKD patients. Despite this, some advantages include being free and brief to administer.

2.2.2.4 Sleep Disorders

As mentioned above, sleep apnea can only be diagnosed through polysomnography. Typically, a physician's referral to a sleep medicine specialist is required to facilitate this assessment. Fortunately, sleep apnea risk level can be easily assessed using the STOP-BANG questionnaire [8]. STOP-BANG is an acronym composed of letters representing various risk factors for sleep apnea: loud *s*noring, feeling *t*ired, fatigued or sleepy during the day, been *o*bserved choking/gasping or stop breathing during sleep, high blood *p*ressure, *B*MI of >35 kg/m^2, *a*ge > 50, large *n*eck size (shirt collar 16 inches/40 cm or larger), and *g*ender = male (this last item actually refers to biological sex rather than gender). An affirmative response to 5 or more questions is indicative of high risk of sleep apnea, and patients should be referred for further evaluation via polysomnography. Patients who are male, have a BMI > 35 kg/m^2, or have a large neck circumference must only score 2 out of 4 STOP items to be considered high risk for sleep apnea. Scores of 0–2 and 3–4 are indicative of low and intermediate sleep apnea risk, respectively. The STOP-BANG is free to use and easily accessible online.

The Insomnia Severity Index (ISI) is a 7-item self report questionnaire that assesses a patient's subjective insomnia severity over the past 2 weeks [11]. Each item is scored on a 5-point Likert-type scale ranging from 0 (least problematic) to 4 (most problematic) with higher scores indicating greater insomnia severity. The ISI explores problems falling asleep, staying asleep, and waking up too early, as well as dissatisfaction with sleep, worry/distress about the sleep problem, interference in daily activities, and how noticeable the sleep problem is to others. Cutoff scores of ≥8, ≥ 15, and ≥ 22 are indicative of subthreshold, moderate, and severe insomnia, but in community samples a score of ≥10 is typically used as the cutoff indicative of subthreshold insomnia severity [24]. Although the ISI is a widely used measure, it has not been validated with CKD patients. Advantages include being brief and free to use.

2.2.3 Case Vignette Analysis: "An Unfortunate New Beginning"

During Mr. Wilson's next clinic visit, he noticed that they had implemented a new intake form that he had to complete, which only took a few seconds. There were some graphical scales to fill out that looked like thermometers, and he decided to be completely honest about how he had been feeling recently – Distress "7", Anxiety "5", Depression "7", Need to Talk to Someone "9". The nurse reviewed these with him and the nephrologist, and after a brief safety assessment, he readily accepted a consultation with the psychiatrist and psychologist in the clinic. During his next visit with the psychiatrist and psychologist, he completed the PHQ-9. This took him just a few more minutes, but he had some difficulty deciding which answer to circle for some of the questions. His score on this questionnaire fell in the range indicative of severe depression (scale score of 20/27), including that the endorsement of item 9 – "Thoughts that you would be better off dead or of hurting yourself" as "*several days* over the past 2 weeks." The psychiatrist noticed that he indicated daily problems with fatigue, poor appetite, trouble falling asleep, and difficulty concentrating, in addition to less frequent problems feeling down and depressed, losing interest in most activities, and thinking he would be better off dead.

Wondering if his score was an accurate reflection of his depression severity, or if it was artificially elevated due to physical symptoms common to dialysis patients, he more thoroughly assessed his symptoms and determined that Mr. Wilson did in fact meet criteria for major depressive disorder and noted that while fatigue, poor appetite, trouble falling asleep, and difficulty concentrating are common in dialysis patients, his poor appetite and trouble falling asleep only started around the same time that his mood worsened, and his fatigue and difficulty concentrating, which had already been present, worsened considerably around that same time. A trial of an antidepressant, such as a selective serotonin reuptake inhibitor, was recommended in addition to cognitive behavioral psychotherapy (CBT); however, Mr. Wilson favored initiating psychotherapy with the clinical psychologist for the time being, declining medication. Again, ruling out acute safety concerns, the psychologist offered a brief series of bi-weekly CBT sessions to Mr. Wilson. The PHQ-9 was administered at every visit to monitor progress. His scale scores gradually decreased, and he no longer endorsed item 9 ("Thoughts that you would be better off dead or of hurting yourself"). By the end of the series of visits, his PHQ-9 score was in the mild severity range (9/27), mostly driven by the somatic items that he experienced rather chronically, but less severely and frequently.

2.2.4 When to Refer for Psychological Assessment

Some of the screening tools presented above provide guidelines for nephrology clinicians on when to refer patients for psychiatric consultation and psychological testing that can aid the clinical psychiatric diagnosis and treatment. On the PHQ-9, psychotherapy or pharmacotherapy is suggested for patients who score $\geq$ 10, and a combination of psychotherapy *and* pharmacotherapy is suggested for patients who score $\geq$ 20. As mentioned previously, on the C-SSRS, patients who report suicidal ideation as well as thinking about *how* they might go about killing themselves should be referred for a more thorough consultation with a mental health specialist such as a psychiatrist, psychologist, or social worker, and safety precautions should be considered. Patients who furthermore report some intent on acting on suicidal thoughts, or who have begun working out the details of a plan, or who have enacted some type of suicidal behavior in the past should receive further consultation with a mental health specialist, and safety precautions should be implemented; if urgent, the patient is asked to go to the emergency department for prompt evaluation.

Patients who score $\geq$ 15 on the GAD-7 should be referred for psychiatric assessment and treatment.

Patients who score high risk for sleep apnea on the STOP-BANG should be referred for polysomnography to diagnose sleep apnea. The gold standard treatment for sleep apnea is continuous positive airway pressure (CPAP) treatment [7]. Patients who exhibit nonadherence to CPAP treatment should be referred for psychiatric/psychological evaluation and intervention. Reasons for nonadherence that may be amenable to treatment include anxiety (e.g., claustrophobia, panic disorder), poor understanding of the rationale for CPAP compliance and health impact of untreated sleep apnea, comorbid insomnia, or unhelpful beliefs about CPAP use (e.g., "I don't notice any difference when I use it").

Patients who report experiencing sleep disturbance at least three nights per week and who score above the cutoff on the ISI would likely benefit from further assessment and treatment. A sleep medicine specialist can work with the patient to prospectively monitor sleep parameters using a sleep diary and further assess sleep disturbance and suitability for treatment. The gold standard treatment for insomnia is cognitive behavioral therapy for insomnia (CBT-i), which has considerable empirical support. Many CKD patients prefer not to add any more medications to their daily regimen, which makes this a desirable treatment for many patients.

In the absence of established guidelines for when to refer patients for further psychological assessment, the clinician should take into consideration symptom severity, level of distress reported by the patient, and degree of impairment in the patient's life, including interpersonal relationships, adherence to treatment recommendations, attendance at dialysis or other medical appointments, and general self-care. Symptoms that are believed to interfere with health-related behaviors that could precipitate more rapid progression of CKD, reduce efficacy of dialysis, or increase risk of transplant graft failure should be addressed immediately. Some examples of treatment-interfering behaviors include nonadherence to dialysis appointments, fluid restrictions, medications, and/or dietary recommendations. Renal programs will often have pathways in place for referring patients who require psychiatric intervention. In the absence of such pathways, renal care providers may explore community resources such as psychiatric services, counseling services through family health teams, not-for-profit community organizations, community crisis outreach teams, hospital-based programs, or private practice psychotherapy (for patients who can afford to pay for services).

Recommendation

- Sudden changes to a patient's behavior or appearance should be explored.
- Referral for psychiatric consultation, psychological testing, and psychiatric management should be considered if there is any concern for the patient's welfare.

2.3 Neuropsychological Assessment

Neuropsychological assessment is a performance-based method to specifically assess cognitive functioning. This section will begin by reviewing common cognitive difficulties or impairments observed among renal patients. It will present some useful screening tools that can be used by frontline medical staff and will identify when patients should be referred for more specialized psychiatric and/or neuropsychological assessment.

2.3.1 Case Vignette: "Worsening Cognitive Changes in a Renal Transplant Patient"

Mr. Smith was a 42-year-old man with a remote history of renal transplant at 25 years of age secondary to end-stage renal disease due to glomerulonephritis. He presented to hospital with a 2-week history of increasingly worsening general malaise, problems with short-term memory, and episodes of confusion. By history, he had responded well to the transplant with no significant complications and went on to complete his college degree and maintain employment. Medical conditions also include hypertension, dyslipidemia, and depressive disorder. He was prescribed sertraline 100 mg per day for depressive disorder by his primary care physician in addition to immunosuppressants, corticosteroids, and a lipid lowering agent. On admission, extensive medical evaluations including blood work, lumbar puncture, and brain MRI were non-significant. He denied a history of significant alcohol or substance use or acute intoxication prior to his recent decompensation. In terms of his baseline cognition, Mr. Smith described himself as "a bit forgetful – more than average." He denied any functional difficulties at work or home secondary to his forgetfulness. However, his employer had recently implemented a new computer system and he was taking longer to learn compared to his co-workers, suggesting potential cognitive impairment prior to his recent worsening.

2.3.2 Common Cognitive Difficulties

Cognitive impairment is common in CKD and is increasingly being recognized as a major cause of chronic disability in those affected with this illness. CKD may be an independent risk factor for cognitive impairment that has a broad effect across most areas of cognition. There is evidence that cognitive impairment can be present across all stages of CKD, is independent of age-related changes, and exists for both lower-order and higher-order cognitive abilities that increase between stages of CKD suggesting a cumulative effect [25]. In this regard, cognitive impairment in CKD can be conceptualized as broad, transcending in stages with no signature neuropsychological profile that can nonetheless serve as a useful marker for the early identification of CKD.

The neurobiological mechanisms that lead to cognitive impairment in CKD have not been clearly defined. Several potential mechanisms have been suggested (see [26] for review), a vast majority of which relate to higher levels of inflammation, oxidative stress, anemia, and uremic toxins that build up in the blood due to compromised and inefficient kidney function. Additionally, CKD has been associated with vascular comorbidities such as diabetes mellitus, hypertension, and cardiovascular disease: conditions which in and of themselves are associated with cognitive impairment in similar areas of cognition and may contribute to a higher risk and severity of cognitive impairment in those presenting with these comorbidities and which may represent comorbid vascular dementia. CKD patients are also at high risk for delirium. (For more information on the neurocognitive ramification of kidney disease, see Chap. 12.)

2.3.3 Cognitive Impairment across Disease Course

Decreased kidney function increases susceptibility to changes in cognitive functioning in individuals affected with CKD. The degree of impaired kidney filtration rate is used as the metric to categorize stage of kidney disease with the estimated glomerular filtration rate (eGFR) representing kidney efficiency in filtering waste from the blood from early (stages 1 and 2) and moderate (stages 3 and 4) to end (stage 5) stages of the disease process. Because of the increased prevalence and severity of CKD in older populations, the majority of studies examining cognitive changes have been focused on later stages of the disease process. This has mistakenly led to a common assertion that cognitive impairment in CKD is relatively asymptomatic in younger individuals at early stages of illness only manifesting at later/end stages of illness [27]. There is increasing evidence that cognitive deficits are already present in the earlier stages of renal impairment and decline at different rates for different cognitive domains as CKD progresses and eGFR declines [1]. For example, a systematic review and meta-analysis revealed that orientation and attention and language ability might be particularly affected in earlier stages of illness and more prone to decline across illness progression, while impairments in memory and executive functioning become more prominent at moderate stages of CKD illness progression [1]. Language skills unlike other cognitive abilities have been identified as the only cognitive domain that demonstrates a linear relationship with eGFR decline. The earlier impact of CKD on attentional processes and language ability likely negatively impacts higher-order cognitive skills such as memory and executive functioning with illness progression.

A more recent systematic review of cognitive impairment in CKD reviewed studies in non-older adults with CKD (under age 65 years) undergoing hemodialysis who were not posttransplant to establish the impact of age-related cognitive changes to cognitive impairment across different stages of CKD [25] (see Table 2.2). Only reviewing studies in individuals younger than 65 years informed whether cognitive impairment in CKD is consequent to the disease process or potentially exacerbated by natural age-related cognitive changes. These findings are summarized below.

Table 2.2 Summary of findings from Brodski et al. systematic review and meta-analysis [25]

CKD stage	Number of studies reviewed	Cognitive impairments identified
1–2	3	• Processing speed • Response speed • Attention • Short-term memory • Set shifting
3–5	9	• Executive functioning • Concentration • Sequencing • Orientation • Working memory • Processing speed continues to decline
5 (end stage)	10	• Most cognitive impairments that initially manifested in earlier stages are exacerbated and progress • Verbal fluency • Visuospatial abilities • Further memory impairment progresses

Early-stage CKD In stages 1 and 2, significant decreases were noted in speed of processing, response speed, attention, short-term memory, and set shifting. These findings are consistent with the notion that the bulk of cognitive deficits in the early stages of CKD comprise the more basic cognitive abilities (attention, processing speed) that are important for higher-order cognitive functions. This is also consistent with reports of reduced mental sharpness, general cognitive slowness, or haziness as early symptoms or indicators of CKD and dispels the myth that early CKD is relatively asymptomatic [27]. It has been proposed that the attention deficits identified in patients with CKD are mediated by altered monoamine-prefrontal cortical circuity [26].

Moderate-stage CKD In individuals with CKD in moderate stages of illness, impairments were shown in processing speed, verbal fluency, memory (recall, short term), orientation, and concentration. While inhibition and switching deficits were also observed, these domains were not more severely impaired than in earlier stages of renal impairment. In general, cognitive performance was substantially poorer among stage 4 compared to stage 3, with almost double the severity of memory and concentration difficulties. As CKD progresses, memory and speed of processing continue to decline. Impairments in higher-order impairment such as concentration and orientation begin to emerge.

End-stage CKD In end stage of illness, most of the cognitive impairments that manifested in earlier and moderate stages continue to exacerbate with progression into end-stage CKD, with significant reduction noted in executive function, memory, and global cognitive functioning. Speed of processing and memory continues to decline with disease progression. Impairments in general cognition at stage 5 compared to stage 4 are more pronounced than those between stage 3 and 4. Although impairments in language have previously been identified in earlier stages of the disease process, language ability was found to be the least impacted area of cognitive impairment compared to other domains in end stages of illness in younger CKD patients. This finding likely reflects different trajectories of decline across different cognitive domains relative to eGFR decline. Additionally, language compared to other cognitive domains might be less impacted in younger patients with CKD at end stages of the illness compared to those who are older and over the age of 65 years.

Clinical Pearl

- Cognitive impairment in CKD has no signature neuropsychological profile and is broad, affecting multiple cognitive domains that transcend across illness progression.

2.3.4 Case Vignette: "Worsening Cognitive Changes in a Renal Transplant Patient" (Continued)

Bedside cognitive screening conducted 2 weeks into his admission following clinical optimization and ruling out reversible causes of delirium revealed that Mr. Smith remained disoriented to date and day. Cognitive screening with the Montreal Cognitive Assessment (MoCA) revealed performance well below what would be expected given his age and educational attainment, for example, with zero out of five words on recall, and a MoCA total score of 23/30. He was unable to recall or describe events immediately leading up to his hospitalization. At the time of testing, he rated his memory at about "75%" returned to baseline. Given Mr. Smith's relatively young age, and his good functional status prior to a rapid decline in cognition, formal neuropsychological assessment was requested to clarify his current level of cognitive functioning and provide input into discharge and medical follow-up planning.

2.3.5 Impact of Kidney Transplantation on Cognition

Evidence for the impact of kidney transplantation on cognition has been mixed. While some studies have suggested improvements in cognition, others have indicated the potential for cognitive decline exacerbated by adverse effects of immunosuppressant medications required after transplantation or by the presence of comorbid depressive disorders [28, 29]. A recent meta-analysis examined which cognitive domains were impacted following kidney transplantation and how their cognition compared to non-transplanted CKD patients and healthy controls [30]. Cognitive performance in the domains of verbal and visual memory, spatial reasoning, processing speed, and general cognitive status was better in patients who had received a transplant compared to those who were on dialysis. Following transplant, significant improvements were apparent in the domains of general cognitive function, information and motor speed, spatial reasoning, and verbal and visual memory. In studies reporting cognitive improvements following kidney transplant, these improvements remained stable at 1-year and 2-year follow-up [31, 32]. Despite these improvements, transplant patients still performed significantly below healthy matched controls/normative data in three cognitive domains (executive function, verbal fluency, and language). Moreover, cognition in some domains (attention, executive function, verbal fluency, and language) did not improve after transplantation (even with long-term follow-up) compared with pre-transplant levels and was not superior compared with dialysis patients.

Overall, the results from this meta-analysis indicate that while domain-specific cognitive improvement can occur for CKD individuals following successful transplantation, impairments persist in executive functioning, verbal fluency, and language where performance remains significantly below standardized normative performance of healthy controls. This would support the idea that neurocognitive disorders such as delirium and/or vascular major neurocognitive disorder (vascular dementia), both commonly encountered in CKD patients, are not impacted by transplantation, at least in these cognitive domains. (For more information on the neurocognitive ramification of kidney disease, see Chap. 12.)

2.3.6 Cognitive Screening Tools

Given the high prevalence of cognitive impairment among patients with CKD that can impact decision-making and compliance, screening for cognitive impairment should ideally start in the early stages of CKD to establish a reference point of baseline functioning that can be monitored across illness progression. Several screening tests are available with a range of administration times and diagnostic accuracy. Many of the available screening tests have not been specifically designed to assess CKD populations which may limit their utility. Nonetheless, in previous studies in hemodialysis patients the Mini-Mental State Examination (MMSE) [33], the Montreal Cognitive Assessment (MoCA) test [34], and the Modified Mini-Mental State (3MS) test [35] have been applied using established cutoffs. San et al. conducted a scoping review of studies summarizing the evidence on cognitive impairment in dialysis populations and identified that these were indeed the most common screening measures consistently used in CKD populations (in order of most common was the MMSE, the 3MS, and the MoCA) [36]. Despite the convenience of administering global cognitive screening measures, clinicians should keep in mind that these measures lack specificity and might be less useful for clinicians who may want to direct care toward specific areas of cognitive impairment that need attention. Additionally, global screening measures of cognition are limited in measuring specific cognitive functions that might be more affected than others in CKD as described elsewhere in this section.

MMSE The MMSE is the most frequently used screening tool for cognitive impairment in the general population and appears to have been the most frequently used screening measure in CKD populations [33, 36]. However, the MMSE may be limited in detecting more subtle degrees of cognitive impairment in CKD as normal performance on the MMSE (greater or equal to 24) does not preclude impaired cognitive function. Indeed, Sarnak et al. found that CKD individuals scorning above cutoff for cognitive impairment on the MMSE demonstrated a high frequency of poor cognitive performance using more detailed measures of multiple cognitive domains [37]. In this regard, the MMSE appears to be limited in identifying the subtle cognitive impairments that can occur in the early stages of CKD. Additionally, clinicians considering use of this screening measure should also keep the following limitations in mind: (1) the MMSE is susceptible to age, literacy/education, socioeconomic, and cultural differences, and (2) it is generally insensitive with respect to identifying mild, and/or focal impairments. Additionally, while it is suitable for older individuals presenting with suspected delirium or major neurocognitive disorder, clinicians are cautioned against using it as a sole diagnostic tool. Finally, clinicians should consider that this test is no longer available in the public domain but is commercially available for purchase from Psychological Assessment Resources (http://parinc.com) who is the copyright owner.

3MS Compared to the MMSE, the 3MS test assesses a broader variety of cognitive functions and covers a wider range of difficulty levels and thus enhances the reliability and validity of test scores; hence, it is also more sensitive for detecting mild neurocognitive disorder compared to the MMSE. With a maximum score of 100, score < 80 has been reported to have a sensitivity of 91% and a specificity of 97% for detecting major neurocognitive disorder in the general population. There do not appear to be any studies that have identified different cutoff scores for CKD populations than the established test cutoff score that has been used.

MoCA The MoCA is a widely used screening measure for the assessment of general cognitive function specifically designed to identify mild neurocognitive disorder. The MoCA appears to be the preferred screening tool for cognitive impairment in the dialysis population and is more sensitive than the MMSE based on a study in which 43 hemodialysis patients with an average age of 58 years were assessed with the MoCA, the MMSE, and a detailed neuropsychological test battery [38]. While the standard MoCA cutoff score is 26, in this study, a MoCA cutoff of ≤24 identified patients with cognitive impairment with a sensitivity of 77% and a specificity of 79% in contrast to the MMSE that only discriminated weakly between groups. Another study sought to establish new MoCA cutoff scores for hemodialysis patients based on their global scores on the Clinical Dementia Rating (CDR) scale [39]. The optimal score to differentiate between cognitively normal and impaired CKD patients was determined to be 23.5 points which corresponds to the cutoff reported by Tiffin-Richards [38]. In this study, MoCA score of <22 was associated with cognitive impairment in contrast to a MoCA score of >28 which rules out cognitive impairment.

Recommendation

- The MoCA is the preferred screening tool for cognitive impairment in the dialysis population.
- The MoCA is a suitable screening measure for any individual who is experiencing memory difficulties but whose MMSE score falls within the normal range.

Clinical Pearl

- Consider using the MoCA instead of the MMSE because of its greater sensitivity to detect more subtle cognitive impairment in earlier stages of CKD.

2.3.7 When to Refer for Neuropsychological Assessment

A number of factors contribute to a decision to refer for specialized neuropsychological assessment. Prior to considering neuropsychological assessment, patients should be medically stabilized with all relevant medical investigations completed and screened for alcohol or substance use and have completed cognitive screening. As outlined in this chapter, it is expected that patients with CKD will have cognitive difficulties relative to their healthy peers. These impairments are often detected on cognitive screening, but interpreting the results of cognitive screening can be complicated by the presence of individual difference factors, psychological symptoms, and/or sleep disorder. Determining when a referral for neuropsychological assessment is in order requires consideration of these factors.

First, assess for the presence of one or more individual difference characteristics that may impact cognitive screening, including specific aspects of educational and occupational attainment, age, and language or cultural factors. For example, individuals with low educational attainment, history of learning disability, or poor literacy often perform poorly on cognitive screening, but it is difficult to ascertain if this is reflective of their long-standing low level of performance or reflective of a decline. Relatedly, individuals who were previously at the top end of the normal distribution in terms of educational achievement and above average intellectual ability may experience cognitive decline, but this will be undetectable by most screening tools and will require specialized assessment. When patients are screened in a second language or are unable to be screened due to language barriers, formal assessment by a neuropsychologist with specialized training and experience with assistance of an interpreter or use of alternative non-language biased testing is recommended.

When screening has been completed appropriately and significant impairment is noted more than what would be expected given the medical condition and/or individual difference factors, or when impairment persists following medical stabilization, the nephrology clinician should consider referring the patient for a psychological/psychiatric assessment. In such cases, a neuropsychological assessment can be further requested by the psychiatrist/psychologist to evaluate the nuances of these impairments and evaluate the impact these may have on the patient's ability to function independently. Finally, formal neuropsychological assessment is also recommended when the presence of significant psychiatric comorbidities precludes the ability to determine the extent to which cognitive difficulties detected on screening may be static or malleable in response to psychiatric intervention and/or psychotherapy.

2.3.8 Case Vignette Analysis: "Worsening Cognitive Changes in a Renal Transplant Patient"

Neuropsychological assessment revealed that Mr. Smith's level of general intellectual ability fell in the average range, consistent with his educational and occupational attainment. Most areas of cognitive ability were commensurate with this level, including attention and concentration for both auditory-verbal and visual information, reasoning and conceptualization, mental set shifting, language, and visual spatial skills. In contrast, significant impairments were noted across all tests of learning and memory; his ability to take in and immediately recall information presented to him either verbally or visually fell at or below the fourth percentile for his age and below the second percentile after a delay. Recognition cues were somewhat helpful, more in prompting visual memory (recognition of shapes – tenth percentile) versus verbal material (recognition of list words – fourth percentile). These findings likely reflect significant declines over previous levels of ability and would be expected to have a profound negative impact on his ability to function adaptively in his workplace and at home in terms of his ability to independently manage his medical condition/medication regimen.

As discussed in this chapter, CKD is often associated with cognitive impairment with most research focused on patients undergoing long-term dialysis, and cognition often improves following transplant [30, 39]. Although long-term follow-up of cognition after renal transplant has not been well-documented, long-term use of immunosuppressants has been linked to cognitive dysfunction [40], though this does not typically present as a rapid decline as noted in Mr. Smith's case. Other possible contributors to consider include alcohol or substance use (see Chap. 11), although Mr. Smith denied these as potential contributors, in addition to his diagnosis of depressive disorder and treatment with sertraline. Although depressive disorder is often associated with memory impairment, the severity of impairment noted here is out of the range normally seen in the context of depressive disorder alone especially for a relatively young, previously high-functioning individual. Clinical monitoring including repeat neuropsychological assessment as an outpatient is recommended in Mr. Smith's case to assist in differential diagnosis of his greater than expected memory impairment.

Recommendation

- Consider patient's age, educational and occupational attainment, and prior level of functioning when interpreting results of cognitive testing.
- Consider presence of comorbid psychiatric symptoms such as depression which may also interfere with cognitive function.

Clinical Pearl

- Most significant cognitive impairments are usually seen among patients undergoing long-term dialysis.
- Long-term use of immunosuppressants following transplant has been linked to cognitive dysfunction including working memory impairment.

2.4 Key Takeaways

- Patients with CKD are at increased risk of a number of neuropsychiatric symptoms including cognitive impairment.
- Depressive disorder is the most common psychiatric disorder among CKD patients, and its presence is associated with poorer clinical outcomes, including more frequent hospital admissions, lengthier hospital stays, higher rates of dialysis withdrawal, and increased risk of morbidity and mortality.
- Anxiety disorder is also common in CKD, and certain types of anxiety disorders/phobias may interfere with patients' ability to engage in treatment, leading to worsening clinical status.
- Decision-making regarding referral for specialized psychological assessment and treatment include consideration of symptom severity, level of distress, and degree of impairment in the patient's life, including interpersonal relationships, adherence to treatment recommendations, attendance at dialysis or other medical appointments, and general self-care.
- Early and routine screening for depression and anxiety with respective treatment, where indicated, may help improve the patient's health-related quality of life and clinical outcomes.
- Sleep disorders are common in CKD including sleep apnea, insomnia, restless legs syndrome, and excessive daytime sleepiness.
- The presence of a sleep disorder may lead to psychological and/or cognitive impairments with a synergistic negative impact on engagement in treatment and clinical outcomes.
- Cognitive deficits most common in CKD include orientation, attention, executive functions such as reasoning and concept formation, and memory.
- Cognitive changes occur early in the course of renal disease and worsen over time.
- Cognitive impairments negatively impact patients' ability to follow treatment protocols and make informed healthcare decisions.
- Routine screening and monitoring of cognition using appropriate tools is important in CKD patients, to inform addition of increased home-based support and advance care directives.
- Referral for specialized neuropsychological assessment is recommended when validity of screening is hampered by individual differences such as very low or very high educational attainment or intellectual ability, language barriers, significant psychiatric comorbidities, or when impairment on screening is greater than expected.

References

1. Berger I, Wu S, Masson P, et al. Cognition in chronic kidney disease: a systematic review and meta-analysis. BMC Med. 2016;14:206–16.
2. Goh ZS, Griva K. Anxiety and depression in patients with end-stage renal disease: impact and management challenges – a narrative review. Int J Nephrol Renovasc Dis. 2018;11:93–102.
3. Palmer S, Vecchio M, Craig JC, et al. Prevalence of depression in chronic kidney disease: systematic review and meta-analysis of observational studies. Kidney Int. 2013;84:179–91.

4. American Psychiatric Association. Diagnostic and Statistical Manual of Mental Disorders. 5th ed. Arlington (VA); 2013.
5. Liu CH, Yeh MK, Weng SC, et al. Suicide and chronic kidney disease: a case-control study. Nephrol Dial Transplant. 2017;32(9):1524–9.
6. Huang CW, Wee PH, Low LL, et al. Prevalence and risk factors for elevated anxiety symptoms and anxiety disorders in chronic kidney disease: a systematic review and meta-analysis. Gen Hosp Psychiatry. 2021;69:27–40.
7. Maung SC, El Sara A, Chapman C, et al. Sleep disorders and chronic kidney disease. World J Nephrol. 2016;5(3):224–32.
8. Chung F, Yegneswaran B, Liao P, et al. STOP questionnaire: a tool to screen patients for obstructive sleep apnea. Anesthesiology. 2008;108(5):812–21.
9. Schutte-Rodin S, Broch L, Buysse D, et al. Clinical guideline for the evaluation and management of chronic insomnia in adults. J Clin Sleep Med. 2008;4(5):487–504.
10. Carney CE, Buysse DJ, Ancoli-Israel S, et al. The consensus sleep diary: standardizing prospective sleep self-monitoring. Sleep. 2012;35(2):287–302.
11. Morin C. Insomnia: psychological assessment and management. Guilford: New York (NY); 1993.
12. Kondo K, Antick JR, Ayers CK, et al. Depression screening tools for patients with kidney failure: a systematic review. Clin J Am Soc Nephrol. 2020;15(12):1785–95.
13. Kroenke K, Spitzer RL, Williams JB. The PHQ-9: validity of a brief depression severity measure. J Gen Intern Med. 2001;16(9):606–13.
14. Watnick S, Wang PL, Demadura T, Ganzini L. Validation of 2 depression screening tools in dialysis patients. Am J Kidney Dis. 2005;46(5):919–24.
15. Kroenke K, Spitzer RL, Williams JB. The patient health Questionnaire 2: validity of a two-item depression screener. Med Care. 2003;41(11):1284–92.
16. Bruera E, Kuehn N, Miller MJ, et al. The Edmonton symptom assessment system (ESAS): a simple method for the assessment of palliative care patients. J Palliat Care. 1991;7(2):6–9.
17. Collister D, Rodrigues JC, Mazzetti A, et al. Single questions for the screening of anxiety and depression in hemodialysis. Can J Kidney Health Dis. 2019;6:1–7.
18. Bjelland I, Dahl AA, Haug TT, Neckelmann D. The validity of the hospital anxiety and depression scale. An updated literature review. J Psychosom Res. 2002;52(2):69–77.
19. Preljevic VT, Østhus TBH, Sandvik L, et al. Screening for anxiety and depression in dialysis patients: comparison of the hospital anxiety and depression scale and the Beck depression inventory. J Psychosom Res. 2012;73(2):139–44.
20. Beck AT, Steer RA, Brown, GK. Manual for the Beck Depression Inventory-II. San Antonio (TX). Psychological Corporation; 1996.
21. Posner K, Brown GK, Stanley B, et al. The Columbia-suicide severity rating scale: initial validity and internal consistency findings from three multisite studies with adolescents and adults. Am J Psychiatry. 2011;168(12):1266–77.
22. Ng CW, How CH, Ng YP. Depression in primary care: assessing suicide risk. Singap Med J. 2017;58(2):72–7.
23. Spitzer RL, Kroenke K, Williams JBW, Löwe B. A brief measure for assessing generalized anxiety disorder: the GAD-7. Arch Intern Med. 2006;166(10):1092–7.
24. Morin CM, Belleville G, Bélanger L, Ivers H. The insomnia severity index: psychometric indicators to detect insomnia cases and evaluate treatment response. Sleeps. 2011;34(5):601–8.
25. Brodski J, Rossell SL, Castle DJ, Tan EJ. A systematic review of cognitive impairments associated with kidney failure in adults before natural age-related changes. J Int Neuropsychol Soc. 2019;25(1):101–14.
26. Viggiano D, Wagner CA, Martino G, et al. Mechanisms of cognitive dysfunction in CKD. Nat Rev Nephrol. 2020;16(8):452–69.
27. Levey AS, Coresh J, Balk E, et al. National Kidney Foundation practice guidelines for chronic kidney disease: evaluation, classification, and stratification. Ann Intern Med. 2003;139:137–47.
28. Troen AM, Scott TM, Anci KED, et al. Cognitive dysfunction and depression in adult kidney transplant recipients: baseline findings from the FAVORIT ancillary cognitive trial (FACT). J Ren Nutr. 2012;22(2):268–76.

29. Martínez-Sanchis S, Bernal MC, Montagud JV, et al. Effects of immunosuppressive drugs on the cognitive functioning of renal transplant recipients: a pilot study. J Clin Exp Neuropsychol. 2011;33:9:1016–24.
30. Joshee P, Wood AG, Wood ER, Grunfeld EA. Meta-analysis of cognitive functioning in patients following kidney transplantation. Nephrol Dial Transplant. 2018;33:1268–77.
31. Harciarek M, Biedunkiewicz B, Lichodziejewska-Niemierko M, et al. Continuous cognitive improvement 1 year following successful kidney transplant. Kidney Int. 2011;79(12):1353–60.
32. Radić J, Ljutić D, Radić M, et al. Kidney transplantation improves cognitive and psychomotor functions in adult hemodialysis patients. Am J Nephrol. 2011;34:399–406.
33. Folstein MF, Folstein SE, McHugh PR. Mini-mental state. A practical method for grading the cognitive state of patients for the clinician. J Psychiatr Res. 1975;12(3):189–98.
34. Nasreddine ZS, Phillips NA, Bédirian V, et al. The Montreal cognitive assessment, MoCA: a brief screening tool for mild cognitive impairment. J Am Geriatr Soc. 2005;53(4):695–9.
35. Teng EL, Chui HC. The modified mini-mental state (3MS) examination. J Clin Psychiatry. 1987;48:314–8.
36. San A, Hiremagalur B, Muircroft W, Grealish L. Screening of cognitive impairment in the dialysis population: a scoping review. Dement Geriatr Cogn Disord. 2017;44:182–95.
37. Sarnak MJ, Tighiouart H, Scott TM, et al. Frequency of and risk factors for poor performance in hemodialysis patients. Neurology. 2013;80:471–80.
38. Tiffin-Richards FE, Costa AS, Holschbach B, et al. The Montreal cognitive assessment (MoCA) – a sensitive screening instrument for detecting cognitive impairment in chronic hemodialysis patients. PLoS One. 2014;9:e106700.
39. Angermann S, Baumann M, Steubl D, et al. Cognitive impairment in hemodialysis patients: implementation of cut-off values for the Montreal cognitive assessment (MoCA)-test for feasible screening. PLoS One. 2017;12(10).
40. Bösche K, Weissenborn K, Christians U, et al. Neurobehavioral consequences of small molecule-drug immunosuppression. Neuropharmacology. 2015;96(Pt A):83–93.
41. Meyer TW, Hostetter TH. Uremia. N Engl J Med. 2007;357:1316–25.

Current State, Knowledge Gaps, and Management Strategies of Kidney Disease for the Psychiatrist

3

Meera Joseph and Azim S. Gangji

3.1 Case Vignette

Mr. Pratt was a 60-year-old gentleman referred to the nephrology clinic for evaluation of chronic kidney disease. He had a past medical history of type 2 diabetes mellitus since the age of 40, complicated by diabetic retinopathy, neuropathy, and hypertension for the last 15 years. He also had a remote history of peptic ulcer disease. He smoked half a pack of cigarettes per day but did not drink alcohol or use other drugs. His current medications are amlodipine 10 mg daily, ramipril 5 mg daily, metformin 1000 mg BID, linagliptin 5 mg daily, and pantoprazole 20 mg daily. He felt well with no symptoms to report. On examination, his weight was 95 kg; blood pressure was 150/80 mm Hg and heart rate of 75 beats per minute. Cardiovascular exam revealed normal heart sounds with no murmurs. His chest was clear. He had no edema. The remainder of his examination was unremarkable. Mr. Pratt's bloodwork demonstrated a hemoglobin of 105 g/L and creatinine 170 umol/L with an eGFR of 39 mL/min per 1.73 m^2. Electrolytes and acid balance were within normal range. Hemoglobin A1c was 8.0%. Urine albumin-to-creatinine ratio measured 60 mg/mmol. There was no blood seen in urine microscopy. Continue reading for clues for diagnosis and management. A case analysis is also presented in Sect. 3.4.

M. Joseph (✉) · A. S. Gangji
Division of Nephrology, Department of Medicine, McMaster University, St. Joseph's Healthcare Hamilton, Hamilton, ON, Canada
e-mail: meera.joseph@medportal.ca; gangji@mcmaster.ca

A. Hategan et al. (eds.), *Psychonephrology*,
https://doi.org/10.1007/978-3-030-84740-1_3

3.2 Chronic Kidney Disease (CKD)

3.2.1 Defining CKD

Chronic kidney disease arises from disease pathways that irreversibly alter the function and structure of the kidney over months to years. The diagnosis of CKD is made if there is evidence of reduced kidney function and evidence of structural kidney damage (e.g., albuminuria, proteinuria, hematuria). The best available indicator of overall kidney function is glomerular filtration rate (GFR), which equals the total amount of fluid filtered through all the functioning nephrons per unit of time. Table 3.1 shows KDIGO (Kidney Disease Improving Global Outcomes) GFR categories in CKD [1]. Current guidelines define CKD as a GFR less than 60 mL/min per 1.73 m^2, or markers of kidney damage, or both, of at least 3-month duration, regardless of underlying etiology. Markers of kidney damage are identified in Table 3.2. End-stage kidney disease (ESKD), or kidney failure, is defined as stage 5 CKD, where GFR is less than 15 mL/min per 1.73 m^2. At this stage, the kidneys are no longer able to sustain life in the long run, and the patient must decide to either proceed with renal replacement therapy (dialysis or transplant) or opt for comprehensive conservative medical care (non-dialytic care).

Clinical Pearl

- Chronic kidney disease (CKD) is defined as glomerular filtration rate (GFR) less than 60 mL/min per 1.73 m^2 or markers of kidney damage or both for at least 3 months in duration.

3.2.2 Epidemiology of CKD

The incidence and prevalence of CKD varies throughout the world. In high-income countries, the prevalence of CKD is reported to be around 11%. Within countries, those living in the lowest socioeconomic quartile have a 60% higher risk of progressive CKD compared to those in the highest quartile. There is also variation between ethnic groups; in Canada, Indigenous people are at a higher risk of developing CKD and disease progression. Although socioeconomic status plays a specific role in the

Table 3.1 GFR categories in CKD [1]

GFR category	GFR (mL/min per 1.73 m^2)	Terms
G1	Greater than or equal to 90	Normal or high
G2	60–89	Mildly decreased
G3a	45–59	Mildly to moderately decreased
G3b	30–44	Moderately to severely decreased
G4	15–29	Severely decreased
G5	Less than 15	Kidney failure

Note: In the absence of kidney damage, neither GFR category G1 or G2 fulfill the criteria for CKD

Table 3.2 Markers of kidney damage [1]

Albuminuria >30 mg/day
Urine sediment abnormalities (e.g., hematuria, red cell casts)
Electrolyte and other abnormalities due to tubular disorders
Abnormalities detected by histology
Structural abnormalities detected by imaging
History of kidney transplantation

incidence and prevalence of CKD, it does not fully explain the increased risk for racial or ethnic minorities [2]. (See also Chap. 21, Cultural Considerations when Caring for Racial and Ethnic Minority Patients with End-Stage Renal Disease.)

Diabetes mellitus and hypertension are the main causes of CKD in all high-income and middle-income countries, as well as in many low-income countries. Diabetes mellitus accounts for 30–50% of all CKD and affects 285 million (6.4%) adults worldwide; this number is expected to increase by 69% in high-income countries and 20% in low-income and middle-income countries by 2030 [2]. With regard to hypertension, more than a quarter of the adult population was estimated to have hypertension in 2000; this proportion is projected to increase by approximately 60% by 2025 [2].

In Asia, India, and sub-Saharan Africa, CKD from glomerulonephritis and unknown causes are more common. Potential contributors are nephrotoxic effects of infections, herbal medicines used by rural populations, and environmental pollution of water by heavy metals and soil by organic compounds (including pesticides) [2].

According to WHO global health estimates, 864,226 deaths (or 1.5% of deaths worldwide) were attributable to CKD in 2012. Ranked 14th in the list of leading causes of death, CKD accounted for 12.2 deaths per 100,000 people. Since 1990, only deaths from complications of HIV infection have increased at a faster rate than deaths from CKD. Projections from the Global Health Observatory suggest that although the death rate from HIV will decrease in the next 15 years, the death rate from CKD will continue to increase to reach 14 per 100,000 people by 2030 [2].

Clinical Pearl

- In high- and middle-income countries, diabetes mellitus and hypertension are the main causes of CKD.
- CKD is a common cause of death and the mortality rate is expected to rise further.

3.2.3 Evaluation of CKD

Like in any evaluation of a patient, the diagnosis of CKD is based on a combination of a history from the patient, physical examination, and investigations.

A carefully gathered, targeted history can give the clinician many clues about the etiology of a patient's CKD. As long-standing diabetes mellitus and hypertension are the most common causes of CKD, it is important to determine duration, control of disease, and complications (e.g., retinopathy, neuropathy, cardiovascular disease). For diabetic patients, those who have diabetic retinopathy have a higher likelihood of having diabetic nephropathy. Due to their associations with CKD, patients should also be asked about (1) risk factors for renovascular disease (history of peripheral and coronary arterial disease, dyslipidemia, resistant hypertension, history of smoking); (2) history of acute kidney injury; (3) history of infections, including those complicated by urinary tract infections, and risk factors for infections such as hepatitis B or C and HIV; (4) history, screening compliance, and symptoms of malignancy; and (5) history and symptoms of autoimmune conditions. Many kidney diseases are inheritable, so it is also important to ask about any family members with a history of kidney disease and needing dialysis or transplantation. Medications, including over-the-counter medications (specifically NSAIDs) and herbal supplements, should also be carefully reviewed as many can be nephrotoxic.

A targeted physical examination should be performed to assess for hypertension and its complications (e.g., arteriovenous nicking on funduscopic examination); signs of volume overload (indicating possible heart failure, cirrhosis or nephrotic syndrome) and depletion; enlarged kidneys that are palpable on exam (query polycystic kidney disease); abnormal abdominal bruits and diminished distal pulses (query renal artery stenosis); and rashes, skin lesions, skin thickening, oral ulcers, and joint swelling (query autoimmune conditions such as vasculitis, scleroderma, or lupus). The physical examination will often be guided by the history and investigations.

Initial laboratory testing for all patients should include a basic metabolic panel that includes serum electrolytes and extended electrolytes, creatinine, and eGFR; complete blood count; urinalysis and urine microscopy; quantification of urine protein with either urine protein-to-creatinine ratio (UPCR) or urine albumin-to-creatinine ratio (UACR). In some cases, a 24-hour urine protein measurement may be warranted. A renal ultrasound is also recommended to assess structural abnormalities and chronicity of the disease. Depending on the history and results of the initial investigation, further work-up such as infectious screen, autoimmune work-up, serum protein electrophoresis (to look for multiple myeloma), and kidney biopsy may be indicated.

Clinical Pearl

- Diabetic patients with diabetic retinopathy have a higher likelihood of developing diabetic nephropathy.
- The causes of CKD are broad, and history and physical examination will guide further assessment and management.

3.2.4 Complications and Management of CKD

Anemia Anemia is a common feature of CKD and prevalence increases as GFR declines. Clinicians should start to think about anemia of CKD when GFR drops to below 60 mL/min per 1.73 m^2. Patients with CKD develop anemia because the kidney is the main source of erythropoietin (EPO), a hormone which stimulates red blood cell production in the bone marrow and drives hemoglobin homoeostasis. Although erythropoietin concentrations can be normal or slightly increased in people with anemia of CKD, they are usually considered inappropriately normal, with similarly anemic patients without CKD having EPO concentrations 10–100 times higher. Uremia-induced inhibitors of erythropoiesis, blood loss, shortened red blood cell survival, and iron deficiency can also contribute to the anemia of CKD [3]. Anemia in CKD is associated with poor outcomes including reduced quality of life, increased incidence of cardiovascular disease, higher rates of hospital admission, cognitive impairment, and mortality [3].

For patients with kidney disease, the target hemoglobin is 95–110 g/L. Iron and recombinant erythropoietin and its synthetic derivatives, known as erythropoiesis-stimulating agents, are widely used to treat anemia and have been shown to reduce the need for blood transfusion in people with CKD. A target higher than 115 g/L is not recommended due to increased risk for stroke, hypertension, and vascular access thrombosis compared with a lower hemoglobin target. Treatment response with erythropoiesis-stimulating agents is often limited by iron deficiency, which is common in patients with CKD. Oral iron is less expensive and more commonly used in early stages of CKD; as CKD progresses and as patients are started on dialysis, greater response has been shown with intravenous iron [3].

Clinical Pearl

- Anemia increases in prevalence and severity as renal function decreases, becoming much more common when the glomerular filtration rate approaches 60 mL/min/1.73 m^2 or less.
- It is a risk factor associated with worse prognosis.

CKD-Mineral Bone Disease In a healthy individual, the kidneys play an important role in maintaining serum calcium and phosphate concentrations through intestinal absorption (by converting vitamin D to calcitriol) and renal tubular excretion (under the negative feedback control of parathyroid hormone (PTH)). Bone mineral disease is a common complication of CKD and is defined as a systemic disorder of bone and mineral metabolism manifested by either one or a combination of the following: (1) abnormalities of calcium, phosphorus, PTH, or vitamin D metabolism; (2) abnormalities in bone turnover, mineralization, volume, linear growth, or strength; or (3) vascular or other soft-tissue calcification. All three of these processes are closely interrelated and account for the significant morbidity and mortality in patients with CKD.

Current recommendations are to lower serum phosphate levels toward the normal range (low-phosphate diet and use of phosphate binders) and to avoid hypocalcemia. It is also recommended that PTH levels be maintained in the range of 2 to 9 times the upper limit of normal for the assay. This can be accomplished with the use of calcimimetics, calcitriol, or vitamin D analogs and phosphate binders [4].

Metabolic Acidosis This is a result of the reduced capacity of damaged kidneys to synthesize ammonia and excrete hydrogen ions. Bone disease, skeletal muscle wasting, and progressive GFR loss are thought to be consequences of chronic metabolic acidosis. Current guidelines recommend serum bicarbonate be maintained at a concentration of 22 mEq/L to lessen these complications [5]. To date, based on a meta-analysis, low-to-moderate evidence suggests that oral bicarbonate therapy or reduced dietary acid intake may decrease the rate of progression of renal function decline [6].

Cardiovascular Disease Mortality from cardiovascular disease is estimated to be 57% higher in individuals with a GFR less than 60 mL/min per 1.73 m^2 and 63% higher in people with micro-albuminuria compared with those without CKD. The risk of having a non-fatal myocardial infarction is increased by 33% when GFR is less than 60 mL/min per 1.73 m^2 and by 48% with micro-albuminuria, with risk of both myocardial infarction and cardiovascular death increasing as GFR declines and quantity of albuminuria increases. Similarly, for cerebrovascular disease, there is an inverse linear association between GFR and risk of stroke and a dose-response association between albuminuria and stroke risk. Stroke risk increased by 7% for every 10 mL/min per 1.73 m^2 decrease in GFR and by 10% for every 25 mg/mmol increase in albumin-creatinine ratio [2].

Clinical practice guidelines recommend antiplatelet treatment approaches similar to that of the general population in individuals with CKD and acute coronary syndromes. For hyperlipidemia, variations between international guidelines reflect uncertainties in the effectiveness of statins among people with CKD. No trials have demonstrated significant harm with statin use in patients with CKD. Therefore, reduction in non-fatal events provides a rationale for the use of statins in CKD patients [7].

A new class of medication, SGLT-2 (sodium-glucose cotransporter-2) inhibitors (a glucose-lowering agent), has demonstrated significant reduction in the rates of cardiovascular death and hospitalization for heart failure. It has also demonstrated decreased rate of progression of proteinuric CKD (diabetic and non-diabetic). It should be strongly considered for those patients with a) an eGFR of at least 25 mL/min per 1.73 m^2 and evidence of type 2 diabetes mellitus and CKD or cerebrovascular disease, b) no diabetes mellitus but with heart failure with reduced ejection fraction, and c) no diabetes mellitus but CKD with proteinuria [8].

Nutrition Elevated protein catabolism and protein malnutrition are common in patients with CKD and ESKD. The underlying etiology includes, but is not limited to, metabolic acidosis intestinal dysbiosis, systemic inflammation, anabolic hormone resistance, energy expenditure elevation, and uremic toxin accumulation. These derangements can further worsen kidney function, leading to poor patient outcomes. Active nutritional measures can mitigate many of the metabolic and hormonal derangements in CKD and ESKD. For patients with relatively stable health conditions and absence of active medical events and not on dialysis, a nutritional assessment every 3–6 months is advisable. Dietary energy provision for both dialysis and non-dialysis CKD patients should be 30–35 kcal/kg (ideal body weight)/day. The recommended amount of protein intake for non-dialysis CKD patients is 0.6 to 0.8 g/kg/day. For patients on peritoneal dialysis and hemodialysis, dietary protein intake in the range of 1.0–1.2 g/kg/day is advised [9, 10]. (See also Chap. 19, Physical Activity and Nutrition in Chronic Kidney Disease.)

3.2.5 Predicting Progression of CKD to ESKD

It is often useful for both the nephrologist and the patient to have an awareness and understanding of the likelihood of progressing from CKD to ESKD in the upcoming few years. This helps guide the timing of planning for renal replacement therapy. In 2011, the Kidney Failure Risk Equation (KFRE), a model to predict the progression of CKD to kidney failure, was developed and validated [11]. It is a model that uses age, sex, eGFR, urine albumin-to-creatinine ratio, and patient location (North America versus not) to predict the progression of CKD to dialysis in patients with CKD stages 3 to 5. The results are presented as a percentage of risk of progression to kidney failure in 2 or 5 years where 3% is considered low risk and 10% is considered intermediate risk over 5 years. As of 2016, the KFRE had been validated in 31 cohorts, including participants with CKD stages 3 to 5 in more than 30 countries spanning 4 continents. It has been demonstrated to be accurate within these diverse populations [12].

Recommendation

- The KFRE (Kidney Failure Risk Equation) model should be used to predict likelihood of progression to ESKD in the next 2 years and 5 years and guide timing of discussion around renal replacement modalities.

3.3 Renal Replacement Therapies

Discussion around renal replacement therapies should ideally occur before a patient reaches ESKD. Most of these modalities require planning in advance, such as creation of an arteriovenous fistula for hemodialysis, insertion of a peritoneal dialysis catheter, or work-up for living-donor pre-emptive transplantation. This section describes the four different modalities. Transplantation and comprehensive conservative management are discussed in greater detail elsewhere in this book.

3.3.1 Hemodialysis

Hemodialysis is a process that acts in lieu of the kidneys to remove metabolic waste products and excess fluid from the body. During the treatment, blood is pumped through a plastic dialyzer at flow rates of 300 to 500 mL per minute, while dialysate (dialysis fluid) flows in the opposite direction at 500 to 800 mL per minute. Diffusion allows molecules move from area of high concentration to low concentration; this results in both clearance of toxins and excess electrolytes (movement from blood to dialysate), along with replenishment of body buffers (movement from dialysate to blood). To remove fluid from the body, a transmembrane pressure is created across the dialyzer to mobilize fluid from the plasma into the dialysate.

Patients on hemodialysis require "dialysis access" in the form of an arteriovenous fistula, graft, or central venous catheter to remove blood from the body for dialysis and then a return mechanism back to the body. A fistula is created by shunting blood from an artery to a vein, which results in growth and thickening of the venous wall; this can then tolerate repeated cannulation. The preferred fistula is created from the anastomosis of the arm's cephalic vein to the radial artery. For those who do not have the ideal anatomy for fistula creation, a graft may be a possibility. This involves interposing a prosthetic graft material between an artery and vein. Unfortunately, grafts have a higher risk of clotting and infection, which is why they are inferior to fistulas.

When dialysis is urgently required, a double-lumen dialysis catheter is used. Insertion into the jugular vein is the preferred location. Temporary access can be used for 2 to 3 weeks, but clotting, low blood flow, and infection limit the life of the catheter. Implantation of a dual-lumen cuffed catheter is a good option for patients who have delayed recovery from acute renal failure, who require access for dialysis until a fistula matures, or who lack any other suitable site for graft placement [13].

There are different options when it comes to hemodialysis. Most commonly, it is performed in-center, at a hospital-based hemodialysis unit, typically 3 times a week for 3.5 to 4 hours per session. For patients who are independent, there is the option of home hemodialysis, where patients do their own treatment at home for approximately 3 to 5 hours a day or 8 hours overnight, 4 to 7 days a week. For some patients, home-dialysis provides more flexibility in scheduling. In-center nocturnal hemodialysis provides patients with the option of coming in overnight for approximately 8 hours, 3 times a week.

3.3.2 Peritoneal Dialysis

Peritoneal dialysis is another form of home-dialysis which uses the patient's own peritoneum as a dialysis membrane. Vascular access for peritoneal dialysis is established by inserting a peritoneal dialysis catheter into the patient, with one end in the abdomen and the other end protruding from the skin. Dialysis solution containing physiologic amounts of sodium, calcium, magnesium, and (usually) lactate as the buffer is infused through the catheter into the peritoneum and remains in place for a determined period called "dwell time." During that time, diffusion occurs across the peritoneal membrane until fresh fluid is exchanged for the old. Glucose added to the dialysate in concentrations of 1.5 to 4.25% provides an osmotic gradient that facilitates movement of fluid from the body into the dialysate. After the dwell time is complete, the dialysate is drained out through the catheter, and fresh dialysis solution is reintroduced.

There are two common modalities of peritoneal dialysis: continuous ambulatory peritoneal dialysis (CAPD) and automated peritoneal dialysis (APD). CAPD is done during the day, where the patient manually performs the exchanges. Frequently, CAPD uses four exchanges of 2 L each of dialysate daily, with an expected drainage volume of approximately 10 L, including ultrafiltration. APD is done overnight with an automated cycler/machine that instills and drains dialysate over the course of 8 to 10 hours, while the patient is asleep. Typically, APD involves five cycles of filling and draining overnight.

Like hemodialysis, peritoneal dialysis comes with its own set of complications. Non-infectious complications include pleural effusions from pleuroperitoneal leaks, hemoperitoneum, pain on dialysate infusion, and catheter migration. Infectious complications include peritoneal dialysis-related peritonitis, exit-site infections, and tunnel infections.

3.3.3 Transplantation

Kidney transplantation is often the renal replacement therapy of choice for patients who reach ESKD. However, although it is superior to dialysis, there are certain patients in which the risks of transplantation may not outweigh the benefits. Therefore, renal transplantation requires a thorough pretransplantation assessment to see if the patient is a suitable candidate. For those who undergo transplantation, they must be carefully monitored for multiple factors including immunosuppressant drug levels and medication toxicities, infections, and higher risk of malignancies. Renal transplantation, including the process of evaluation, donors, immunosuppression, and complications posttransplantation, is discussed in great detail in Chap. 4, Renal Transplant Essentials.

3.3.4 Conservative Kidney Care

Comprehensive conservative care is planned holistic patient-centered care for patients with ESKD. Table 3.3 highlights key elements of comprehensive conservative care. Comprehensive conservative care does not include dialysis [14]. Please refer to Chap. 18 where comprehensive conservative care is discussed in greater detail.

Table 3.3 Key elements of comprehensive conservative care [14]

Interventions to delay progression of kidney disease and minimize risk of complications
Shared decision-making
Active symptom management
Detailed communication
Psychologic support
Social and family support
Cultural and spiritual domains of care

3.4 Case Vignette Analysis

Mr. Pratt was a gentleman with a long-standing history of hypertension and diabetes mellitus. He had evidence of stage 3 proteinuric CKD. The most likely etiology of his CKD is diabetic nephropathy, especially given his history of diabetic retinopathy. There is nothing else on history, physical examination, or investigations to point toward another cause of CKD. We may consider screening for multiple myeloma given his age and obtain an ultrasound of the kidneys. There is no indication for a kidney biopsy currently.

In terms of management, Mr. Pratt was hypertensive. As a diabetic with CKD, his target blood pressure should be less than 130/80 mmHg. He is currently on a calcium channel blocker and an ACE inhibitor. The dose of his ACE inhibitor can be titrated upward. It is likely that he will require a third agent such as a diuretic. With regard to his diabetes mellitus, he is not at his target A1c of 7% or less. With type 2 diabetes mellitus, proteinuric CKD, and an eGFR greater than 25 mL/min per 1.73 m^2, he would be an excellent candidate for an SGLT-2 inhibitor such as dapagliflozin. This will decrease his risk of having a cardiovascular event, slow down the progression of his CKD, and improve his glycemic control. The diuretic effect of SGLT-2 inhibitors may also contribute to lowering his blood pressure. Mr. Pratt also had evidence of anemia. He is not a candidate for erythropoiesis-stimulating agent treatment at this time, but he should be screened for iron deficiency and started on oral replacement if deficient (along with screening for colon cancer, if not done). Finally, Mr. Pratt should be counseled on smoking cessation.

It is useful to know Mr. Pratt's risk of progressing to ESKD. According to the Kidney Failure Risk Equation (KFRE) [11], his risk of progressing to ESKD is 4.2% in the next 2 years and 12.5% in the next 5 years.

3.5 Key Takeaways

- The diagnosis of CKD is made if there is evidence of reduced kidney function, evidence of structural kidney damage, or both.
- There are five stages of CKD.
- Assessment of CKD should involve a targeted history, physical examination, and investigations, including a basic metabolic work-up, CBC, creatinine, eGFR, UPCR/UACR, and renal ultrasound.
- The Kidney Failure Risk Equation (KFRE) is a useful tool in predicting the 2- and 5-year risk of progression to ESKD and aids in educating and preparing the individual for ESKD therapies.
- Renal replacement therapy for those who reach stage 5 CKD includes hemodialysis, peritoneal dialysis, kidney transplantation, and comprehensive conservative care.

References

1. Levey AS, Eckardt KU, Tsukamoto Y, et al. Definition and classification of chronic kidney disease: a position statement from kidney disease: improving global outcomes (KDIGO). Kidney Int. 2005;67(6):2089–100.
2. Webster AC, Nagler EV, Morton RL, Masson P. Chronic kidney disease. Lancet. 2017;389(10075):1238–52.
3. Nurko S. Anemia in chronic kidney disease: causes, diagnosis, treatment. Clevel Clin J Med. 2006;73(3):289.
4. Ketteler M, Block GA, Evenepoel P, Fukagawa M, Herzog CA, McCann L, Moe SM, Shroff R, Tonelli MA, Toussaint ND, Vervloet MG. Executive summary of the 2017 KDIGO chronic kidney disease–mineral and bone disorder (CKD-MBD) guideline update: what's changed and why it matters. Kidney Int. 2017;92(1):26–36.
5. Kraut JA, Madias NE. Metabolic acidosis of CKD: an update. Am J Kidney Dis. 2016;67(2):307–17.
6. Navaneethan SD, Shao J, Buysse J, Bushinsky DA. Effects of treatment of metabolic acidosis in CKD: a systematic review and meta-analysis. Clin J Am Soc Nephrol. 2019;14(7):1011–20.
7. Herzog CA, Asinger RW, Berger AK, Charytan DM, Díez J, Hart RG, Eckardt KU, Kasiske BL, McCullough PA, Passman RS, DeLoach SS. Cardiovascular disease in chronic kidney disease. A clinical update from kidney disease: improving global outcomes (KDIGO). Kidney Int. 2011;80(6):572–86.
8. Cherney DZ, Verma S. DAPA-CKD: the beginning of a new era in renal protection. J Am Coll Cardiol Basic Trans Sci. 2021;6(1):74–7.
9. Zha Y, Qian Q. Protein nutrition and malnutrition in CKD and ESRD. Nutrients. 2017;9(3):208.
10. Ikizler TA, Burrowes JD, Byham-Gray LD, Campbell KL, Carrero JJ, Chan W, Fouque D, Friedman AN, Ghaddar S, Goldstein-Fuchs DJ, Kaysen GA. KDOQI clinical practice guideline for nutrition in CKD: 2020 update. Am J Kidney Dis. 2020;76(3):S1–07.
11. Tangri N, Stevens LA, Griffith J, Tighiouart H, Djurdjev O, Naimark D, Levin A, Levey AS. A predictive model for progression of chronic kidney disease to kidney failure. JAMA. 2011;305(15):1553–9.
12. Whitlock RH, Chartier M, Komenda P, Hingwala J, Rigatto C, Walld R, Dart A, Tangri N. Validation of the kidney failure risk equation in Manitoba. Can J Kidney Health Dis. 2017;4:2054358117705372.
13. Pastan S, Bailey J. Dialysis therapy. N Engl J Med. 1998;338(20):1428–37.
14. Murtagh FE, Burns A, Moranne O, Morton RL, Naicker S. Supportive care: comprehensive conservative care in end-stage kidney disease. Clin J Am Soc Nephrol. 2016;11(10):1909–14.

Renal Transplant Essentials

4

Meera Joseph and Azim S. Gangji

4.1 Renal Transplant Statistics

The need for renal replacement therapy is growing. In 2017, there were 124,500 newly reported cases of end-stage kidney disease (ESKD) in the United States. The unadjusted (crude) incidence rate was 370.2 per million/year in the US population. The number of prevalent ESKD cases has continued to rise by about 20,000 cases per year. In 2017, 86.9% of incident ESKD patients began renal replacement therapy with hemodialysis, 10.1% started with peritoneal dialysis, and 2.9% received a preemptive kidney transplant [1]. In Canada, the rate of new patients per million population starting renal replacement therapy increased on average by 1.6% per year between 2010 and 2019. The number of patients receiving dialysis nearly doubled over 20 years, from 11,601 in 2000 to 23,125 in 2019. Of the 23,125 patients on dialysis in 2019, three-quarters were receiving institutional hemodialysis [2].

The development of ESKD is associated with a substantial reduction in health-related quality of life and premature death. The unadjusted 5-year patient survival for patients on hemodialysis and peritoneal dialysis are 42.8% and 50.6%, respectively [2]. Kidney transplantation is the treatment of choice for ESKD as it prolongs survival, improves quality of life, and is less costly than dialysis [3].

In the United States, after remaining relatively stagnant for many years, the number of kidney transplants increased each year starting in 2015, reaching the highest annual count to date of 24,273 in 2019 [4]. In Canada, the proportion of patients with ESKD living with a functioning transplant increased from 40% in 2010 to 43%

M. Joseph (✉) · A. S. Gangji
Division of Nephrology, Department of Medicine, McMaster University, St. Joseph's Healthcare Hamilton, Hamilton, ON, Canada
e-mail: meera.joseph@medportal.ca; gangji@mcmaster.ca

A. Hategan et al. (eds.), *Psychonephrology*,
https://doi.org/10.1007/978-3-030-84740-1_4

in 2019. The number of kidney transplants performed per year increased by 41%. Also, the number of patients who received a preemptive kidney transplant (i.e., received a transplant prior to starting dialysis first) increased from 136 in 2010 to 178 in 2019 [2].

Patients who have had a kidney transplant may have the option to receive dialysis when their allograft fails; therefore, allograft survival is commonly measured. In the United States, 5-year graft survival in deceased donor kidney transplants ranged between 64.6 and 84.9% depending on the characteristics of the donor. Among living donor transplants, 5-year graft survival ranged between 80.2 and 90.7% depending on the age of the donor [4]. According to the latest available data from Canadian Organ Replacement Register (CORR), unadjusted 5-year allograft survival is 79.8% for patients who received a kidney from a deceased donor, compared with 92.4% for patients who received a kidney from a living donor [2].

4.2 Case Vignette

Mr. Doyle, a 45-year-old man, was being followed in the multidisciplinary kidney care clinic for chronic kidney disease secondary to type 2 diabetes mellitus. His kidney function had been declining gradually for the previous 10 years. On this visit, his eGFR was measured at 19 mL/min/1.73 m^2 with an albumin-creatinine ratio of 150 mg/mmol. Four months ago, it was 22 mL/min/1.73 m^2. His risk of developing kidney failure, requiring dialysis or transplantation, was predicted to be 50% in 2 years. He was previously in denial about his diagnosis and did not want to discuss dialysis modalities or transplantation. He told you that his sister was interested in donating her kidney to him and asked you what the transplant process would be like. Continue reading to understand the process of kidney transplantation, work-up of recipients and donors, and what Mr. Doyle could expect posttransplantation.

4.3 Pretransplant Considerations

The pretransplant period is often a very anxious time, during which patients face the decision to pursue transplant, the process of transplant evaluation, and the subsequent waiting period. Additionally, candidates may experience fears about the procedure, the possibility of being told that they are not a suitable candidate, that their potential donor is not suitable, and the possibility of dying on the waitlist or from a complication of the transplant [5]. This section aims to broadly describe the assessment process for the recipient, the types of donors and assessment of living donors, and the process of being listed for transplantation. Understanding the pretransplant period in broad strokes will assist in understanding the process a patient may experience at the time of psychological or psychiatric assessment.

4.3.1 Transplant Recipient Assessment

Although, in general, transplant is superior to dialysis, there are certain patients in which the risks of transplantation may outweigh the benefits. Therefore, careful evaluation of each potential recipient is completed by a multidisciplinary and multi-specialty team to decide if a patient is an eligible candidate and what steps need to be taken prior to listing.

Cardiovascular disease is a major cause of graft loss and the leading cause of death in renal transplant recipients. By 36 months after transplantation, nearly 40% of patients will have experienced a cardiovascular disease-related event [6]. Therefore, a careful cardiovascular work-up is completed under the care of a dedicated cardiologist for each recipient. Depending on their risk factors and presence of pre-existing disease, the work-up can range from an exercise stress test to coronary angiography.

Other considerations in pretransplantation include (1) peripheral arterial disease, as disease in the iliac arteries may make the surgery difficult and reduce perfusion to the new kidney; (2) age-appropriate malignancy screening, as the incidence of cancer is higher in transplant recipients than in the general population and is one of the major causes of death in this patient group [7]; and (3) infectious complications and exposures, including screening for tuberculosis, hepatitis B and C, HIV, Epstein Barr virus, and cytomegalovirus (discussed in Sect. 4.5.2). Depending on the patient's comorbidities and past medical history, other screening and evaluations may also be warranted.

Immunologic testing screens the patient for antibodies that may attack the donor kidney and result in rejection of the organ. A patient with donor-specific antibodies, or antibodies against histocompatibility antigens expressed on the donor kidney, is not a suitable match. Some patients who have had previous "sensitizing events" such as a previous transplant may have a large number of antibodies to histocompatibility antigens, making it difficult to find a suitable match.

Psychosocial issues can have a significant impact on transplant outcomes. This includes social determinants (relationships and support systems, finances, transportation, housing), psychological health (personality factors, congnitive function), and lifestyle factors (independence, substance misuse).Therefore, patients with a history of psychosocial issues should undergo evaluation by a social worker and/or a psychologist.

Previously diagnosed or undiagnosed psychiatric conditions may also raise issues of concern such as capacity and consent or adherence to transplant medications. Adherence to medications, as will be discussed later, is crucial for ensuring allograft longevity and survival, and patients who demonstrate neuropsychiatric decompensation may be less adherent to medications, routine blood work, and follow-up. In circumstances such as these, involvement of a psychiatrist is recommended.

From the time a referral is received, the transplant assessment can take between 3 and 9 months for recipients with a living donor and 6 and 12 months for recipients hoping for a deceased donor to enter the wait-list. This assessment time depends on the medical complexity of the patient or kidney donor and the patient's availability to attend appointments. For patients who come forward with a living donor prior to starting dialysis, the assessment is ideally completed in time for transplantation prior to the patient needing dialysis (preemptive transplantation).

Clinical Pearl

- Transplant recipient assessment requires thorough evaluation in various domains to ensure that the benefits of transplantation outweigh the risks.
- The assessment also includes a psychological evaluation if the patient has a comorbid psychiatric illness that may affect the longevity of the allograft.

4.3.2 Transplant Donors

Kidney donors can be either deceased donors or living donors. The terminology used to describe deceased donors is an "alphabet soup" of sorts [8]. Firstly, a deceased donor is either a standard criteria donor (SCD) or an extended criteria donor (ECD). ECD donors are either aged 60 or older at the time of death or aged 50–59 with any two of the following three criteria: (1) cause of death is a cerebrovascular accident (i.e., stroke); (2) pre-existing history of hypertension; and (3) terminal serum creatinine greater than 1.5 mg/dL. Any donor that does not meet ECD criteria is an SCD donor. The criteria for ECD donors are based on variables that increase the risk of graft failure by 70% compared with an SCD kidney [8]. Together with their transplant nephrologist, patients can decide if they want to be on the ECD wait-list at the time of listing. For patients who are older, receiving an ECD kidney in a timelier fashion can be more beneficial than remaining on dialysis and waiting for an SCD kidney given their higher risk of dying on the wait-list.

After the determination of SCD versus ECD is made, the cause of death is described as donation after cardiac death (DCD) or neurologic determination of death (NDD). DCD donors do not meet the criteria for brain death, and therefore the heart must stop prior to organ retrieval. Depending on how quickly the donor expires after discontinuation of life support, perfusion to the donor kidney may be decreased for some time if blood pressure is not maintained; this increases the likelihood of delayed graft function, defined as the need for dialysis in the first week posttransplantation (discussed further in Sect. 4.5.3). In contrast, for NDD donors who are diagnosed with brain death, cardiac circulation is artificially maintained during organ retrieval, thereby maintaining good perfusion to the donor kidney and reducing the incidence of delayed graft function.

Living donation occurs when an individual freely decides to donate one of their two kidneys to a person in need of a transplant. Kidney donation is the most common type of living organ donation and tends to be very successful. To donate a kidney, the donor must be in good health with no history of high blood pressure, diabetes mellitus, heart disease, kidney disease, or hepatitis. Like recipients, a series of tests are carefully done to try and ensure that living donation will not result in any harm to the donor. This again can include both physical and psychological evaluations. Investigations are completed to ensure that the donor who has come forward is an appropriate immunologic match for the recipient they wish to donate to. If the donor is not a match, both the recipient and the donor may wish to enter a "paired exchange program" in which both the donor and recipient are entered into a pool and matched with suitable partners.

There are many advantages to considering living donor transplantation. First, transplantation can be done preemptively, meaning at a time when the patient has reached ESKD, but before they start dialysis. This has associated improved long-term patient survival and spares patients time on dialysis and the associated adverse health outcomes. Second, living donor kidneys tend to be healthier than deceased donor kidneys and, on average, tend to last longer (15–20 years, as opposed to 10–15 years for a deceased donor kidney).

Living kidney donation is not without its risks. It is ultimately an irreversible surgery with the potential for serious complications and even death. Therefore, it is important that the donor must be the one to freely approach the healthcare team showing interest in donation, and both the donor and recipient must be fully informed of the benefits and risks involved, so that an informed decision can be made freely and without coercion.

Recommendation

- It is important that living donation is introduced early to patients while considering modalities for renal replacement therapy and that living donation is done freely without coercion.
- If there is any doubt in the clinician's mind that the donor is not coming forward freely or that donation may have a negative psychological impact, a pre-donation psychiatrist assessment is recommended.

4.3.3 Transplant Listing

In the United States, organ allocation is managed nationally by the United Network for Organ Sharing (UNOS), which uses a complex computer algorithm to distribute organs in a fair manner. Factors that are taken into consideration in the algorithm for kidney transplants include waiting time, donor/recipient immune status, prior living donor, distance from donor hospital, survival benefit, and pediatric status. In Canada, if the recipient is approved for transplant, he or she may be added to the provincial wait-list for a deceased donor kidney. The wait time in Ontario is 3–9 years, depending on the patient's blood group, antibody level, and availability of organs. Each patient's position on the wait-list is determined by an allocation point system that considers the patient's dialysis vintage (time spent on dialysis) and the patient's antibody levels. For patients who were once kidney donors, they will move to the top of the list, as will pediatric patients. In the United States, for example, patients with ESKD who were wait-listed in 2013; the median wait time for a transplant was 4.2 years [9]. Patients with ESKD in Canada who receive a transplant from a deceased donor will spend an average of 3.7 years on dialysis before receiving a transplant [2]. For recipients with a living donor, surgery is usually scheduled 6–12 weeks after both the recipient and donor have been cleared. If the patient develops an acute medical illness after being listed for transplantation, they will be placed on hold until the acute issues are resolved and the patient is once again fit for transplantation.

4.4 Immunosuppression

4.4.1 Common Immunosuppressive Agents

Immunosuppressive drugs are the key to successful allograft function. Immunosuppressive agents are used for induction (i.e., intense immunosuppression in the initial days after transplantation), maintenance, and reversal of diagnosed rejection. Immunosuppression can be achieved by depleting lymphocytes, diverting lymphocyte traffic, or blocking lymphocyte response pathways.

The most common induction agents are high-dose glucocorticoids (e.g., methylprednisolone) with either an agent that depletes T cells (anti-thymocyte globulin (ATG)) or one that inhibits T-cell replication and B-cell activation (basiliximab). Both medications will typically only be given over the first few days posttransplantation. The patient will not be discharged home on these induction agents.

Maintenance immunosuppression typically involves a cocktail of three classes of immunosuppressive agents, calcineurin inhibitors, anti-metabolites, and glucocorticoids, which are highlighted below.

Calcineurin Inhibitors (CNIs). The most common CNIs used are cyclosporine and tacrolimus. Cyclosporine is a cyclic polypeptide of fungal origin, whereas tacrolimus is a macrolide antibiotic compound isolated from *Streptomyces tsukubaensis*. CNIs impair the expression of several critical cytokine genes that promote T-cell activation. It is important to know that, while they are staple of transplant maintenance immunosuppression, CNIs can be nephrotoxic and can lead to enhancement of early posttransplant graft dysfunction, dose-related reversible renal vasoconstriction, chronic interstitial fibrosis, acute microvascular disease, hypertension, and electrolyte abnormalities. Non-renal side effects are outlined in Table 4.1 [10]. CNIs have a narrow therapeutic index and require careful monitoring to ensure drug levels are within the therapeutic range and not toxic.

Anti-metabolites The most commonly used anti-metabolites are mycophenolate mofetil (MMF) and mycophenolic acid (MPA). MMF is a prodrug having MPA as active compound. MPA is a reversible inhibitor of the enzyme inosine

Table 4.1 Common side effects of calcineurin inhibitors [10]

System	Side effects
Renal	Enhancement of early posttransplant graft dysfunction; dose-related reversible renal vasoconstriction; chronic interstitial fibrosis; acute microvascular disease; hypertension; electrolyte abnormalities
Metabolic	Dyslipidemia; glucose intolerance; new-onset diabetes mellitus
Neuropsychiatric	Headaches, tremors, dysesthesias, seizures, leukoencephalopathy, insomnia, memory impairment, delirium, mood instability, anxiety, psychosis
Gastrointestinal	Hepatic dysfunction; cholelithiasis; anorexia; vomiting; diarrhea; abdominal discomfort
Cosmetic	Hypertrichosis; gingival hyperplasia; gynecomastia; hair loss or frank alopecia
Other	Malignancy; infection; thromboembolism; cardiomyopathy

monophosphate dehydrogenase and a selective anti-metabolite. It blocks the proliferation of T and B cells, inhibits antibody formation and the generation of cytotoxic T cells, downregulates the expression of adhesion molecules, and impairs their binding to vascular endothelial cells. Anti-metabolites also come with side effects. MMF (CellCept) and the enteric-coated MPA (Myfortic) most commonly have gastrointestinal side effects such as diarrhea, nausea, dyspepsia, vomiting, esophagitis, and gastritis. Most of these side effects resolve with dose reduction. They may also result in hematologic side effects such as leukopenia, anemia, and thrombocytopenia, which also require a dose reduction [10].

Glucocorticoids Glucocorticoids were one of the first classes of medications used to prevent rejection after solid organ transplantation in the 1960s. Methylprednisolone and prednisone are used frequently as part of the immunosuppressive regimen, both for induction and maintenance. Corticosteroids have immunosuppressive, anti-inflammatory, and lympholytic effects. The most important complications of glucocorticoids are cosmetic changes (hirsutism, weight gain), bone related such as osteonecrosis and osteoporosis, metabolic changes including dyslipidemia and steroid-induced diabetes mellitus, impaired wound healing, cataracts, and dose-related psychiatric side effects (restlessness, irritability, anxiety, depression, and psychosis) [10]. (For further details on psychiatric effects of these medications, see Chap. 14, Psychotoxicity of Immunomodulators.)

4.4.2 Adherence to Immunosuppression

Adherence is important in all chronic disease states, but it is especially important in transplant recipients because of the risk of graft rejection and premature graft loss, increased health complications, healthcare costs, death, and the scarcity of organ donation. Non-adherence to immunosuppressive medications can take many forms, ranging from taking medications at the wrong time to not taking medications at all. Canadian consensus guidelines state that "patient non-adherence to therapy is a contraindication to kidney transplantation" [11]. At the time of transplant assessment, it is essential to inform patients about the importance of adhering to medical therapy, as well as attending appointments and completing blood work in a timely fashion. For those who have demonstrated non-adherence to dialysis, there is a weaker recommendation that kidney transplantation should be delayed until the patient has demonstrated adherence to therapy for 6 months.

Several barriers have been identified to not adhering to taking immunosuppressive medications: cost, male sex, non-White race/ethnicity, use of mycophenolate mofetil or tacrolimus, lack of social support, medication side effects, psychological distress, and lifestyle factors.

One survey demonstrated that patients who are non-adherent tended to be more forgetful and missed doses of their medications when they were diverted from their daily routines or were financially constrained [12]. They also believed that immunosuppressive medications disrupted their lives and felt that they had less control over their lives and that their immunosuppressive medications were not necessary. The study also found that the recipients who did adhere to their medication regimens had greater life satisfactions, including the relationship they had with their healthcare providers [12].

Recommendation

- Improving interactions with healthcare providers, increasing access to healthcare, and ensuring understanding of health-related information received may contribute to knowledge of the importance of immunosuppressive medications and thereby improve adherence.

4.4.3 Psychiatric and Psychological Reactions to Immunosuppression

Although this section is detailed elsewhere in the book, with the introduction of low-dose corticosteroid therapy and newer calcineurin inhibitors, florid psychiatric responses to immunosuppression are less common. Mania may be observed in some patients treated with corticosteroids. Low-dose corticosteroids (equivalent of daily dose of 30 mg of prednisone or less) can be, however, associated with mood changes and irritability in the early post-transplant period. These changes may not always be noticed by the patient, but brought to the patient's or the physician's attention by family and friends. (For more details on psychiatric side effects, see Chap. 14, Psychotoxicity of Immunomodulators.)

4.5 Posttransplant Complications

Recipient expectations after transplantation are understandably high. Patients expect to be off dialysis, in better physical health, notice an improvement in their quality of life, and be able to return to activities such as work, study, travel, and parenting. The expectation of transplantation is sometimes "freedom from the sick role." For most transplant recipients, transplantation goes well with little or no significant complications, and expectations are met or exceeded. A minority, however, will face associated complications that can either have short- or long-term impacts on their physical and psychological well-being.

4.5.1 Surgical Complications

Surgical complications of renal transplantation include hemorrhage and thrombosis, vascular complications (e.g., renal artery thrombosis, renal artery stenosis, renal vein thrombosis, venous thromboembolism, aneurysm, fistula), urinary complications (e.g., urine leaks, obstruction, hematuria), and wound-related complications (e.g., infectious and non-infectious). The overall incidence of surgical complications after kidney transplant is low, especially when compared to extrarenal transplants such as liver or pancreas. Many centers report an incidence in the 5–10% range. However, monitoring for surgical complications is critical [13].

4.5.2 Infections

Infections are a common cause of morbidity and mortality after transplantation, and infections rank as second leading cause of death in patients with allograft function. Patients are more susceptible to routine viruses and microorganisms and opportunistic infections, such as cytomegalovirus, Epstein-Barr virus, and BK viremia, which are highlighted below.

Cytomegalovirus Infection Cytomegalovirus (CMV) infection is the most common opportunistic infection in kidney transplant recipients, occurring in 8% of patients. Transplant recipients are at greater risk of CMV infection if the donor is seropositive for CMV and the recipient is seronegative; the use of T-cell depleting agents for transplant induction; simultaneous kidney-pancreas transplant; donors over the age of 60; the presence of allograft rejection; and the concurrent infection with other viruses.

It is important to distinguish between CMV infection and CMV disease. CMV infection is defined as evidence of CMV replication, regardless of symptoms. To be diagnosed with CMV disease, the patient must have evidence of infection along with symptoms such as fever, fatigue, and manifestation of organs affected (e.g., diarrhea) as well as laboratory evidence of leukopenia, thrombocytopenia, or evidence of tissue invasion.

CMV has been associated with diminished patient and graft survival. Infection within 100 days of transplant is an independent risk factor for overall recipient mortality, and early CMV disease is associated with increased cardiovascular mortality beyond 100 days. Therefore, depending on donor and recipient serology, and whether or not a T-cell depleting agent is used at the time of induction, CMV prophylaxis with valganciclovir is used for a minimum of 3–6 months posttransplantation [14].

Epstein-Barr Virus (EBV) Infection and Posttransplant Lymphoproliferative Disorder Although less common than CMV, Epstein-Barr virus (EBV) is a significant cause of posttransplant morbidity and mortality because of its association with the development of posttransplant lymphoproliferative disorder (PTLD). PTLD is defined as lymphoid proliferation arising in transplant recipients and may present in many different organs, including the allograft. Approximately 62–79% of PTLD cases have been associated with EBV. They are most common in patients who are seronegative for EBV and who receive an EBV-seropositive organ.

EBV-associated PTLD usually occurs in the first year after transplant. EBV disease may present with a nonspecific febrile syndrome, lymphadenopathy, hepatosplenomegaly, and atypical lymphocytosis. Other manifestations include organ-specific disease (gastroenteritis, hepatitis, or pneumonitis) and hematologic disorders, including leukopenia, thrombocytopenia, hemolytic anemia, and hemophagocytosis. Primary EBV infection in EBV-seronegative recipients usually occurs in the first 3–6 months, and there is often an elevated EBV viral load. PTLD typically follows the primary infection.

Observational studies have shown 50% mortality from EBV-associated PTLD. Currently there is no consensus regarding the treatment of PTLD, but reduction of immunosuppression is routinely used and can lead to remission in 23–86% of patients. Current therapy for lymphoproliferative disorders including rituximab is often utilized. Although antiviral therapy has been used alone or with immunoglobulin, no evidence supports its efficacy.

Patients with isolated allograft involvement have a 5-year survival rate of 68% compared with 36–38% in kidney transplant recipients with PTLD extending beyond the allograft. There is no standardized therapy to prevent PTLD; however, effective prevention of CMV may prevent EBV disease by limiting immunomodulation by CMV infection.

The Kidney Disease: Improving Global Outcomes (KDIGO) guidelines propose monitoring EBV viral load by nucleic acid testing (NAT) in the first posttransplant week, then monthly for the first 3–6 months, and then every 3 months until the end of first posttransplant year; viral load should also be monitored after acute rejection therapy in high-risk groups [14].

BK Viremia and Nephropathy BK polyoma virus (BKV) is a member of the polyoma family of viruses that has been associated with polyoma virus-associated nephropathy and polyoma virus-associated hemorrhagic cystitis. BK nephropathy affects up to 10% of kidney transplant recipients, and the rate of renal allograft loss varies from 10% to 80%. BK nephropathy will usually be preceded by BK viremia by approximately 8 weeks. In half of those who develop BK viremia, it will be within 3 months posttransplantation. Most BKV nephropathy occurs in the first 2 years after transplant. BK nephropathy will most often manifest with renal dysfunction; less commonly, patients may develop ureteric obstruction from stenosis or stricture.

Risk factors for BK nephropathy can be divided into high levels of immunosuppression and recipient and donor characteristics. BK nephropathy is more common in patients who are induced with potent immunosuppressive agents including T-cell depleting agents and the combination of tacrolimus and mycophenolate. Recipient characteristics predisposing to BK nephropathy are older age and male sex, whereas donor characteristics include female sex, deceased donation, increased cold ischemia time, and African-American ethnicity.

The KDIGO guidelines recommend routine screening of plasma for BK virus after transplantation. Treatment options for BKV replication and disease range from switching immunosuppression, decreasing the overall dose of immunosuppression, and consideration of discontinuing certain immunosuppressive agents [14].

4.5.3 Delayed Graft Function and Graft Loss

Delayed graft function is a form of acute kidney injury that results in the need for dialysis within 1 week posttransplantation. There are many known risk factors for delayed graft function. These include (1) factors associated with procurement of the organ, such as donation after cardiac death; (2) donor factors such as age over 55 or pre-existing diabetes mellitus or hypertension or an elevated serum creatinine; and (3) recipient factors that can be classified as pre-renal (i.e., hypovolemia), renal (i.e., acute tubular necrosis), and post renal (i.e., leak or obstruction of the ureter).

During a period of delayed graft function, the patient needs to balance emotions of hope that the graft will start working, with emotions of fear or potential fear of graft loss and return to dialysis. Emotional responses to this difficult situation can vary from anxiety to anger to depression. Those who do not seem concerned may be using denial to suppress their feelings of concern. These patients may be misinterpreted by the care team as being unaware of the situation or having little or poor insight. In fact, these patients are aware, but are unable to face the possibility of graft failure and the grim possibility of returning to dialysis.

4.5.4 Posttransplant Delirium

Delirium is a well-known postoperative medical complication and the most common surgical complication among older adults; however, little research has been done on postoperative delirium in kidney transplant recipients per se. In one cohort study of 893 postoperative kidney transplant recipients, 4.7% developed delirium; 19% were of the hypoactive subtype, 16.7% were of the hyperactive subtype, and 64.3% were of the mixed subtype [15]. The incidence of delirium increased with age (2% for those aged 18–49 versus 13.8% for those aged 75 and older). For patients who were both aged 75 and older and frail, the incidence increased to 20%. For 81% of patients, the cause of delirium was not listed; for those in which the etiology was identified, it included stroke (ischemic and embolic), sepsis, hyponatremia, and adverse drug reactions. Risk factors for delirium identified in this study included advanced age, frailty, increased comorbidity burden, pre-existing cognitive impairment, dialysis vintage, and disability in either activities of daily living or instrumental activities of daily living [15]. Deceased donor recipients were also more likely to experience delirium when compared to living donor recipients. Postoperative delirium had an impact on length of stay in hospital (2.49-fold higher length of stay for recipients with delirium) and discharge destination (22.41-fold increased risk of institutional discharge for recipients who experienced delirium) [15]. Those who experienced delirium were also at a 2.73-fold increased risk of death-censored graft loss and 3.12-fold increased risk of posttransplant mortality [15].

Research in other surgical settings has shown that delirium is preventable in up to 40% of patients. Delirium post-renal transplant is even more complicated, given not only the surgical risk factors but also the medical, metabolic, and medication-associated risks, which warrants further investigation and attention, especially given the associated risks of poor outcomes. (For further details, see Chap. 12, Neurocognitive Ramifications of Renal Disease.)

4.5.5 Posttransplant Cognitive Impairment

Cognitive impairment is prevalent in as many as 50% to 87% of dialysis patients, most commonly attributed to vascular changes, including vascular dementia. Not much is known about cognition and brain changes after kidney transplantation. Although cognition may improve after kidney transplantation, a cross-sectional study of kidney transplant recipients demonstrated that the majority of transplant patients, with a mean age of 54 years, had cognitive impairment, with the overall prevalence being more than two times the prevalence in those 65 years or older in the general population [16]. Lower scores on the Montreal Cognitive Assessment (MoCA) testing were associated with older age, male sex, and a lower level of education [16]. Those authors noted a higher prevalence of cognitive impairment with older age, a trend that is similar to that seen in the general population but occurring at a much younger age in kidney transplant recipients [16]. This suggests that cognitive impairment in dialysis patients may not be entirely reversible. Despite improvement in kidney function after transplantation, prolonged exposure to comorbid medical conditions including metabolic and vascular changes that are associated with kidney disease may result in non-reversible cerebrovascular disease that persists after successful transplantation. Alteration of the microbiome, immunomodulation, and neurotoxicity from medications such as calcineurin inhibitors or corticosteroids may also contribute to cognitive impairment in transplant recipients [15].

4.6 Case Vignette Analysis

Mr. Doyle's sister came forward as a potential living donor for Mr. Doyle and was found to be a good immunologic match. She went through appropriate screening, and there were no concerns about her being a kidney donor. Mr. Doyle was worked up for renal transplant, and he was deemed fit to proceed. Once his eGFR reached 11 mL/min/1.73 m^2, he was scheduled for a preemptive transplant, before needing to start dialysis. His transplant induction comprised basiliximab and methylprednisone. His maintenance immunosuppression is now tacrolimus, mycophenolic acid (Myfortic), and prednisone. Because his serology was negative for CMV and his sister's serology was positive for CMV (CMV mismatch), he was also started on valganciclovir posttransplant to prevent CMV infection. He was discharged 5 days after his surgery with no postoperative complications and was scheduled to be followed up in the transplant clinic for ongoing monitoring of his renal function, drug levels, and possible complications.

4.7 Key Takeaways

- In general, renal transplantation is considered superior to dialysis; however, a thorough pretransplant assessment must be completed to ensure that the risks of transplantation do not outweigh the benefits.
- Transplant donors can be living or deceased. Deceased donors are classified as standard or extended criteria donors (SCD vs ECD); organ retrieval occurs in two situations: in donation after cardiac death (DCD) donors, organ retrieval occurs after the heart has stopped beating, whereas neurologic determination of death (NDD) donors are determined to be brain-dead and, therefore, circulation is maintained during retrieval.
- Transplant immunosuppression includes medications for induction and maintenance. Maintenance typically includes a calcineurin inhibitor (CNI), an antimetabolite, and a glucocorticoid. All three classes can have adverse effects.
- Transplant recipients must be carefully monitored for complications including cardiovascular events, infection, and malignancy.
- Posttransplant recipients can experience delirium; one major risk factor is the high prevalence of cognitive impairment in those patients previously on dialysis and who are now recipients of kidney transplants.
- To provide optimal care for these complex patients, it is important for the psychiatrist, psychologist, and transplant physician to co-manage the care of transplant patients with psychological and psychiatric concerns.

References

1. U.S. Renal Data System 2019 Annual Data Report: Epidemiology of Kidney Disease in the United States. [Internet]. https://www.usrds.org/media/2371/2019-executive-summary.pdf. Accessed 5 April 2021.
2. Annual Statistics on Organ Replacement in Canada Dialysis, Transplantation and Donation, 2010 to 2019. [Internet]. https://www.cihi.ca/en/organ-replacement-in-canada-corr-annual-statistics-2020. Accessed 5 April 2021.
3. Overbeck I, Bartels M, Decker O, Harms J, Hauss J, Fangmann J. Changes in quality of life after renal transplantation. Transplant Proc. 2005;37(3):1618–21.
4. OTPN/SRTR 2019 Annual Data Report: Kidney. [Internet]. https://srtr.transplant.hrsa.gov/annual_reports/2019/Kidney.aspx. Accessed 5 April 2021.

5. Olbrisch ME, Benedict SM, Ashe K, Levenson JL. Psychological assessment and care of organ transplant patients. J Consult Clin Psychol. 2002;70(3):771–83.
6. Shirali AC, Bia MJ. Management of cardiovascular disease in renal transplant recipients. Clin J Am Soc Nephrol. 2008;3(2):491–504.
7. Morath C, Mueller M, Goldschmidt H, Schwenger V, Opelz G, Zeier M. Malignancy in renal transplantation. J Am Soc Nephrol. 2004;15(6):1582–8.
8. Rao PS, Ojo A. The alphabet soup of kidney transplantation: SCD, DCD, ECD – fundamentals for the practicing nephrologist. Clin J Am Soc Nephrol. 2009;4(11):1827–31.
9. USRDS End Stage Renal Disease: Chapter 6, [Internet]. https://adr.usrds.org/2020/end-stage-renal-disease/6-transplantation
10. Muntean A, Lucan M. Immunosuppression in kidney transplantation. Clujul Med. 2013;86(3):177–80.
11. Knoll G, Cockfield S, Blydt-Hansen T, Baran D, Kiberd B, Landsberg D, Rush D, Cole E. Canadian Society of Transplantation: consensus guidelines on eligibility for kidney transplantation. CMAJ. 2005;173(10):S1–25.
12. Chisholm-Burns M, Pinsky B, Parker G, et al. Factors related to immunosuppressant medication adherence in renal transplant recipients. Clin Transplant. 2012;26(5):706–13.
13. Karam G, Maillet F, Braud G, et al. Surgical complications in kidney transplantation. Ann Urol (Paris). 2007;41(6):261–75.
14. Karuthu S, Blumberg EA. Common infections in kidney transplant recipients. Clin J Am Soc Nephrol. 2012;7(12):2058–70.
15. Haugen CE, Mountford A, Warsame F, et al. Incidence, risk factors, and sequelae of post-kidney transplant delirium. J Am Soc Nephrol. 2018;29(6):1752–9.
16. Gupta A, Mahnken JD, Johnson DK, et al. Prevalence and correlates of cognitive impairment in kidney transplant recipients. BMC Nephrol. 2017;18(1):1–8.

5 Overview of Psychopharmacology Principles in Nephrology

Poh Choo How and Glen Xiong

5.1 Introduction

The kidneys play an important role in the elimination of drugs from systemic circulation. Renal function as measured by glomerular filtration rate (GFR) naturally declines with age due in part to intrinsic factors such as vascular changes, decrease in renal perfusion rates, and cellular senescence [1]. In healthy individuals, GFR can decline by up to 50% between the age of 30 and 80 years, and a GFR of 30–60 mL/min/1.73 m^2, equivalent to stage 3 CKD, has been observed in 15–30% of individuals aged 65 and above. Chronic medical conditions such as diabetes mellitus and hypertension are further risk factors for chronic kidney disease (CKD). Many psychotropic drugs can also directly or indirectly affect renal function in the long term [2]. Given the kidney's function in elimination of drugs, GFR monitoring in those who are at risk for and who have CKD should be part of our psychiatric clinical practice so that appropriate adjustments of psychotropic and other medications can be made for patients with impaired renal function. (See Table 5.1 for categorization of CKD stages.)

P. C. How (✉) · G. Xiong
Department of Psychiatry and Behavioral Sciences, University of California, Davis, Sacramento, CA, USA
e-mail: phow@ucdavis.edu; gxiong@ucdavis.edu

A. Hategan et al. (eds.), *Psychonephrology*,
https://doi.org/10.1007/978-3-030-84740-1_5

Table 5.1 Summary of chronic kidney disease (CKD) stages

CKD stages		GFR (mL/min/1.73 m^2)	Creatinine clearance (mL/min)	Complications
1	Presence of kidney damage with normal GFR	≥ 90	90–120	Potential markers for kidney damage: hypertension due to kidney disease, asymptomatic lab abnormalities/urinalysis (microalbuminemia)/radiologic and histologic abnormalities
2	Presence of kidney damage with mild decrease in GFR	60–89	45–60	
3	Moderate decrease of GFR	30–59	20–60	Anemia, hyperparathyroidism (leading to bone/mineral disorder), cardiovascular disease (due to hypertension), low serum albumin
4	Severe decrease in GFR	15–29	10–25	
5	Kidney failure (end-stage renal disease, or ESRD)	< 15	< 10	Worsened symptoms of all the above and uremia

Clinical Pearl

– Glomerular filtration rate (GFR) is the best overall indicator of renal function and can be decreased even if creatinine levels are normal.

Recommendation

– Obtain baseline GFR prior to starting medications when possible, or start medications at 30–50% of the usual starting dose in patients at high risk of CKD such as patient with hypertension and diabetes mellitus.

5.2 Case Vignette

A 56-year-old man with long history of schizoaffective disorder, hypertension, diabetes mellitus, and tobacco use (60-pack-years) presented with manic symptoms, including pressured speech, and refusing to leave a local restaurant. He was brought into the psychiatric emergency services because he had told the police that he owned the restaurant and he demanded that they serve him dinner without him having to pay. The psychiatrist reviewed the medical records and saw that he was last seen by the emergency services 8 years ago. He was prescribed lithium 600 mg twice daily, valproic acid 750 mg twice daily, and olanzapine 20 mg nightly. His blood pressure was 180/95, and blood glucose was 350 mg/dL (19.4 mmol/L). What is a reasonable starting dose of psychiatric medications for this patient? We will return to his case later in this chapter for further analysis.

5.3 Pharmacokinetics and the Kidney

Pharmacokinetics is defined as the means by which the body processes drugs and other substances. These processes include absorption, distribution, metabolism, and elimination and are affected by changes in renal function.

5.3.1 Absorption

The rate of absorption of orally administered drugs is influenced by gastrointestinal factors such as motility, pH, expression of epithelial drug transporters, and intestinal CYP450 activity [3]. Low gut pH favors absorption of slightly acidic drugs, whereas higher pH favors absorption of slightly basic drugs. Epithelial transporters (e.g., OATP and P-glycoprotein family of transporters) are the "workhorses" of the absorption process, and a balance between uptake and efflux transporter activity and expression in gut epithelia is crucial for drug absorption. Intestinal CYP450 enzymes function to metabolize drug molecules, making them more difficult to absorb through epithelial transporters due to additional polarization of the drug molecules. Changes in gut motility affect the rate of drug absorption but not necessarily the amount of drug absorption.

In moderate to severe CKD, urea retention results in increased ammonia levels, which contribute to increased gut pH, altering the absorption of weakly acidic drugs [4]. Animal studies indicate that accumulation of uremic toxins decrease the expression and activity of efflux transporters in gut membranes. Uremic toxins have also been implicated in decreased activity of intestinal CYP450, tipping the balance to less polarized parent drugs that are more easily absorbed through epithelial transporters. In addition, accumulation of uremic toxins affects the expression of tight junction proteins that help to maintain the integrity of the epithelial lining of the gut, allowing drug moieties to leak into the plasma via paracellular transport. Overall, gut/intestinal absorption is increased with CKD and ESRD.

Clinical Pearl

- Intestinal absorption of orally administered medications is usually increased with CKD.

Recommendation

- Be cautious when dosing medication in patients with CKD, even for medications that may not be renally cleared.

5.3.2 Distribution

Drug plasma concentrations depend on the volume of distribution (Vd) of drugs in hydrophilic, lipophilic, and other compartments. With aging, the percentage of body water decreases, while body fat increases, thereby decreasing the Vd of hydrophilic drugs and increasing the Vd of lipophilic drugs, with a prolonged half-life [3].

Another compartment or factor to consider is that many drugs are extensively bound to plasma proteins and only unbound or free drugs are available for receptor binding. For example, albumin binds weakly acidic drugs, and alpha-1-acidic glycoprotein binds weakly basic drugs.

In moderate to severe CKD, albuminuria results in decreased plasma concentrations of albumin, leading to an increased free drug fraction of weakly acidic drugs [4]. At the same time, there are increased levels of alpha-1-acidic glycoprotein in response to inflammation, decreasing the free drug fraction of weakly basic drugs. Uremic toxins also compete for plasma protein binding sites leading to further increase of free drug fractions of weakly basic drugs. Altogether, there is increased free drug concentration due to decreased albumin through proteinuria and competition for protein binding with uremic toxins. Vd is increased for many drugs due to decreased protein binding, increased tissue binding, and alterations in fluid dynamics such as fluid overload.

Clinical Pearl

- In CKD, volume of distribution is increased for many drugs due to fluid overload, and drug-protein binding is decreased due to hypoalbuminemia.

Recommendation

- Water-soluble medications such as lithium may have large volume of distribution, therefore requiring higher doses (or longer time) to establish steady state.

5.3.3 Metabolism

About 70% of drugs undergo phase I metabolism prior to excretion, mediated by intestinal and hepatic CYP450 enzymes [3]. Intestinal metabolism decreases absorption of a drug, leading to excretion of drugs along with fecal matter, whereas hepatic metabolism contributes to downstream elimination via the kidneys. CYP 3A4 and 2C9 metabolize nearly 40% of clinically used drugs. Phase II glucuronidation and acetylation further increases aqueous solubility of drugs to facilitate renal elimination. In moderate to severe CKD, there is decreased expression and activity of hepatic CYP450 and phase II enzymes in response to the accumulation of uremic toxins, leading to an increase in the ratio of parent drug/metabolite and increased half-life of the parent drug [4]. This also has implications on the activity of the drug depending on whether the parent drug or the metabolite is actively involved in the pharmacodynamic action of the drug. Overall, the ability of the body to metabolize drugs is decreased in CKD.

Clinical Pearl

- Drug metabolism is decreased in CKD.

Recommendation
- Avoid polypharmacy and use of drugs that inhibit CYP450 enzymes.

5.3.4 Elimination

A majority of drugs are eliminated through the kidney following hepatic metabolism. However, CKD also affects non-renal drug excretion of orally administered drugs that occurs via the biliary system, mediated by hepatic efflux drug transporters. In normal aging and CKD, decreases in GFR lead to decreased rates of excretion of parent drugs and their metabolites [3]. In CKD, uremic toxins and nephrocyte cell death affect the expression of renal drug transporters that facilitate the excretion of metabolites via the kidney [4]. Overall, there is a decreased rate of renal and biliary drug excretion with CKD, increasing the elimination half-life of drugs and their metabolites.

Table 5.2 summarizes the pharmacokinetic changes with CKD.

Table 5.2 Pharmacokinetic changes with chronic kidney disease

	Factors	Changes in CKD
Absorption	Gut pH (low pH favors absorption of slightly acidic drugs; higher pH favors absorption of slight basic drugs	Urea retention results in increased ammonia leading to increased gut pH, altering the absorption of weakly basic drugs
	Balance between uptake and efflux transporter activity and expression in gut epithelia	Decreased expression of efflux transporter proteins leads to increased overall uptake of drugs across gut epithelia
	Intestinal CYP450 enzyme levels and activity	Decreased activity of intestinal CYP450 enzymes
	Paracellular transport	Decreased expression of tight junction proteins in intestinal epithelia in response to higher urea levels increases absorption via paracellular transport (rodent model) Overall: increased absorption due to increased paracellular transport, decreased intestinal CYP450 activity, decreased activity of efflux transporters
Distribution	Volume of distribution	Overall increase in Vd of lipophilic compartment (fat) and decrease of Vd of hydrophilic compartment (aqueous) with increased age
	Protein binding – many drugs are extensively bound to plasma protein, while unbound/free drugs are available for receptor binding (e.g., albumin binds weakly acidic drugs, and alpha-1-acidic glycoprotein binds weakly basic drugs)	Decreased albumin levels as a result of albuminuria increases free drug fractions of weakly acidic drugs Increased levels of alpha-1-acidic glycoprotein in ESRD due to chronic inflammation decreases free drug fractions of weakly basic drugs Uremic toxins compete for plasma protein binding sites leading to increase in free drug fractions Overall: increased free drug concentration due to decreased albumin through proteinuria and competition for protein binding with uremic toxins, potential increased Vd of hydrophilic drugs with fluid retention

(continued)

Table 5.2 (continued)

	Factors	Changes in CKD
Metabolism	73% of drugs undergo phase I metabolism prior to excretion, mediated by intestinal and hepatic CYP450 enzymes. CYP 3A4 and 2C9 metabolize ~43% of clinically used drugs. Phase II glucuronidation and acetylation increase aqueous solubility and facilitate elimination by kidneys	Decreased expression and activities of hepatic CYP450s and phase II enzymes in moderate to severe CKD in response to accumulation of uremic toxins in the bloodstream. Overall decreased metabolism of drugs with increased Cmax and medication levels Overall: decreased phase I and phase II metabolism due to decreased expression/activities of these enzymes
Elimination	Non-renal drug excretion occurs via the biliary system, mediated by hepatic drug transporters	Decreases in GFR decreases rate of excretion of parent drugs and their metabolites Kidney disease decreases expression of renal drug transporters that facilitate excretion of metabolites, via uremic toxins Decreased expression of transporters secondary to uremic toxins leads to decreased biliary excretion of drugs Overall: decreased renal and biliary drug excretion

Clinical Pearl
- Both renal and non-renal drug excretion are decreased in CKD.

Recommendation
- Consider lower starting and maximum doses of medications in patients with CKD.

5.3.5 Acute Kidney Injury

Acute kidney injury (AKI) can occur due to pre-renal (e.g., dehydration, hypoperfusion secondary to trauma), intrinsic (e.g., acute tubular necrosis in response to nephrotoxic drugs, infection), or post-renal (e.g. outflow obstruction). In the setting of AKI in critically ill patients in the medical inpatient or intensive care unit, GI absorption is often affected by minimal oral intake of food and liquids, with a reliance on intravascular fluid repletion and nutrition [5]. Proton pump inhibitors and H2-antagonists for stress ulcer prophylaxis lead to increase in gastric pH, affecting the GI absorption of weakly acidic drugs. Slow GI motility leads to an increased time to Cmax (maximum plasma drug concentration) but does not alter plasma drug concentration levels. Overall, the intravenous route should be considered for adequate absorption of medications in critically ill patients.

Monitoring of fluid balance (input and output) and blood pressure helps to gauge volume of distribution and guide adjustments of rates and volumes of fluid repletion as needed. Consider also third spacing in the setting of infection as contributing to decreased systemic volume of distribution leading to renal hypoperfusion (e.g., in ascites, accumulation of fluids in the peritoneal space pulls aqueous volume away from systemic circulation, leading to hepatorenal syndrome). Metabolism of drugs does not seem to be affected in AKI in a majority of studies and appears to be more strongly correlated to the accumulation of uremic toxins as a result of CKD.

5.3.6 Hemodialysis

Whether or not a drug can be eliminated via dialysis depends on their molecular weight, protein binding, volume of distribution, the type of dialysis membrane used, and blood and dialysate flow rates [6]. Smaller molecules are more easily cleared by dialysis through diffusion across the dialysis membrane. Drugs that are less extensively bound to plasma proteins are also more easily removed from circulations. In addition, drugs that have a smaller Vd tend to have a higher concentration across the dialysis membrane and thus are more readily removed by dialysis. The properties of the dialysis membrane (e.g., size of pore and surface area) also affect the dialyzability of different drugs. Faster blood and dialysate flow rates also facilitate the clearance of drugs by dialysis. The Renal Pharmacy Consultants' publication *Dialysis of Drugs* provides a reference for the dialyzability of drugs [7]; however, there continues to be little or no data regarding the dialyzability of most psychotropic medications. Interestingly, metabolism of drugs is recovered in patients on hemodialysis as regular removal of uremic toxins removes their ability to affect the expression and activity of CYP450 metabolic enzymes [5].

Clinical Pearl

- Most drugs cannot be removed by hemodialysis, and most patients on hemodialysis take an average of 9–12 medications.

Recommendation

- Strongly consider non-pharmacological treatment, and avoid initiation of new drugs and high doses of drugs where possible.
- For drugs that can be removed by hemodialysis, determine whether post-hemodialysis supplementation is necessary (see Table 5.3)

Table 5.3 Protein binding, molecular weight, and dialyzability of selected psychotropic drugs

	% plasma protein bound	% renal clearance	Dialyzability (conventional/ high permeability)	Recommendations for dose adjustments in CKD	Other considerations
Antipsychotics					
Chlorpromazine	98	ND	No/unlikely	None	Risk of orthostatic hypotension. Increased risk of lowering seizure threshold
Haloperidol	92	<1	No/unlikely	None	Increased risk of QTc prolongation with intravascular formulation
Aripiprazole	99	25	Unlikely/unlikely	None	Significant interactions with other drugs metabolized by CYP450 2D6 and 3A4
Clozapine	95	50	No/unlikely	None. Titrate to response	Increased risk of metabolic side effects contributing to the development of type 2 diabetes mellitus, leading to CKD. Increased risk of lowering seizure threshold. Risk of orthostatic hypotension
Olanzapine	93	56	No/unlikely	None	Increased risk of metabolic side effects contributing to the development of type 2 diabetes mellitus, leading to CKD
Quetiapine	83	<1	ND/ND	None	Increased risk of metabolic side effects contributing to the development of type 2 diabetes mellitus, leading to CKD
Risperidone	89	10–40	ND/ND	Consider lower starting dose of 0.5 mg BID and lower maximum dose of 1.5 mg BID	Wide variation in renal clearance with parent drug/metabolite clearance reduced by up to 60% in CKD
Ziprasidone	99	ND	ND/ND	Consider lower starting and maximum dose in CKD 1-3. Avoid in CKD 4-5 due to risk of QTC prolongation	Increased risk of QTc prolongation. Poor oral absorption; needs to be administered with 350 kcal meal

Antidepressants					
Sertraline	98	ND	No/unlikely	None	
Fluoxetine	94	ND	No/unlikely	None	Potential for drug-drug interaction due to inhibition of CYP450 enzymes. Risk of SIADH
Paroxetine	95	ND	No/no	Consider lower starting dose of 10 mg/day and lower maximum dose of 30 mg/day	Increased Cmax and half-life in CKD
Citalopram	ND	20%, renal clearance decreases by 40% in CKD	No/no	Consider lower starting dose	May cause prolonged QTc. Monitor QTc in setting of electrolyte abnormalities
Escitalopram	56	ND	ND	Consider lower starting dose	May cause prolonged QTc. Monitor QTc in setting of electrolyte abnormalities
Venlafaxine	< 30	87%	No/unlikely	Lower maximum dose of 112.5 mg/day in CKD	Dose-related increase in blood pressure; may contribute to worsening renal impairment from worsening hypertension
Duloxetine	95	70	Unlikely/unlikely	Consider lower starting dose and gradual titration in CKD3. Avoid in CKD5	Dose-related increase in blood pressure; may contribute to worsening renal impairment from worsening hypertension. Risk of hepatoxicity that can lead to renal dysfunction
Bupropion	88	< 10	No/no	Consider lower starting dose and gradual titration	Monitor electrolytes due to increased risk of reducing seizure threshold

(continued)

Table 5.3 (continued)

	% plasma protein bound	% renal clearance	Dialyzability (conventional/ high permeability)	Recommendations for dose adjustments in CKD	Other considerations
Mirtazapine	85	< 10 renal clearance decreased by 50% in CKD3	ND/ND	Consider lower starting dose of 7.5 mg/day and lower maximum dose of 22.5 mg/day	
Trazodone	90	No data	No/unlikely	None	
Mood stabilizers					
Lithium	0	100%	Yes/yes	Consider lower starting dose (150 mg/day) and lower maximum dose (450 mg/day) in CKD 1-3. Relatively contraindicated in CKD 4-5	Serum drug monitoring. Drug-drug interactions with thiazide diuretics, NSAIDs. Removed by hemodialysis, administration of single dose after dialysis is recommended to restore therapeutic levels
Valproic acid	93	1–3	No/yes	No	Check *free* serum valproic acid levels in CKD with hypoalbuminemia. Potential to cause pancreatitis in CKD. Some removal by hemodialysis
Carbamazepine	76	1	No/yes	None	Drug-drug interactions with valproic acid, felbamate, digoxin, cyclosporin. Serum drug monitoring is required; risk of SIADH
Oxcarbazepine	40	50	ND/ND	Decrease dose or start at 50% in CKD 3, no data for CKD5	Serum drug monitoring, risk of SIADH

Lamotrigine	ND	10	No/ND	Decrease dose by 25% in CKD 3–4. Maximum of 100 mg daily in CKD stage 5	
Benzodiazepines/non-benzodiazepines					
Alprazolam	80	15	No/ND	None	
Chlordiazepoxide	97	ND	No/unlikely	Consider lower initial starting dose (7.5 mg/day) and lower maximum dose (50mg/day) in CKD	
Clonazepam	86	ND	No/ND	None	
Diazepam	99	ND	No/ND	None	
Lorazepam	91	33% decreased renal clearance with CKD	No/ND	Consider lower initial starting dose and maximum daily dose of 4mg/day	
Zolpidem	92	67	No/unlikely	Decrease dose by 50% in CKD	
Cognitive enhancers					
Donepezil	96	57%	Unlikely/ND	None	
Memantine	45	Primarily renal	ND/ND	Consider lower initial starting dose and maximum daily dose by half (maximum of 10 mg/day) in CKD3-5	
Rivastigmine	40–50	ND	ND/ND	None	

Data compiled from [5–8, 10, 12, 13, 15, 16]
Abbreviations: *ND* no data, *BID* twice a day

5.3.7 Renal Transplantation

Renal transplantation is associated with improved eGFR and renal clearance of drugs. However, many renal transplant recipients have an eGFR of < 60 mL/min/1.73 m^2 1 year after receiving their graft, equivalent to CKD stage 3 [8]. Factors influencing posttransplantation renal function including the health of the donor kidney, degree of match, immunosuppression regimen, adherence to medications, renal diet, and other aspects of posttransplant care. The same precautions in dosing of medications should apply to renal graft recipients.

5.4 Recommendations for Dosage Adjustment of Psychotropic Drugs in Patients with Renal Impairment

Pharmacokinetic changes resulting from renal function impairment significantly contribute to increased half-life and systemic accumulation of drugs. This is further complicated by data showing that patients with CKD take and average of 9–12 medications to treat various comorbidities, placing patients at further risk for adverse drug reactions and drug-drug interactions [5]. Despite numerous studies on changes in pharmacokinetics in CKD, there are many challenges in translating these data into clinical application and dosing guidelines. In the case of psychotropic medications, the use of the lowest effective doses of medications, minimizing polypharmacy, and use of non-pharmacologic interventions are general guiding principles for the prescription of medications/therapies in patients. In patients with renal impairment, safe and effective doses of psychotropic medications may need to be adjusted on an individual level depending on the severity of functional/behavior impairment, goals of therapy, degree of renal impairment, and the risks and benefits of specific medication therapies [9]. Ongoing monitoring of adverse events, changes in renal function, and, in some cases, serum drug levels can help guide dose adjustments such as decreased starting dose, slow titration with smaller incremental increases in dose, and lower maximum dose. Large-scale studies of pharmacokinetic changes in psychotropic medications in the setting of moderate to chronic kidney disease have not been done. The following description reflects data from review of smaller-scale studies and is summarized in Table 5.3.

Clinical Pearl

- GFR decreases with age.

Recommendation

- Monitor GFR as patients age.
- Review and reconsider medication dosing in patients with renal impairment (see Table 5.3).
- Check renally cleared medications more frequently such as checking lithium levels every 4–6 weeks in clinical scenarios where fluid shift and GFR change is likely.

5.4.1 Antipsychotics

While many medications require renal clearance, most antipsychotics are predominantly cleared through the hepatic/biliary pathway [4]. However, in moderate to severe CKD, dose adjustments have been recommended for risperidone and ziprasidone due to decreased renal clearance of their metabolites. Antipsychotics can cause many adverse events that cause or interact with the effects of renal impairment. Second-generation antipsychotics such as olanzapine, quetiapine, and clozapine contribute to the development of metabolic syndrome, increasing the risk for developing type 2 diabetes mellitus which contributes to renal impairment. Chlorpromazine, clozapine, and other antipsychotics that lower the seizure threshold present additional risk of seizures to individuals with electrolyte abnormalities associated with CKD. Similarly, some antipsychotics (e.g., ziprasidone) contribute to the risk of developing QTc prolongation and arrhythmias. Theoretically, there is a risk of orthostatic hypotension as a side effect of antipsychotics contributing to worsening renal disease due to renal hypoperfusion as well as augmenting drop in blood pressure associated with hemodialysis. Antipsychotics are highly protein bound; however, assays for free drug levels have not been developed or are not widely available; therefore, it is recommended to titrate antipsychotics to clinical efficacy rather than to a specific plasma level. There are some case reports associat ing risperidone with the development of syndrome of inappropriate antidiuretic hormone (SIADH) secretion though this side effect appears to be rare.

Clinical Pearl
- Second-generation antipsychotics can cause metabolic syndrome and can lead to the development of type 2 diabetes mellitus, which is a risk factor for CKD.

Recommendation
- Monitor hemoglobin A1c levels and GFR in patients on second-generation antipsychotics.
- Treat hyperlipidemia, diabetes mellitus, and hypertension that may develop as a result of the use of psychotropic medications.

5.4.2 Antidepressants

Depressive disorders are highly comorbid in patients with CKD and on hemodialysis (20–30%) [10]. Depressed mood is the most frequent psychiatric symptom among renal transplant recipients (25%) and is associated with non-adherence to immunosuppressant medication, graft failure, general poor outcomes, and all-cause mortality. Treatment of depressive disorders in CKD, hemodialysis, and renal transplantation is associated with improved adherence to medication, diet, hemodialysis, and immunosuppressant regimens [11]. In addition to non-pharmacological interventions, selective serotonin reuptake inhibitors (SSRIs) have been shown to be generally safe for the treatment of depressive disorders in CKD with recommendations for lower starting and maximum doses in cases of CKD (see Table 5.3). Some SSRIs are strong inhibitors of CYP450 enzymes and can worsen the metabolism of other drugs in CKD. SSRIs also have an antiplatelet effect, and renal transplant recipients are at a theoretical risk of GI bleeding due to the concurrent use of antiplatelet agents and steroids, which also impair platelet function. Citalopram can prolong the QTc interval and should be used with greater caution in severe renal impairment with electrolyte abnormalities. SSRIs also carry some risk for syndrome of inappropriate antidiuretic hormone (SIADH) secretion, and regular monitoring of sodium levels is prudent in moderate to severe CKD (approximately every 3 months).

The serotonin and norepinephrine reuptake inhibitors (SNRIs) venlafaxine and duloxetine cause a dose-dependent increase in blood pressure which in the long run can worsen renal function. Duloxetine metabolite levels are 7–9 times higher in CKD compared to normal renal function and should be avoided in severe CKD and hemodialysis patients. Although bupropion (a norepinephrine-dopamine reuptake inhibitor) is eliminated to a large extent via the liver, severe renal impairment can affect non-renal elimination as previously discussed. Therefore, caution is called for in the use of bupropion, which carries a risk of lowering seizure threshold especially in the setting of electrolyte abnormalities. The half-life of tricyclic antidepressants (TCAs) is markedly increased in CKD, and therapeutic drug monitoring can help with dosage adjustments in CKD, though TCAs should be reserved for treatment-resistant depressive disorders given the availability of alternative antidepressant medications with better safety profiles. Monoamine oxidase inhibitor (MAOI) use is discouraged in CKD due to lack of safety data and orthostatic hypotension effects in this population. Antidepressants are also highly protein bound, and dosage adjustments should be considered in the case of CKD-related hypoalbuminemia.

Clinical Pearl

- QTc prolongation and decreased seizure threshold are some pharmacodynamic interactions between antipsychotics/antidepressants and electrolyte abnormalities seen in CKD.

Recommendation

- Monitor ECGs in patients with CKD on medications that may also prolong QTc.
- Consider alternative therapies if QTc prolongation is a concern.

5.4.3 Mood Stabilizers

Lithium has been shown to be an efficacious treatment for bipolar disorder and its renotoxicity has been well documented. There is a 15% decrease in GFR associated with taking lithium alone [12]. Lithium is not protein bound and is excreted unmetabolized solely by the kidney. Treatment of bipolar disorder with lithium should be accompanied by regular monitoring of lithium levels and GFR to monitor for the development of CKD. Dose reduction in CKD is important to avoid lithium toxicity. Lithium is a small molecule and can be removed by hemodialysis; hence, administration of a supplemental dose post-hemodialysis is recommended to restore therapeutic levels. Given the renotoxicity of lithium, use of other mood stabilizing agents should be considered in patients developing CKD in response to lithium. Lithium therapy can be continued in CKD stages 1–3 if the patient does not respond to other mood stabilizers or second-generation antipsychotics, but with appropriate dose adjustments and monitoring of levels and renal function. Lithium is relatively contraindicated in CKD stages 4–5.

Valproic acid is predominantly excreted via the hepatobiliary pathway. With moderate to severe CKD, protein-bound valproic acid levels will give a falsely lower drug level in the setting of hypoalbuminemia, and it is important to obtain *free* and total valproic acid levels to determine accurate drug concentrations [12, 13]. Carbamazepine is metabolized almost entirely by CYP450, and there are no recommendations for dose adjustment with renal failure. However, it also carries a risk of SIADH and contributes to significant drug-drug interactions due to its ability to both induce and inhibit CYP 3A4. With the availability of other mood-stabilizing agents, it is best to avoid the use of carbamazepine in patients with multiple comorbidities and polypharmacy. Oxcarbazepine is a safer option in this population with lower inhibition of CYP450 activity though it also carries a risk for SIADH. A fraction of valproic acid and carbamazepine can be removed during HD, but there are no recommendations for post-hemodialysis repletion.

Clinical Pearl

- Many medications, including valproic acid, are highly protein bound, and the free drug fraction of medications changes as a result of hypoalbuminemia associated with CKD.

Recommendation

- Check *free* and total valproic acid levels to get an accurate level in patients with hypoalbuminemia.

5.4.4 Benzodiazepines/Non-benzodiazepines

Anxiety is also highly comorbid with CKD (see Chap. 11). Benzodiazepines and non-benzodiazepines are metabolized by the liver for the most part though dose adjustments in the setting of CKD are recommended for some. Dose reduction is recommended for chlordiazepoxide, lorazepam, and zolpidem. AKI and CKD patients with electrolyte abnormalities are at risk for delirium, and benzodiazepines should be used judiciously in this population due to their deliriogenic properties [5, 12].

5.4.5 Cognitive Enhancers

The cognitive enhancers donepezil, memantine, and rivastigmine are primarily renally cleared [14–16]. The pharmacokinetics of donepezil and rivastigmine do not appear to be altered with renal impairment. The half-life and concentration of memantine do increase in moderate to severe CKD, and a dose adjustment to half initial and maximum doses is recommended.

5.5 Case Vignette Analysis

This 56-year-old with a history of hypertension, diabetes mellitus, and tobacco use disorder was at high risk for CKD. His GFR should be measured based on his age, ethnicity, and weight. He is at high risk of lithium toxicity, and his lithium should not be started at prior dose from 8 years ago. A dose of 300 mg twice daily or at most 900 mg per day may be considered, assuming that diuretics and ACE inhibitors or angiotensin reuptake blockers (ARB) are also initially avoided. In the inpatient setting, he may require more frequent lithium levels each time his medications are adjusted. Similarly, due to hypoalbuminemia from CKD, he may also not tolerate the higher dose of valproate that he used to take. A reasonable starting dose for valproate may be 500 mg twice daily (usual range 10–20 mg/kg/24h). Olanzapine dose may also need to be lowered by 5–10 mg depending on his current weight. However, because of diabetes mellitus, olanzapine is avoided for this patient. Nevertheless, medication choice will also depend on the severity of his psychiatric illness and experience with other antipsychotic medications.

5.6 Key Takeaways

- Glomerular filtration rate (GFR) is the best overall indicator of renal function and can be decreased even if creatinine levels are normal. GFR declines with age.
- Obtaining a baseline GFR prior to starting medications when possible, or starting medications at 30–50% of the usual starting dose in patients at high risk for CKD such as patients with hypertension and diabetes mellitus, is recommended.
- Absorption of orally administered medications is increased in CKD. Lower starting and maintenance doses of medications may be required.

- Volume of distribution (Vd) of hydrophilic medications is increased with CKD due to fluid accumulation. Some medication doses will need to be increased to achieve therapeutic levels (e.g., lithium).
- Vd of protein bound drugs is decreased due to hypoalbuminemia. Check for free drug levels of highly protein bound drugs (e.g., valproic acid).
- Metabolism and elimination of drugs are decreased in CKD. Use the minimum effective dose of medications.
- Most drugs cannot be removed by hemodialysis.

References

1. Weinstein JR, Anderson S. The aging kidney: physiological changes. Adv Chronic Kidney Dis. 2010;17(4):302–7.
2. McIntyre RS, Baghdady NT, Banik S, Swartz SA. The use of psychotropic drugs in patients with impaired renal function. Prim Psychiatry. 2008;15(1):73–88.
3. Aymanns C, Keller F, Maus S, Hartmann B, Czock D. Review on pharmacokinetics and pharmacodynamics and the aging kidney. Clin J Am Soc Nephrol. 2010;5(2):314–27.
4. Naud J, Nolin TD, Leblond FA, Pichette V. Current understanding of drug disposition in kidney disease. J Clin Pharmacol. 2012;52(S1):10S–22S.
5. Matzke GR, Aronoff GR, Atkinson AJ Jr, et al. Drug dosing consideration in patients with acute and chronic kidney disease – a clinical update from Kidney Disease: Improving Global Outcomes (KDIGO). Kidney Int. 2011;80(11):1122–37.
6. Velenosi TJ, Urquhart BL. Pharmacokinetic considerations in chronic kidney disease and patients requiring dialysis. Expert Opin Drug Metab Toxicol. 2014;10(8):1131–43.
7. Bailie GR, Mason NA. Dialysis of drugs. Saline: Renal Pharmacy Consultants; 2020.
8. Chilcot J, Spencer BW, Maple H, Mamode N. Depression and kidney transplantation. Transplantation. 2014;97(7):717–21.
9. Baghdady NT, Banik S, Swartz SA, McIntyre RS. Psychotropic drugs and renal failure: translating the evidence for clinical practice. Adv Ther. 2009;26(4):404–24.
10. Nagler EV, Webster AC, Vanholder R, Zoccali C. Antidepressants for depression in stage 3–5 chronic kidney disease: a systematic review of pharmacokinetics, efficacy and safety with recommendations by European Renal Best Practice (ERBP). Nephrol Dial Transplant. 2012;27(10):3736–45.
11. Huang Y, Tilea A, Gillespie B, Shahinian V, Banerjee T, Grubbs V, Powe N, Rios-Burrows N, Pavkov M, Saran R. Understanding trends in kidney function 1 year after kidney transplant in the United States. J Am Soc Nephrol. 2017;28(8):2498–510.
12. Cohen LM, Tessier EG, Germain MJ, Levy NB. Update on psychotropic medication use in renal disease. Psychosomatics. 2004;45(1):34–48.
13. Zhang F, Xue J, Shao J, Jia L. Compilation of 222 drugs' plasma protein binding data and guidance for study designs. Drug Discov Today. 2012;17(9-10):475–85.
14. Moritoyo T, Hasunuma T, Harada K, Tateishi T, Watanabe M, Kotegawa T, Nagai M, Kumagai Y, Fujitani T, Okura T, Fukuoka T. Effect of renal impairment on the pharmacokinetics of memantine. J Pharmacol Sci. 2012;119(4):324–9.
15. Nagy CF, Kumar D, Cullen EI, Bolton WK, Marbury TC, Gutierrez MJ, Hutman HW, Pratt RD. Steady-state pharmacokinetics and safety of donepezil HCl in subjects with moderately impaired renal function. Br J Clin Pharmacol. 2004;58:18–24.
16. Lefevre G, Callegari F, Gsteiger S, Xiong Y. Effects of renal impairment on steady-state plasma concentrations of rivastigmine: a population pharmacokinetic analysis of capsule and patch formulations in patients with Alzheimer's disease. Drugs Aging. 2016;33(10):725–36.

Renal Toxicity of Psychotropic Medications

6

Poh Choo How and Glen Xiong

6.1 Introduction

The kidneys play an important role in the elimination of most psychotropic drugs. Psychotropic drugs can have direct and/or indirect renotoxic effects on kidney function. Notably, lithium's renotoxicity has been well characterized. Some antipsychotics can worsen renal function indirectly through metabolic dysregulation and the development of diabetes mellitus, which affects renal function mainly through vascular changes related to advanced glycation end products on renal microvasculature. Antidepressants, antipsychotics, and anti-epileptic agents also cause SIADH, indirectly increasing the renal workload of maintaining plasma osmolality. While many cases of renal injury are reversible with discontinuation of the causal agent, psychotropic therapy usually involves chronic use, exposing patients to renal side effects in the long term. Close monitoring of renal function, health conditions, drug-drug interactions, and, in some cases, medication levels, along with the use of the lowest effective doses of medications, can help decrease adverse events related to psychotropic drug therapy.

P. C. How (✉) · G. Xiong
Department of Psychiatry and Behavioral Sciences, University of California, Davis, Sacramento, CA, USA
e-mail: phow@ucdavis.edu; gxiong@ucdavis.edu

A. Hategan et al. (eds.), *Psychonephrology*,
https://doi.org/10.1007/978-3-030-84740-1_6

6.2 Case Vignette

A 45-year-old woman with bipolar disorder presented with confusion and tremors. She stumbled and fell while she was walking to the bathroom resulting in right hip fracture. She apparently has been having cough, fever, and fatigue. She had not been eating or drinking as usual over the last 5 days. She took lithium 900 mg/day, risperidone 2 mg/day, and ibuprofen 800 mg 2–3 times per day in the last week for fever. In the emergency room, she is found to have lithium of 6.3 mmol/L (normal level: 0.5–1.2 mmol/L, or mEq/L). We will return to her case later in this chapter for further analysis.

6.3 Lithium and Chronic Renal Impairment

Lithium is widely recognized as the most effective long-term therapy for bipolar disorder, with efficacy for the treatment of manic and depressive episodes, and additional evidence demonstrating reduced suicide risk in long-term users. The use of lithium is complicated by its narrow therapeutic range, requiring frequent drug level monitoring. Additionally, long-term lithium use can lead to side effects such as chronic renal impairment, nephrogenic diabetes insipidus (discussed later in the chapter), hypothyroidism, hyperparathyroidism, and weight gain.

Broadly, systematic review and meta-analysis of the effects of lithium on glomerular filtration rate (GFR) shows that use of lithium is associated with a reduction of GFR by 6.22 mL/min/1.73 m^2 (95% CI − 14.65 to 2.20, $p = 0.148$) compared to non-users [1]. Retrospective analysis of laboratory data of ~500,000 patients of the National Health Services in the United Kingdom over the course of 20 years demonstrated that after adjusting for age, sex, and comorbid diabetes mellitus, lithium use was associated with development of stage 3 or higher chronic kidney disease (CKD), which is defined as a GFR below 60 mL/min/1.73 m^2 (HR 1.93 [1.76–2.12; $p < 0.0001$]) [2]. Women were at greater risk of developing renal impairment compared to men, and younger women (< 60 years of age) were at greater risk than older women. Overall, a higher than median serum level (0.6 mmol/L) was associated with an increased risk of renal impairment (HR 1.62 [1.41–1.85; $p < 0.0001$]). The length of time taking lithium itself was not associated with an increase in renal impairment (HR 0.50 [0.44–0.58; $p < 0.0001$]).

Monitoring of adverse effects of lithium should take place at every follow-up appointment and serum drug levels obtained each time the dosage of lithium is changed and at least every 3–6 months if the patient is taking the same dose chronically [3]. GFR and thyroid function tests should also be tested at least every 3–6 months and the dose of lithium adjusted in cases of decreased GFR. Specific changes in dosing have not been defined, and the general recommendation is to titrate doses slowly with more frequent monitoring of serum levels and avoid the use

Table 6.1 Recommended monitoring for patients taking lithium

	Baseline	5–7 days after dose initiation or dosage change	Every 3–6 months	Every office visit
Vital signs	✓		✓	✓
Health history	✓			✓
Current medications	✓			✓
Lithium level		✓	✓	
BMP	✓		✓	
CBC	✓		✓	
TSH	✓		✓	
Urinalysis	✓			
Pregnancy test	✓			
ECG if cardiac history or age > 40	✓		✓	
Review: Risk of lithium toxicity, thyroid dysfunction, blood dyscrasia, cardiac abnormalities, teratogenicity, drug interactions, contraception use if female of reproductive age	✓			✓

of lithium in stage 5 CKD. Psychiatrists should endeavor to use the lowest effective dose of lithium given that higher serum levels are associated with a greater degree of renal impairment. See Table 6.1 for recommended monitoring for patients taking lithium.

Clinical Pearl

- Development of CKD is associated with higher steady-state lithium levels above 0.6 mmol/L.

Recommendation

- Use the lowest effective dose of lithium therapy and closely monitor lithium levels and renal function (see Table 6.1).
- Check lithium levels with each dose escalation (usually after 4–5 days), initiation of medications that affect GFR (NSAIDS, ACE inhibitors, angiotensin reuptake blockers, diuretics), and conditions that cause dehydration (extreme heat, excessive caffeine intake, and respiratory and other infections).

Table 6.2 Symptoms of lithium toxicity

Symptoms	Acute	Chronic
Gastrointestinal	Nausea, vomiting, diarrhea	
Neurological	Mild: postural fine tremor, dysphoria, memory problems, slow reaction time, irritability	Gradual development of sluggishness, ataxia, confusion, agitation
	Moderate: ataxia, dizziness, slurred speech, lethargy, increased deep tendon reflexes, peripheral neuropathy, dysarthria	
	Severe: convulsions/seizures, delirium, stupor, coma, SILENT (syndrome of irreversible lithium-effected neurotoxicity)	
Musculoskeletal	Mild: coarse tremor, muscle twitching	Fine tremor, muscle twitching
	Moderate: Severe: muscle weakness, ataxia	
Renal	Acute renal failure	Nephrogenic diabetes insipidus, chronic renal failure, polyuria/polydipsia
Endocrine	Transient hyperglycemia, hypercalcemia	Hypothyroidism, hyperparathyroidism/ hypercalcemia
Cardiovascular	Moderate: T wave inversion, SA/AV node dysfunction, bradycardia, sinoatrial block, peripheral edema, hypotension, acute heart failure	T wave flattening
Hematological	Leukocytosis (elevated neutrophil and eosinophil counts)	Leukocytosis (elevated neutrophil and eosinophil counts)
Dermatological	Acute dermatitis	Psoriasis, dermatitis, edema
Ophthalmological	Nystagmus, blurred vision	Nystagmus, burning, tearing, exophthalmos, papilledema

6.3.1 Acute Lithium Toxicity

Lithium has a narrow therapeutic range, with a desirable range in serum lithium concentration of 0.5–1.2 mmol/L at steady-state levels. Since the half-life of lithium is about 24 h, steady-state levels should be obtained after 5 days of initiation of lithium or a change in dose. Any steady-state level above 1.2 mmol/L is defined as lithium toxicity, which manifests with a range of symptoms, the severity of which depends on the degree of lithium toxicity [3]. Often, even when toxic serum concentrations are reached, there is a latent effect with a delay of 1 or 2 days before symptoms of toxicity appear. Severe acute lithium toxicity is characterized by delirium, confusion, tremor, ataxia, dysarthria, renal insufficiency, and seizures. Table 6.2 summarizes the signs and symptoms of acute lithium toxicity as compared to chronic effects of lithium.

Clinical Pearl

- Symptoms of moderate to severe lithium toxicity often manifest 1–2 days after toxic serum concentrations are reached.

Recommendation
- Monitor closely for symptoms of mild lithium toxicity upon lithium initiation and dose increase.

Acute lithium toxicity can occur due to accidental or intentional intake of excessive amounts of lithium, drug-drug interactions that increase serum lithium concentration, or secondary to acute renal failure (e.g., with dehydration from decreased oral intake or from infections such as gastroenteritis with diarrhea and vomiting). Lithium in the form of a salt (commonly, lithium carbonate and lithium citrate [liquid]) is rapidly and completely absorbed after oral administration, is not metabolized, and is excreted unchanged by the kidneys [3]. As a result, any changes in renal function or lithium intake can result in lithium toxicity. Accidental increases in lithium concentration is often a result of drug-drug interactions with drugs that reduce lithium renal clearance, such as thiazides and ACE inhibitors, nonsteroidal anti-inflammatory drugs (NSAIDs) such as ibuprofen and naproxen, and other drugs that alter sodium balance (more discussion under nephrogenic diabetes insipidus and SIADH) (see Table 6.3).

Treatment of acute lithium toxicity should always begin with the basics of assessing and maintaining airway, breathing, and circulation (ABCs). With intentional or unintentional excessive intake of lithium, gastric decontamination is recommended with gastric lavage or whole bowel irrigation with a balanced electrolyte fluid such as polyethylene glycol, especially in the case of overdose of sustained-release formulation of lithium. Activated charcoal does not absorb lithium but may help by removing other possible substances that were ingested in overdose.

The goals of treatment of lithium toxicity is, firstly, to decrease serum lithium concentration to <1.0 mmol/L and, secondly, to correct fluid and electrolyte imbalance to prevent the potential neurologic sequelae of lithium toxicity [3]. In mild cases of lithium toxicity, discontinuation of lithium and rehydration with normal saline is usually sufficient to reverse the toxicity. More aggressive hydration may be needed in cases of moderate lithium toxicity to facilitate renal clearance of lithium, and finally, hemodialysis should be considered in severe lithium toxicity. Hemodialysis is recommended for toxic lithium levels of 4.0 mmol/L and above to facilitate removal of lithium from circulation but should also be considered at lower toxic

Table 6.3 Lithium drug-drug interactions

Drugs that increase lithium toxicity even at therapeutic doses	Amitriptyline
	Pancuronium
	Antipsychotics
	Succinylcholine
Drugs that reduce lithium renal clearance	Diuretics: thiazide diuretics
	K+ sparing diuretics (e.g., spironolactone)
	ACE inhibitors
	NSAIDs: ibuprofen, ketoprofen, naproxen
	Others: tetracycline, methyldopa, phenytoin, steroids

Table 6.4 Recommended management of lithium toxicity

	Serum concentration (mmol/L)	Recommended management[a]
Mild	1.2–1.5	Discontinue lithium, ABCs, rehydration with normal saline
Moderate	1.5–2.5	Discontinue lithium, ABCs, aggressive fluid resuscitation with normal saline
		Monitor lithium levels, electrolyte levels, renal function
		Correct electrolyte abnormalities
		Monitor cardiac function
Severe	> 2.5	Discontinue lithium, ABCs, aggressive fluid resuscitation with normal saline
		Monitor lithium levels, electrolyte levels, renal function
		Correct electrolyte abnormalities
		Monitor cardiac function
		Strongly consider hemodialysis

[a]Gastrointestinal decontamination should also be performed in the case of ingestion of excessive amounts of lithium. *ABC* airway, breathing, circulation

lithium levels in patients not responding to aggressive fluid hydration. A BUN/creatinine ratio of 20:1 indicates uremia (azotemia), and the patient is likely to respond to extensive fluid hydration. Patients exhibiting BUN/creatinine ratios of 10:1 are less likely to improve with intravascular hydration and will likely require hemodialysis. In addition to monitoring and correcting electrolyte levels and renal function, close monitoring of cardiac function with electrocardiograms or telemetry is necessary [4]. See Table 6.4 for a summary of recommended management of lithium toxicity.

6.3.2 Diabetes Insipidus

Nephrogenic diabetes insipidus (NDI) is a common side effect of lithium use, occurring in about 20% of adults aged 18–64 and 30% percent of adults aged 65 and above who have been treated with lithium for 5 or more years [5, 6]. NDI is defined as either having a urine volume of more than 3 L/24 h or decreased urine osmolality of less than 300 mOsm/kg. The symptoms of NDI include polydipsia, polyuria, and also nocturia, which then lead to secondary symptoms such as orthostatic hypotension/syncope, hypernatremia, lethargy, and irritability. Serum sodium in patients with normal thirst mechanisms is often in the high normal range, while hypernatremia can develop in those whose thirst is impaired or cannot be expressed (e.g., neurologically impaired adults who cannot independently access free water). NDI is characterized by the inability of renal cells to sense and respond to the stimulus of vasopressin, also known as antidiuretic hormone, whose function is to facilitate the reabsorption of excess water filtered in the urine.

The etiology of lithium-induced diabetes insipidus is multifactorial. (1) Lithium (even normal, non-toxic levels of lithium) competes with sodium for reuptake at the cortical collecting tubules, leading to natriuresis. With decreased sodium reabsorption, water reuptake from filtered urine is also compromised, leading to increased urination. (2) Lithium also more directly reduces the expression of sodium reuptake channels in the kidney by decreasing the activity and levels of the second messenger, cyclic AMP. (3) Lithium decreases the responsiveness of renal tubular cells to aldosterone, a hormone that is upregulated in response to low sodium levels and is responsible for upregulating the expression of renal epithelial sodium channels. (4) Lithium decreases the expression of Aquaporin 2, an epithelial water channel that functions to reabsorb excess water filtered in the urine in response to ADH signaling. Overall, these result in an inability of the kidney to concentrate urine, hence leading to increased urine volume (polyuria) and increased thirst and drinking to replace free water loss (polydipsia).

Older adult patients are more vulnerable to developing NDI in response to lithium therapy due to age-associated renal impairment and longer duration of treatment. They also report less urinary and thirst symptoms [6]. Nocturia is often the first reported symptom related to NDI as urine is normally most concentrated in the morning due to lack of fluid ingestion overnight and increased fluid intake throughout the day. Clinicians should increase their vigilance for decreased urine osmolality in older adults and in those with longer duration and higher doses of lithium therapy to decrease the risk of lithium intoxication, falls, and sequelae of hypernatremia.

Lithium-induced NDI can be treated using diuretics, with the caveat that lithium dosing may need to be adjusted (reduced) to take into the account the resulting plasma volume contraction occurring as a result of increased diuresis. A combination of hydrochlorothiazide and the potassium-sparing diuretic amiloride or monotherapy with acetazolamide have been shown to be effective in treating NDI. Close monitoring of lithium levels and slow titration is recommended in this case due to the increased risk of lithium toxicity with the use of diuretics. Although NSAIDs can also increase recovery of free water in renal tubules by inhibiting the action of prostaglandins that antagonize the action of ADH, long-term use of NSAIDs for this purpose is not recommended.

Clinical Pearl

- Older adult patients with nephrogenic diabetes insipidus (NDI) report less urinary and thirst symptoms compared to younger patients. Nocturia may be the first symptom of NDI reported by patients.

Recommendation

- Review urinary symptoms and fluid intake with patients on lithium therapy.

6.3.3 Syndrome of Irreversible Lithium-Effectuated Neurotoxicity (SILENT)

As previously discussed, lithium toxicity is associated with a variety of neurologic sequelae. While most of the effects of lithium toxicity are reversible with resolution of lithium toxicity to normal therapeutic levels, or cessation of lithium therapy altogether, long-term sequelae of lithium treatment and toxicity are being increasingly recognized. In 1987, the descriptive term of syndrome of irreversible lithium-effectuated neurotoxicity (SILENT) was proposed to describe long-term sequelae of lithium use/toxicity long after cessation of therapy [7]. Analyses of peer-reviewed publications revealed 90 cases of descriptive of SILENT in literature discussing the effects of lithium toxicity. SILENT was more prevalent in women (n = 49) compared to men (n = 35) and adults ranging from 21 to 77 years old with a mean age of 46 years. The average dose of lithium in SILENT cases was 1400 mg/day with average lithium level of 2.28 mmol/L.

Typical presentation of SILENT includes cerebellar dysfunction, extrapyramidal symptoms (EPS), brainstem dysfunction, and major neurocognitive disorder/dementia occurring persistently 2 months beyond cessation of lithium therapy. Atypical symptoms included but were not limited to blindness (from retrobulbar optic neuritis and central pontine myelinolysis), persistent motor and sensory peripheral neuropathy, myopathy, and choreoathetoid movements. SILENT occurred as a result of both lithium monotherapy and in combined therapy with antipsychotics (e.g., haloperidol, chlorpromazine), valproic acid, tricyclic antidepressants (e.g., amitriptyline), diuretics, aspirin, and beta-blockers. The longest case at the time demonstrated a persistence of neurologic sequelae up to 5 years after lithium discontinuation. With a variety of unpredictable and irreversible neurological symptoms and syndromes occurring, the authors proposed lithium-induced demyelination across multiple sites in the central nervous system, including the cerebellum and brainstem, was a putative cause of SILENT [7]. Another case report using MRI studies suggested that loss of gray matter in the cerebellum was also a feature of SILENT [8]. Given the irreversibility of the neurologic sequelae, patients should be managed based on their symptoms, e.g., physical therapy for ataxia, speech training for dysarthria, and cognitive training for symptoms of major neurocognitive disorder/dementia. Preventive measures such as lower lithium dosages and lithium level, as well as aggressive treatment of lithium toxicity, while avoiding rapid correction of lithium levels and abrupt lithium discontinuation, may decrease the risk of the development of SILENT.

Clinical Pearl

- Patients on lithium therapy are at risk for long-term neurological sequelae, even at usual doses of lithium and non-toxic lithium levels.

Recommendation

- Use the lowest effective dose for lithium therapy; avoid abrupt lithium discontinuation.

6.4 Antidepressants

Antidepressant use is considered generally safe with respect to renal function, although dosing adjustments have been recommended in the setting of chronic renal impairment (see Chap. 5). Acute kidney injury can occur with overdose of antidepressants. Although no direct renotoxic effect is known, antidepressant use is associated with the development of chronic kidney disease in older adults. Older adults treated with selective serotonin reuptake inhibitors (SSRIs) and serotonin-norepinephrine reuptake inhibitors (SNRIs) have a relative risk of about 2.5 for developing chronic kidney disease compared to those not taking antidepressants [9]. A greater effect is seen with hyponatremia where older adults taking antidepressants have a relative risk of 4–5 times of being hospitalized with hyponatremia compared to non-users of antidepressants. The incidence of hyponatremia ranges widely from 1% to 40% of SSRI users and up to 70% for venlafaxine users [9]. Hyponatremia (defined as sodium concentration of <135 mmol/L) normally occurs within 30 days of antidepressant initiation and is usually corrected within days to weeks after cessation of the drug. Risk factors for developing hyponatremia include older age, female sex, low body weight (< 60 kg), previous history of hyponatremia, and concomitant use of other medications known to induce hyponatremia [9].

6.4.1 Syndrome of Inappropriate Antidiuretic Hormone Secretion (SIADH)

The hyponatremia seen with SSRI use is associated with SIADH, as serotonin is implicated in the regulation of ADH release. SSRIs and other psychiatric medications (see Table 6.5) appear to enhance ADH secretion or impair the suppression of ADH release, leading to impaired water excretion. SIADH is associated with euvolemic hyponatremia, decreased serum osmolality (< 275 mOsm/kg), increased urine osmolality (> 100 mOsm/kg), and urinary sodium (> 40 mEq/L), normal potassium concentration, without acid-base disturbance. With drug-induced SIADH, patients are euvolemic and have otherwise normal renal, adrenal, and thyroid functions. The clinical presentation of SIADH ranges from asymptomatic to mild with nonspecific symptoms such as fatigue, to acute and severe symptoms such as delirium and seizures if there is an acute change in sodium level and plasma osmolality. SIADH can occur with even low doses of antidepressants, occurring early after initiation of therapy. Monitoring for changes in sodium concentration

Table 6.5 Psychiatric medications that can induce SIADH

Antidepressants	SSRIs (e.g., fluoxetine, paroxetine, sertraline, citalopram, escitalopram)
	SNRIs (e.g., venlafaxine)
	TCAs (e.g., amitriptyline)
Antipsychotics	Haloperidol
Mood stabilizers	Carbamazepine
	Oxcarbazepine
	Valproic acid

with a basic metabolic panel is suggested at baseline, 2 and 4 weeks after initiation and then every 3 months to help detect SIADH especially in groups at higher risk to develop hyponatremia [9]. Drug-drug pharmacodynamic interactions can increase the risk or exacerbate SIADH, e.g., with co-administration with NSAIDs (secondary to inhibition of prostaglandins and potentiation of ADH effect on the tubules), proton pump inhibitors, ACE inhibitors, some antipsychotics and mood stabilizers (see Table 6.5), and morphine. Given the reversibility of drug-induced SIADH with discontinuation of the precipitating drug, alternative medications should be considered in those who develop a SIADH as a result of antidepressant treatment. A small study in older adults suggested that older patients treated with lithium and an antidepressant were less likely to develop hypernatremia associated with NDI (OR 0.14) possibly attributable to the SIADH effects of antidepressants [10].

Clinical Pearl

- Drug-induced SIADH usually occurs within 30 days of drug initiation, and older adults, women, and lower weight individuals are at higher risk for SIADH.

Recommendation

- Monitor for changes in sodium levels with a basic metabolic panel at baseline, 2 and 4 weeks after initiation of therapy and every 3 months for those at higher risk of developing SIADH.
- Screen for drug-drug interactions with other medications that can cause SIADH at follow-up visits.
- Consider alternative antidepressant therapy if the patient develops SIADH.

6.5 Antipsychotics

In a recent Danish population-based case-control study, the use of second-generation antipsychotics was associated with a small increased risk of developing CKD in both current and past users (OR 1.25) [11]. All antipsychotics with both low and high risk of inducing metabolic syndrome (except aripiprazole, which was not evaluated) were implicated in the increased risk for CKD. Among second-generation antipsychotics, clozapine had the highest risk for inducing CKD with an OR of 1.8. The etiology of antipsychotic induced CKD is wide ranging, including interstitial nephritis (from clozapine, olanzapine, quetiapine), but is less well characterized for other antipsychotics. Use of second-generation antipsychotics in adults aged 65 years or younger is also associated with hospitalization for acute kidney injury (RR 1.7) possibly due to hypotension and decreased renal perfusion and/or post-renal syndrome due to urinary retention from anticholinergic effects of the medications. Antipsychotics can also indirectly cause acute kidney injury as an indirect effect of neuroleptic malignant syndrome due to the overwhelming of glomeruli with creatinine kinase released from muscle cells and CKD through the development of diabetic nephropathy as a result of metabolic syndrome and diabetes mellitus. Some antipsychotics can also cause SIADH (Table 6.5) and NDI (olanzapine).

Clinical Pearl

- Antipsychotics are associated with the development of AKI and CKD.

Recommendation

- Monitor renal function in patients treated with antipsychotics and adjust dosages according to guidelines.

6.6 Other Psychotropic Drugs

Although rare, case reports of acute kidney injury with other psychotropic drugs have been reported. Lamotrigine is associated with acute interstitial nephritis [12]. Haloperidol, valproic acid, carbamazepine, and oxcarbazepine are associated with SIADH, and olanzapine is associated with NDI [13, 14]. Valproic acid and carbamazepine can also cause subclinical renal glomerular and tubular dysfunctions [15]. Topiramate is associated with renal stones. To date there is no known association between benzodiazepines, non-benzodiazepines, and cognitive enhancers with acute kidney injury and chronic kidney disease.

6.7 Case Vignette Analysis

The patient described previously in the case scenario presented with classic signs and symptoms of lithium toxicity. Due to upper respiratory infection which is associated with fever-related fluid loss, reduced oral fluid intake, and administration of NSAIDS, all of which lead to reduced GFR and therefore lithium toxicity. This patient's lithium should have been reduced or held as she developed tremor, dysmetria, ataxia, and confusion. This patient presented with moderate to severe lithium toxicity. In the case, treatment should be initiated with aggressive volume resuscitation with intravenous fluids. If symptoms do not improve and lithium level does not lower in the next 24 h, hemodialysis may be indicated.

6.8 Key Takeaways

- Lithium use is associated with a decline in GFR and development of chronic kidney disease.
- Lithium dose and higher than median lithium levels, rather than length of time on lithium therapy, increases the risk of lithium-induced renal impairment.

- Lithium therapy requires regular monitoring of lithium level, renal and thyroid function, and cardiac function for patients above the age of 40.
- Symptoms of lithium toxicity often manifest 1–2 days after toxic serum concentrations are reached.
- Avoid other nephrotoxic drugs in patients treated with lithium (e.g., NSAIDs, ACE inhibitors).
- Lithium therapy can lead to nephrogenic diabetes insipidus (NDI). Older patients are more vulnerable to developing NDI. The most common and earliest symptom reported is nocturia.
- Lithium toxicity can lead to syndrome of irreversible lithium-effectuated neurotoxicity (SILENT), and retrial of lithium should be avoided in these patients.
- SSRI and SNRI use is associated with syndrome of inappropriate antidiuretic hormone secretion (SIADH). Monitor sodium levels at baseline, upon starting therapy, and periodically in patients taking antidepressants.
- Use of antipsychotics is associated with the development of CKD. Clozapine carries the highest risk of causing CKD.

References

1. McKnight RF, Adida M, Budge K, Stockton S, Goodwin GM, Geddes JR. Lithium toxicity profile: a systematic review and meta-analysis. Lancet. 2012;379(9817):721–8.
2. Shine B, McKnight RF, Leaver L, Geddes JR. Long-term effects of lithium on renal, thyroid, and parathyroid function: a retrospective analysis of laboratory data. Lancet. 2015;386(9992):461–8.
3. Oruch R, Elderbi MA, Khattab HA, Pryme IF, Lund A. Lithium: a review of pharmacology, clinical uses, and toxicity. Eur J Pharmacol. 2014;740:464–73.
4. Brahm NC. Lithium-induced bradycardia: a rare but serious adverse effect. Curr Psychiatr Ther. 2017;16(11):41–3.
5. Behl T, Kotwani A, Kaur I, Goel H. Mechanisms of prolonged lithium therapy-induced nephrogenic diabetes insipidus. Eur J Pharmacol. 2015;755:27–33.
6. Rej S, Segal M, Low NC, Mucsi I, Holcroft C, Shulman K, Looper K. The McGill geriatric lithium-induced diabetes insipidus clinical study (McGLIDICS). Can J Psychiatry. 2014;59(6):327–34.
7. Munshi KR, Thampy A. The syndrome of irreversible lithium-effectuated neurotoxicity. Clin Neuropharmacol. 2005;28(1):38–49.
8. Ikeda Y, Kameyama M, Amanuma M, Narita K, Takei Y. Total and regional brain volume reductions due to the Syndrome of Irreversible Lithium-Effectuated Neurotoxicity (SILENT): a voxel-based morphometric study. Prog Neuro-Psychopharmacol Biol Psychiatry. 2010;34(1):244–6.
9. Farmand S, Lindh JD, Calissendorff J, Skov J, Falhammar H, Nathanson D, Mannheimer B. Differences in associations of antidepressants and hospitalization due to hyponatremia. Am J Med. 2018;131(1):56–63.
10. Rej S, Looper K, Segal M. Do antidepressants lower the prevalence of lithium-associated hypernatremia in the elderly? A retrospective study. Can Geriatr J. 2013;16(2):38.
11. Højlund M, Lund LC, Herping JL, Haastrup MB, Damkier P, Henriksen DP. Second-generation antipsychotics and the risk of chronic kidney disease: a population-based case-control study. BMJ Open. 2020;10(8):e038247.
12. Matta A, Assalie NA, Gupta RK, Morales MD, Conti R. A rare case of lamotrigine-induced acute interstitial nephritis. J Community Hosp Intern Med Perspect. 2016;6(6):32976.

13. Hwang YJ, Dixon SN, Reiss JP, Wald R, Parikh CR, Gandhi S, Shariff SZ, Pannu N, Nash DM, Rehman F, Garg AX. Atypical antipsychotic drugs and the risk for acute kidney injury and other adverse outcomes in older adults: a population-based cohort study. Ann Intern Med. 2014;161(4):242–8.
14. Koçer E, Alçelik A, Canan F. Olanzapine intoxication-related transient diabetes insipidus. Ren Fail. 2011;33(8):842–3.
15. Hamed SA, Rageh TA, Mohamad AO, Abou Elnour SM. Renal dysfunctions/injury in adult epilepsy patients treated with carbamazepine or valproate. Expert Rev Clin Pharmacol. 2018;11(8):819–24.

Overview of Psychotherapy Principles for Patients with Kidney Disease

7

Tyler G. Tulloch, Jelena P. King, Joseph R. Pellizzari, and Heather E. McNeely

7.1 Introduction

This chapter will provide a general overview of issues to consider when providing psychotherapy to patients with chronic kidney disease (CKD) and is not intended as an instruction manual for learning how to provide psychotherapy more generally. It will be most helpful for mental health professionals of various disciplines already versed in psychotherapy who may be less familiar with treating kidney disease patients, or for anyone looking to learn how general principles of psychotherapy can be applied to this specific population. This chapter will briefly review psychological disorders commonly experienced by kidney disease patients, which are discussed in more detail in Chap. 2. It will describe the biopsychosocial model, a helpful framework for conceptualizing problems experienced by kidney disease patients. The

T. G. Tulloch (✉)
Kidney Urinary Program, St. Joseph's Healthcare Hamilton, Department of Psychiatry and Behavioural Neurosciences, McMaster University, Hamilton, ON, Canada
e-mail: ttulloch@stjoes.ca

J. P. King
Department of Psychiatry & Behavioural Neurosciences, St. Joseph's Healthcare Hamilton, Clinical Neuropsychology Services, Hamilton, ON, Canada
e-mail: kingj@stjosham.on.ca

H. E. McNeely
Department of Psychiatry and Behavioural Neurosciences, McMaster University, St. Joseph's Healthcare Hamilton, Clinical Neuropsychology Services, Hamilton, ON, Canada
e-mail: hmcneely@stjoes.ca

J. R. Pellizzari
St. Joseph's Healthcare Hamilton, McMaster University, Hamilton, ON, Canada
e-mail: jpellizz@stjosham.on.ca

A. Hategan et al. (eds.), *Psychonephrology*,
https://doi.org/10.1007/978-3-030-84740-1_7

cognitive behavioral model will be introduced and evidence for cognitive behavioral psychotherapy reviewed. Finally, issues specific to patients with CKD will be described, along with potential barriers in providing psychotherapy and some suggestions on how to overcome them.

7.1.1 What Is Psychotherapy?

Psychotherapy, in its most broad definition, refers to the treatment of a psychiatric disorder or condition through psychological rather than somatic means. In more recent years, efforts have been made to regulate the term and practice of psychotherapy, resulting in more precise definitions of the term, which may vary by jurisdiction. Within the Canadian province of Ontario, where the authors of this chapter practice, the controlled act of psychotherapy has been legally defined as treating "by means of psychotherapy technique, delivered through a therapeutic relationship, an individual's serious disorder of thought, cognition, mood, emotional regulation, perception or memory that may seriously impair the individual's judgment, insight, behavior, communication or social functioning" [1]. Depending on the jurisdiction, laws may regulate who is authorized to provide psychotherapy and/or identify themselves as psychotherapists, which may include psychologists, psychiatrists or other physicians, physician assistants, nurses, social workers, occupational therapists, or registered psychotherapists not belonging to any of these disciplines. In this chapter, the term *psychotherapist* will be used to refer generically to the mental health clinician providing psychotherapy.

7.2 Relevance of Psychotherapy for Renal Patients

CKD is both chronic and progressive, and patients often face an uncertain future, not knowing when the disease will progress to the next stage or what symptoms they will experience along the way. Nephrologists and other multidisciplinary care team members provide recommendations for slowing the progression of kidney disease, summarized in Table 7.1 [2], but it is up to patients to follow these recommendations. Adhering to all of these recommendations may be challenging, and poor adherence may result in more rapid progression of CKD.

Even with excellent adherence to all recommendations, unforeseen circumstances or illness (including comorbid illness) may precipitate more rapid progression of CKD. Patients must cope not only with the uncertain future that awaits them but also with the stress and responsibility of managing their health day-to-day. Furthermore, patients must cope with new and worsening symptoms of uremia and comorbid health conditions that arise as CKD progresses toward end-stage kidney disease (ESKD). They must make life-changing health-related decisions about what they will do once their kidneys fail, with each option requiring varying degrees of advance planning and accompanied by phase-specific challenges. These are summarized in Table 7.2.

Table 7.1 Strategies for slowing the progression of CKD [2]

Type of intervention	Treatment targets
Medical management	Control blood pressure
	Reduce albuminuria
	Control blood glucose
Nutritional interventions	Limit sodium intake
	Limit phosphorous and potassium as clinically indicated
	Adequate, but not excessive, protein intake
	Adequate caloric intake
Lifestyle interventions	Smoking cessation
	Physical activity:
	20–30 min daily
	Aerobic *and* strength training

Table 7.2 End-stage kidney disease and treatment options

Goal	Treatment options/ settings	Patient challenges
Renal replacement therapy	Hemodialysis	Fistula surgery
	In facility	Body image concerns (fistula)
	At home	Cannulation
		Fluid/dietary restrictions
		3–6 months' advance notice for fistula creation
	Peritoneal dialysis (PD)	PD catheter insertion
	Continuous ambulatory (CAPD)	Body image concerns (PD catheter)
	Automated (APD)	No swimming/bathing (PD catheter immersion)
		Fluid/dietary restrictions
		Upper BMI limit
		Risk of peritonitis
Kidney transplant	Living donor transplant	Lifetime immunosuppressant medication:
	Deceased donor transplant	Strict adherence
		Side effects
		Finding eligible donor (living donor)
		Waitlist wait time (deceased donor)
Conservative management	Hospice	End of life preparation:
	Home	Psychological
	Hospital	Spiritual
		Social (loved ones)
		Medical (palliative care)
		Financial
		Choosing where to spend final days

The life of a CKD patient is fraught with uncertainty and any number of physical, emotional, and social challenges as symptoms worsen and new treatments are started [3]. This presents an opportunity for growth, and while some patients are able to cope with these challenges, others are overwhelmed and struggle to continue living life the way they would like. Patients may be reluctant to pursue pharmacological treatment for psychological distress due to an already high pill burden for managing CKD or concerns of drug-drug interactions with psychotropic medication. Many kidney patients may never have considered seeking treatment for comorbid psychiatric symptoms or conditions and may be unaware of the benefits of psychotherapy, especially in the absence of a diagnosed psychiatric disorder. Kidney disease treatment programs that can provide access to mental health services should consider normalizing this process early on in the CKD journey by incorporating discussions about mental health and provide consultation with mental health specialists into routine multidisciplinary care. As discussed in Chap. 2, it is recommended to routinely screen for mental health problems such as depressive disorder that may significantly interfere with treatment adherence and progression of CKD. Patients who score above established cutoffs on standardized and validated psychiatric symptom measures may benefit from further assessment and clinical interventions, including psychotherapy to learn effective coping strategies and reduce symptoms/distress.

7.2.1 Common Presenting Concerns

As mentioned above, CKD is a *process,* rather than a single discrete event, and patients may have very different needs at different points along the way. For example, stage 3–4 CKD patients may struggle to adhere to treatment recommendations to slow disease progression; have difficulty adjusting to the idea of a future living with progressive, chronic illness; and/or find health-related decision-making challenging. Stage 5 CKD patients may experience further decline in quality of life and/or impairment in activities of daily living as uremic symptoms become more burdensome. Patients on dialysis may not be able to sufficiently adhere to dietary or fluid restrictions, experience changes in important relationships, and/or find treatments difficult to tolerate. Furthermore, patients at any stage of this journey may experience clinically significant distress or impairment with symptoms that meet diagnostic criteria for a comorbid psychiatric disorder.

Literature on the prevalence and impact of psychiatric disorders in renal patients is reviewed elsewhere in this book. To summarize briefly, the prevalence of depressive disorders is estimated at 22.8% in dialysis patients when measured via clinician-administered interview and 39.3% when assessed via questionnaire [4]. The presence of depressive disorders in renal patients is particularly concerning, given that it is associated with more frequent hospital admissions, longer hospital stays, greater likelihood of withdrawing from dialysis, and greater risk of morbidity and mortality [5]. There is evidence that patients are at significantly increased risk of suicide during their first 3 months after initiating dialysis [6]; therefore, careful monitoring of patients during this critical period is wise. Dialysis patients should be made aware of mental health supports available to them, whether within the dialysis service or elsewhere in the institution or community.

Anxiety is also highly prevalent in kidney disease, with 43% of patients experiencing elevated anxiety and 19% diagnosed with at least one anxiety disorder. It is associated with poorer quality of life, adherence to treatment recommendations, and risk of mortality and progression to ESKD [7]. Furthermore, specific anxiety disorders such as blood-injection-injury (specific) phobia or agoraphobia may cause significant distress and care interference in patients who require hemodialysis and/or dialyze in center with other patients. Sleep disorders, including obstructive sleep apnea and insomnia, are also highly prevalent in kidney disease patients, with estimates ranging from 70% to 80% for sleep apnea and 50% to 75% for insomnia. Screening tips for the above disorders are reviewed in Chap. 2.

Kidney disease patients may well benefit from psychotherapy for any number of concerns, across many different time points on the CKD journey. They need not meet diagnostic criteria for a comorbid psychiatric disorder to benefit substantially from psychotherapy. Rather, one should consider the impact of unhelpful thoughts, emotions, or behaviors on a patient's psychological and physical well-being, including their ability to successfully manage the progression of their illness and make treatment related decisions.

7.2.2 Case Vignette: "One Thing After Another"

Mr. Hastings was a 63-year-old male with multiple health problems, including chronic kidney disease, type 2 diabetes mellitus, hypertension, and obesity. He and his wife had two adult sons and several grandchildren who live a 6-h drive away. He and his wife had had plans to move closer to one of their sons in a few years once he retired to spend more time with their grandchildren. A few years previously he had received education from a nurse educator on renal replacement therapy options and decided to try for a preemptive living donor kidney transplant so that he could avoid having to start dialysis. His two sons completed the pretransplant screening and work-up at their local hospitals, and to everyone's delight, one of them was found to be an ideal donor match. Later however, Mr. Hastings' own transplant nephrologist had expressed concern over his high body mass index (BMI) as well as his very poor adherence to monitoring blood sugars and following a renal diet. As a result, he was told that for the transplant to proceed, he would still need to lose around 20 kg (44 lbs) and improve his diabetic management.

Since then, he had had increasing difficulty managing his blood glucose and has made several trips to the local emergency department due to dangerously high blood glucose levels. Despite ongoing follow-up with his multidisciplinary team consisting of his nephrologist, diabetes nurse educator, dietitian, and others, he had been unable to follow all of their recommendations, which consisted of checking his blood glucose several times daily, managing his insulin doses, following a renal diet and diabetic diet, and taking several blood pressure medications. His estimated glomerular filtration rate (eGFR) dropped from 28 to 15 mL/min/1.73 m^2 over the previous year, and he started to experience some uremic symptoms such as lower limb edema, shortness of breath, and confusion. He had also noticed worsening peripheral neuropathy in his feet, which made it harder for him to get around.

One month previously, at his follow-up in the multidisciplinary kidney care clinic, he met with his team of care providers, who "dropped a bombshell," as he would later put it, that, due to several risk factors that have not been adequately managed (e.g., BMI, poor adherence to blood sugar management), he had run out of time for a preemptive transplant and would need to decide what type of dialysis to start on, likely within the next year. Since then, he had become increasingly discouraged with his numerous failed attempts to manage his health. He wondered if he will ever get to the point where he is eligible for transplant and if there is any point in starting dialysis at all if he is going to spend his future "tied to a machine."

7.3 Biopsychosocial Model

The biopsychosocial model of health sets the stage for the role of psychotherapy in renal patients with its proposed dynamic interplay among biological, psychological, and interpersonal factors [8]. Further elaborations of these relationships can also be found in cognitive behavioral formulations with inter-related domains of cognition, emotion, behavior, and physical sensations. Psychotherapy is fundamentally interpersonal, regardless of the modality. It offers a rich opportunity for learning coping strategies and enhancements to adjustment to many difficult aspects of the renal disease course. It also offers a professional mechanism for social support ("someone to talk to") and self-disclosure around one's medical narrative. Emotional expression and the provision of validation and empathy in an interpersonal context is a potent combination for one struggling with renal disease. All kidney disease patients who present with distress across the continuum from mild to moderate levels to diagnosable comorbid mental health conditions could potentially benefit.

7.3.1 Multidisciplinary Care

The multidisciplinary care model that includes nephrologists, other physicians, nurse specialists, dietitians, social workers, and pharmacists is common in CKD care and is associated with lower risk of all-cause mortality, slower decline in eGFR, lower hospitalization rates, and fewer temporary catheterizations for dialysis patients [9]. In a meta-analysis of 21 research studies that reported using multidisciplinary care teams including at the very least nephrologists and nurses, 67% of teams included a dietitian, 52% included a social worker, and 33% included a pharmacist [9]. A study in the United Kingdom, where mental health services are provided free of charge as part of the National Health Service, psychosocial services in nephrology settings are provided by social workers (36%), psychologists (34%), counselors/psychotherapists (16%), and youth workers (5%) [10]. Given the reciprocal relationship between physical and mental health, psychotherapists working with CKD patients are advised to integrate with the patient's multidisciplinary team rather than work separately in a "silo." In this way, the patient's care team can function efficiently to more quickly identify issues that may impact disease progression and management.

7.3.2 Patient Confidentiality in Multidisciplinary Care

One important issue to consider in working within a multidisciplinary care team is that of confidentiality and informed consent. While regulations may vary by jurisdiction, psychotherapists should typically discuss issues of confidentiality as early as possible in the therapeutic relationship and to obtain informed consent prior to commencing treatment. This involves, among other things, informing patients who will have access to information that they disclose to the psychotherapist, how that information could be used, and when confidentiality must be broken in accordance with the law to ensure safety of the patient and others. The psychotherapist working on a multidisciplinary team must ensure that patients are aware that other team members will have access to information discussed in psychotherapy, given their role in the patient's circle of care. Patients may be less willing to divulge information to a psychotherapist knowing that a full team of care providers may be privy to that information. A psychotherapist working in this setting, therefore, should be prepared to discuss the advantages and disadvantages of participating in psychotherapy with a member of the multidisciplinary team versus referring out to someone in private practice, where confidentiality regulations and practices may be different.

As part of the informed consent process, psychotherapists should also set patient expectations regarding length and frequency of therapy sessions, duration of therapy, and psychotherapeutic techniques likely to be used. While psychotherapists may be trained in any number of theoretical orientations, they should strive to implement evidence-based treatment with empirical support for CKD patients when working with this population. Cognitive behavioral therapy (CBT), an evidence-based treatment for several psychological disorders will be described next, along with preliminary data on its efficacy with CKD patients.

Clinical Pearl

- Some patients will be relieved that their psychotherapist is in regular communication with their other care providers, while others may be uncomfortable with this idea. Discussing this at treatment outset will help to foster a trusting relationship and build therapeutic rapport.

Recommendation

- Ensure that patients understand who else on their multidisciplinary care team will have access to information discussed in psychotherapy and documented in the medical record.

7.3.3 Case Vignette: "One Thing After Another" (Continued)

Mr. Hastings was referred to the nurse educator to review his dialysis options, and after the visit, he was referred to meet with a health psychologist, a recommendation which he found odd. After hearing more about the health psychologist's role on the team, he decided he would like to set up a meeting to see if she could help with some of his challenges managing his health. He was not sure if he wanted his nephrologist and everyone else to know he would be seeing a psychologist, but after discussing the pros and cons, he decided it might make a good impression on his other health-care providers if they saw that he was taking steps to manage things better.

7.4 Cognitive Behavioral Therapy

Cognitive behavioral therapy (CBT), developed by Beck [11] and Ellis [12], is based on the premise that maladaptive cognitions contribute to the maintenance of emotional distress and psychiatric disorders. In CBT, maladaptive cognitions include core beliefs or schemas that individuals hold about the world, the self, and the future which are often manifested as automatic thoughts in particular situations. Within CBT intervention, therapeutic strategies are aimed at changing or balancing these maladaptive cognitions to reduce emotional distress, modify self-defeating behaviors, and increase overall functioning.

CBT is considered to be the gold standard for psychotherapeutic treatment in most clinical contexts [13]. CBT has been the most researched form of psychotherapy and is systematically superior to other models of psychotherapy treatment, and in those cases where systematic differences among psychotherapy models have been identified, they typically favor CBT. Several comprehensive and contemporary reviews of meta-analytic studies have revealed that CBT has been implemented across a wide range of psychiatric conditions [14, 15]. In general, the greatest effect sizes and strongest support for the efficacy of CBT are in anxiety disorders, somatic symptom and related disorders (formerly somatoform disorders), bulimia nervosa, anger control problems, and managing general stress [14]. While studies examining the efficacy of CBT as a sole intervention in depressive disorders have been mixed, CBT in combination with psychotropic medication has been shown to be superior to either alone and has been shown to reduce relapse/recurrence rates [14, 16].

7.4.1 Efficacy of CBT with Kidney Patients

Several studies have examined the efficacy of CBT in kidney patients, with the majority focusing on treatment of depression, anxiety, and insomnia symptoms in hemodialysis patients. Othman et al. summarized these studies in a systematic review and found that in all but one study, CBT was more effective than control conditions at reducing depression and anxiety symptom severity and improving sleep quality and quality of life [17]. The duration of these CBT interventions ranged from 5 weeks to 12 weeks, and one intervention was provided chairside during hemodialysis [18–20]. One intervention was provided in group rather than individual format [20]. Control groups included sleep hygiene education (for patients with insomnia), hemodialysis treatment as usual, and non-direct counseling [21]. Benefits of CBT were maintained during follow-up periods of up to 9 months. A one-arm feasibility study demonstrated that Internet-administered CBT was effective at reducing depressive symptoms in hemodialysis patients [22]. A meta-analysis by Ng et al. further supported the efficacy of CBT in improving symptoms of depression, anxiety, and quality of life in hemodialysis patients [23].

7.4.2 CBT Techniques

CBT refers to a variety of interventions that utilize and combine cognitive, behavioral, and emotion-focused techniques. As emotions are often difficult to change directly, CBT targets emotions by helping individuals increase their awareness of and work on changing thoughts and behaviors that are contributing to distressing emotions such as anxiety, depression, or fear. Figure 7.1 illustrates how the relationship between thoughts, behaviors, emotions, and physical reactions is conceptualized in CBT. Some of the core interventions are briefly reviewed below.

Cognitive Restructuring Sometimes also referred to as cognitive reappraisal, this strategy teaches individuals to recognize dysfunctional thought patterns and develop more rational, balanced, and grounded ways of understanding challenging situations. Cognitive restructuring involves additional approaches to increase awareness of thoughts and improve thinking, which can include tracking thoughts during difficult situations, using thought records to challenge and reappraise unhelpful thinking patterns, identifying cognitive distortions, and engaging in behavioral experiments to test out the accuracy of thinking or likelihood of feared outcome(s).

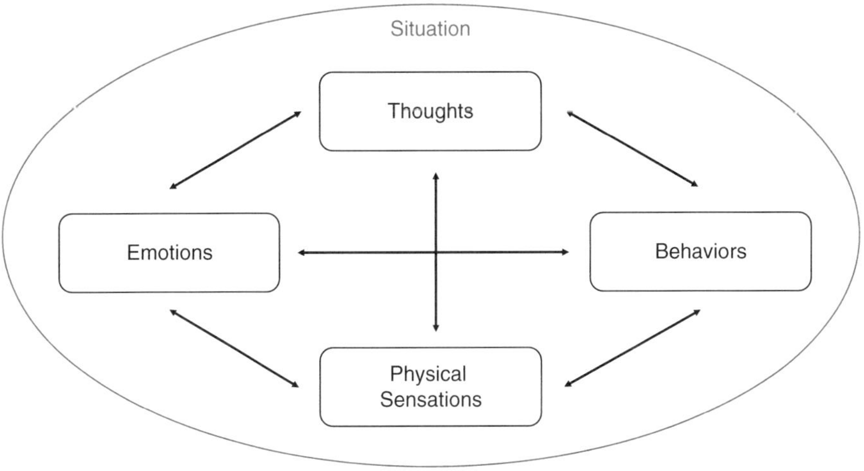

Fig. 7.1 The cognitive behavioral model

Behavioral Activation Within the CBT model, psychological symptoms such as depression and anxiety are often maintained and reinforced through avoidance behaviors and withdrawal from adaptive coping activities. Behavioral activation includes increasing activity and access to reinforcing, pleasurable activities which ultimately improves functioning by decreasing avoidance behavior that was maintaining symptoms, and improving self-confidence/self-efficacy and contributing to a greater sense of purpose.

Exposure According to the cognitive model, fear of objects, activities, or situations is maintained through avoidance behavior. Exposure intervention involves exposing individuals to what is feared, often in a graded manner to break the pattern of avoidance and fear. Within a graded exposure approach, individuals are exposed to their fears in a hierarchical manner, from least to most feared, which facilitates gradual extinction that is less distressing than initial exposure to the most feared item in the hierarchy (which is the flooding approach to exposure).

Problem-Solving Collaborative problem-solving is a core component of CBT that helps individuals create realistic and achievable adaptive coping strategies for a wide range of problems including depression, anxiety, anger, stress management, and coping with medical illness. A structured approach to problem-solving is implemented and can comprise analyzing a problem, identifying options for coping, evaluating the options, deciding upon a plan, and developing strategies for implementing the plan. These problem-solving techniques help individuals learn skills which increase their self-efficacy/sense of control and decrease hopelessness and despair so that life issues that previously felt overwhelming are now manageable.

Relaxation Relaxation techniques are incorporated in CBT to help individuals manage distressing emotions that often arise during active CBT treatment, which in and of itself can be conceptualized as a form of exposure where individuals start confronting their issues. Relaxation techniques include muscle relaxation, deep breathing, or imagery that can be selected based on presenting difficulties and individual preferences. Implementing and teaching relaxation skills can go a long way toward increasing positive treatment expectations and building therapeutic rapport. Helping individuals learn relaxation skills can be conveyed as a method of increasing control that does not necessitate a direct discussion of mental health difficulties, which can be important for those individuals who are concerned about mental health stigma. Because relaxation techniques are generally easy to teach and learn, it is advantageous to teach these techniques early in treatment to give patients an easy-to- learn, yet highly effective, skill set.

7.4.3 Considerations in Evaluating CBT Suitability

Predicting who will benefit from CBT is an important consideration with respect to optimizing treatment outcome and treatment efficacy. Safran et al. have specified ten criteria of suitability that can assist with this determination, published as part of their Suitability for Short-Term Cognitive Therapy Rating Scales [24]. This scale is published with a manual to guide interviewers in probing for the information

Table 7.3 Suitability for short-term cognitive therapy rating scales – criteria to determine CBT suitability [25]

Criteria	Considerations
Accessibility of automatic thoughts	The ability to be aware of and identify automatic thoughts in situations is necessary for restructuring, challenging, and reappraising unhelpful thinking patterns and identifying cognitive distortions
Awareness and differentiation of emotions	The capacity to identify and label different emotions in the past and present is important in CBT despite its cognitive focus. Identifying emotional states as it relates to thoughts and behaviors is a core component of CBT
Acceptance of personal responsibility for change	The ability of individuals to recognize their role in contributing to their personal situations and in their recovery will increase their ability to make effective changes in CBT and work toward their goals
Compatibility with cognitive rationale	The extent that individuals can understand and appreciate the CBT model/therapeutic approach will ultimately impact their facility in making links between thoughts, emotions, and behaviors
Alliance potential (in-session evidence)	The in-session quality of individuals' interaction with the therapist can provide information regarding their ability to form a therapeutic alliance. Stronger therapeutic alliance predicts increased CBT efficacy
Alliance potential (out-of-session evidence)	The patient's history of past meaningful relationships, including previous psychotherapies, can indicate the potential quality of the therapeutic alliance that can be established in CBT
Chronicity of presenting issues	The extent and severity of the patient's presenting issues/symptoms is important to establish as those individuals with unfocused, multiple, or very chronic problems, including those with severe personality disorder, are unlikely to benefit from CBT
Security operations	The extent to which individuals block exploration of anxiety-provoking content with defenses such as intellectualization or avoidance can limit the benefit of CBT
Focality	Those individuals who have greater capacity to remain focused and persistent working on problems/goals will likely be more successful in completing homework and more actively engaged in their CBT treatment
General optimism/ pessimism regarding therapy	The extent that individuals feel they will benefit (or not) from CBT treatment can affect their motivation and engagement for treatment. Those more pessimistic regarding therapy will benefit less from CBT and may be more likely drop out of treatment

required to make these ratings. These are summarized in Table 7.3 with some considerations provided for each criterion to assist clinicians in establishing whether a patient might be suitable for CBT.

Recommendation

– Individuals with substance use disorder comorbidity would likely benefit from targeted substance use disorder treatment prior to initiating CBT. Individuals with a personality disorder diagnosis are less likely to benefit from short-term CBT and might be more suitable for other psychotherapy treatments such as dialectical behavior therapy (DBT) or psychodynamic psychotherapy. Individuals with long-standing interpersonal issues will often require longer CBT treatment durations.

7.5 Applying CBT with Renal Patients

This section will provide some tips on applying CBT with kidney patients; however, it is not an exhaustive guide. A highly recommended resource for anyone looking to increase competency in providing CBT to individuals with chronic illness is *CBT for Chronic Illness and Palliative Care: A Workbook and Toolkit* [25].

7.5.1 Self-Learning

While some CKD patients may seek psychotherapy for long-standing symptoms of a psychological disorder such as depression or insomnia, others may seek therapy for assistance with more CKD-specific concerns, such as adjusting to changes in their health, managing symptoms, or coping with new or existing treatments. For this reason, psychotherapists working with CKD patients should seek to educate themselves about CKD including causes, symptoms, and treatment options, including hemodialysis (at home and in center), peritoneal dialysis (automated and continuous ambulatory), kidney transplant (living and deceased donor), and conservative renal care (palliative care). It is also helpful to have a basic understanding of common comorbid medical conditions including diabetes mellitus, cardiovascular disease, and complications of CKD and poorly managed diabetes mellitus, such as peripheral neuropathy, retinopathy, and hypo- and hyperglycemia. If you are a non-medically trained psychotherapist reading this textbook, you are well on your way to accomplishing this important task of learning more about CKD and the patient experience. Other sources of education include shadowing multidisciplinary team members during outpatient clinics or education/training sessions or accessing reliable online resources.

Clinical Pearl

- Colleagues are a valuable resource. Establish warm, professional relationships with multidisciplinary colleagues to foster a symbiotic relationship that benefits everyone, including shared patients.

7.5.2 Goal Setting

Fundamental to CBT, or any type of psychotherapy, is a shared understanding of what the patient and therapist are working toward or the goal of psychotherapy. This should be identified in *collaboration* with the patient, rather than be *imposed on* the patient by the psychotherapist. That is not to say that the goal cannot change over time as priorities or circumstances change, but it is important that the psychotherapist and patient have a clear and mutual sense of what they are aiming to accomplish. The scope of the goal may be limited by availability of time or resources on the part of the psychotherapist or patient. For example, if therapist can only offer brief psychotherapy to patients (e.g., five sessions) due to program constraints, the psychotherapist/patient duo should consider short- or mid-term goals such as learning a series of coping strategies (e.g., relaxation strategies, assertive communication, problem-solving) or focusing on a specific symptom or problem that may be interfering with dialysis or other treatments (e.g., needle phobia, insomnia, fatigue, adherence to fluid restriction or medications).

Patients may have an upcoming procedure or deadline for health-related decision-making that requires a brief, focused intervention (e.g., choosing a type of dialysis, preparing for an upcoming surgical procedure). Even with no externally imposed time restrictions, it is helpful to set expectations at the outset around how many sessions will be provided, rather than leave the process open-ended. This encourages the patient and psychotherapist to focus on established goals and continue making progress. A lack of collaboratively defined goals or expectations for length of psychotherapy may lead to slow (or no) progress.

Recommendation

– Spend time at psychotherapy outset collaboratively setting treatment goals as well as expectations for duration and frequency of psychotherapy. This will help both patient and psychotherapist gain and keep momentum in psychotherapy.

7.5.3 Case Conceptualization

Behind the scenes, it is helpful to begin formulating a case conceptualization with information gleaned from your patient. This involves considering the biopsychosocial factors that may have contributed to the problem being addressed in psychotherapy, as well as the factors maintaining problematic thoughts, emotions, or behaviors. This will likely include CKD-specific factors such as physical symptoms, illness history, reactions of loved ones to the illness, and illness-related losses (e.g., financial, occupational, social, physical). Case conceptualization can be shared with the patient, particularly if it helps the patient gain insight into the problem, and can be further refined as new information is gleaned. Information about the patient used in case conceptualization is typically obtained early on during initial assessment, which should take place during the first few sessions prior to commencing formal psychotherapy. Chapter 2 presents tips for psychological assessment in CKD, including common screening tools.

7.5.4 Deciding on a Treatment Setting

In traditional psychotherapy, a patient would typically meet the psychotherapist in a quiet, private setting, furnished with comfortable armchairs or sofas. While some psychotherapists may be fortunate enough to have such an environment in which to meet CKD patients, most will offer services in the same setting patients attend other multidisciplinary appointments, such as hospital outpatient clinics, medical offices, examination rooms, or even busy dialysis units. Ideally, and at the very least, psychotherapy should take place in a private setting such that patients are free to speak openly without risk of being overheard. It is usually possible to arrange for a private space such as an examination room or isolation room even in a busy outpatient clinic or dialysis unit, but in some cases, patients may prefer to forego privacy over the convenience of meeting during a scheduled dialysis treatment. For example, hemodialysis patients must typically travel to the dialysis unit three times weekly and spend 4–5 hours on site each visit. It may be inconvenient or undesirable for patients to travel into the clinic on their "off days," particularly if there are transportation or mobility issues that make coming in more challenging. Furthermore, they may not wish to arrive early or stay late on dialysis days, given how much of the day is already consumed by dialysis. Such patients must choose between spending more time at the clinic, coming in on an off day, or multitasking by meeting for psychotherapy while on dialysis. Regardless, the psychotherapist should make every effort to arrange and offer a private space for therapy.

Telepsychology presents a solution to this dilemma for patients who are tech savvy and willing to meet via video or, less ideally, telephone. In some circumstances, psychotherapists may be willing to pay home visits to provide therapy in the patient's own home; however, this is uncommon and presents a specific set of potential ethical concerns to navigate carefully. This type of service may be better suited to psychotherapy with home dialysis patients (hemodialysis or peritoneal dialysis) where nurses and dialysis technologists routinely pay home visits. For home dialysis patients, providing psychotherapy in the patient's home may be a desirable alternative to having patients travel onsite, as renal services are already being provided in that setting. In this case, psychotherapists must carefully consider issues such as maintaining patient confidentiality when traveling with patient information or providing psychotherapy where other family members may be present, maintaining strict professional boundaries, following infection prevention and control procedures to minimize risk to self and patients, and considering common etiquette that is rarely considered in traditional therapy settings (e.g., removing shoes versus leaving them on, accepting versus declining refreshments, and even what to do if nature calls at an inopportune time).

7.5.5 Structure of CBT

As mentioned previously, it is helpful to discuss at treatment outset what the patient can expect in terms of number and frequency of sessions. It may be useful to consider gradually "thinning out" sessions toward the end of a course of psychotherapy, to give the patient time to practice applying strategies with longer periods in between sessions. Given that CKD is a progressive disease, patients who have completed a course of psychotherapy may require additional resources or brief follow-up to review previously learned strategies or how to apply them to new challenges. It may be helpful to address this during the final sessions. The psychotherapist may want to consider offering group rather than individual CBT if a number of patients present with similar concerns, including sleep disturbance, fatigue, depression, or poor adherence to fluid and dietary restrictions. Psychotherapists trained in administering group CBT could offer this format instead of individual CBT to harness the advantages of group therapy and to reach more patients with fewer resources.

7.5.6 Psychotherapist Flexibility

Kidney patients often experience fluctuating health status; as symptoms flare, treatment plans change, or comorbid medical conditions arise. Problems such as fatigue, pain, or nausea may interfere in a patient's ability to keep scheduled appointments. Last-minute medical procedures or physician visits may get scheduled, or as mentioned above, dialysis treatments may limit a patient's availability. Consequently, patients may not always be in a position to provide the standard 24- or 48-h notice to cancel appointments. Furthermore, kidney disease patients may have more frequently shifting priorities in therapy based on new or unexpected symptoms, procedures, or treatment plans. As such, it is helpful to remain as flexible as possible when providing psychotherapy to kidney disease patients. That is not to say that the psychotherapist must completely change course each time a patient's priorities shift, but rather consider returning to the initial case conceptualization for a bird's eye view of how new symptoms or concerns fit into the initial conceptualization. This may provide some continuity to therapy and also help the patient to understand how similar biopsychosocial factors play a role in maintaining seemingly different problems.

7.5.7 Symptom Monitoring

An important part of psychotherapy is ongoing symptom monitoring to determine whether therapy is having the desired effect. Standardized screening tools such as those presented in Chap. 2 have been developed to monitor change in specific symptoms such as depressed mood, anxiety, and insomnia. Sometimes, however, the goal of psychotherapy is not to decrease a specific symptom as much as it is to help a patient cope better with challenges or increase overall well-being or quality of life. In these cases, symptom-specific measures are less useful.

Fortunately, there are measures of well-being and quality of life that can be used to track a patient's general progress. For example, the Outcome Rating Scale (ORS) and Session Rating Scale (SRS) are a set of ultra-brief measures to be used at the beginning and end of each session, respectively [26]. The ORS makes use of a visual analog scale where patients mark an "X" on a line to indicate their well-being across four domains: individual, interpersonal, social, and overall. A total score is calculated and compared against indicators of reliable and clinically significant change. The ORS provides a measure of well-being relative to a general cutoff and can be used to track change in well-being over time.

The SRS also uses a visual analog scale and is completed at the end of each session. Patients mark an "X" on a line to rate four important aspects of the therapy session: relationship, goals and progress, approach or method, and overall rating. The SRS provides an indicator of how the patient feels about each session. It measures therapeutic alliance, an important factor in psychotherapy, and provides an opportunity for the therapist and patient to identify and discuss problems with the therapeutic relationship or focus of therapy that the patient may otherwise not bring up. Visual analog scales require less cognitive effort to complete, which is helpful for renal patients whose cognition may be mildly impaired due to uremia or other factors. The ORS and SRS are free to use in pencil and paper form by individual therapists, but a paid license is required for institutional use or administration in digital/electronic form.

7.5.8 Motivational Enhancement

Behavior change is often a component of psychotherapy with renal patients. For example, increasing activity levels, taking medications as prescribed, and limiting fluid intake may all be relevant treatment targets. Such change is not always easy, despite patients understanding of the importance of it. According to the transtheoretical model, or stages of change model, people move through a series of stages of change ranging from precontemplation to contemplation, preparation, action, maintenance, and termination [27]. Chapter 11, *Substance Use Disorders and the Kidney*, presents this model in Table 11.6. Behavioral interventions should be matched to a person's current stage of change in order to be effective. For example, patients in an early stage such as contemplation will not likely benefit from active interventions encouraging new behaviors, whereas patients who are in the action stage may be ready to start making changes. Patients not yet in the preparation or action phase may benefit from additional motivational enhancement, a technique also known as motivational interviewing.

The goal of motivational enhancement is to enhance a person's intrinsic motivation for change by decreasing ambivalence [28]. Four main processes involved in motivational interviewing include (i) engaging the patient, (ii) focusing in on the relevant issue, (iii) evoking the patient's own motivation for change, and (iv) planning how change will occur (but only once the patient has evidenced some motivation to proceed). Four specific skills involved in motivational interviewing include (i) asking open-ended questions, (ii) affirming what a patient is doing well/correctly, (iii) reflecting on a patient's statements, and (iv) summarizing what you have gleaned from a patient [29]. One helpful tool for exploring a patient's ambivalence around changing problematic behavior is to tabulate in writing the costs and benefits of changing, as well as the costs and benefits of not changing. This is known as a

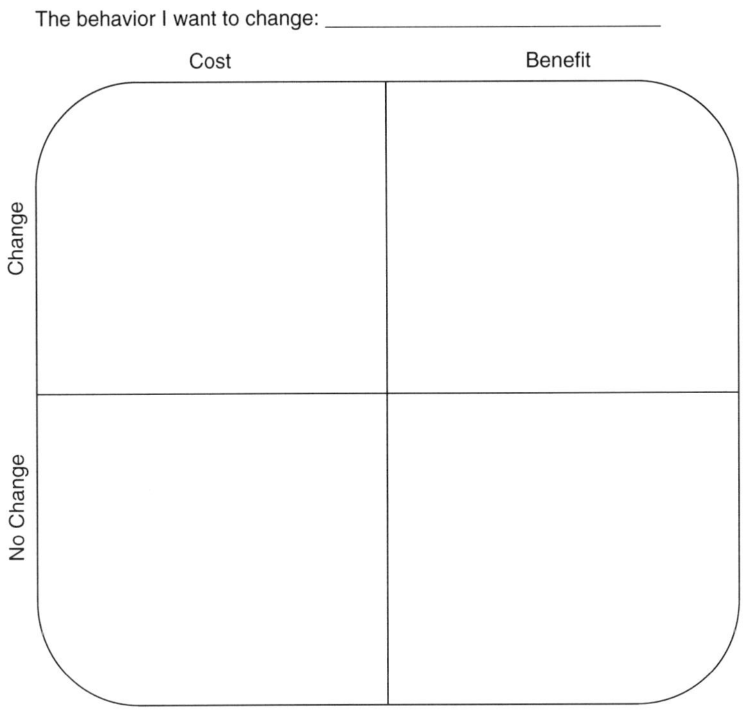

Fig. 7.2 Decisional balance worksheet

decisional balance matrix, and this simple exercise can help patients put their own pros and cons of change into perspective when laid out visually in front of them. A sample decisional balance matrix is presented in Fig. 7.2; however, it can quickly be created with any blank piece of paper or whiteboard.

Recommendation

- When working with renal patients to promote behavior change, consider what stage of change your patient is in before moving ahead.

Clinical Pearl

- If you sense a patient pushing back, stalling, or making "excuses" for not moving forward with change, stop what you are doing and spend time exploring their ambivalence and intrinsic motivation for change.
- Weighing the costs and benefits of changing versus not changing can facilitate exploring and decreasing ambivalence (see Fig. 7.2).

7.6 Challenges in Providing Psychotherapy to Kidney Patients

Some of the challenges in providing psychotherapy to kidney patients have been described previously, including finding time and space to meet with hemodialysis patients who are already spending considerable time coming into the clinic. There are other challenges that are more common in older patients and those with chronic illness that merit consideration, as they may be relevant for renal patients. There may be physical or practical barriers to meeting in person, such as illness or physical disability that limit mobility and make traveling to and from appointments unpleasant, impractical, or generally challenging. Another practical barrier is lack of access to transportation. Some patients may not have a vehicle or family member who can drive them to appointments, which makes meeting in person challenging and could pose a financial burden for patients with limited financial resources who would need to pay for transportation.

As mentioned previously, offering telepsychology through video or, less ideally, telephone may be one way to accommodate patients who have a difficult time getting from home to appointments. Of course, not all patients will have Internet access or access to a smart device or will want to conduct therapy in this manner. Another potential solution is to schedule therapy sessions around preexisting clinic visits so that patients need not make an extra trip to the clinic. One disadvantage of this solution is that patients must stay longer at the clinic, but for many patients, this may be preferred to making an extra trip. Solutions to these barriers should be offered and discussed rather than decided unilaterally by the therapist. Consulting the patient in this process will serve to build rapport and strengthen therapeutic alliance.

Cognitive challenges often encountered in the context of CKD are another consideration when engaging a patient with renal disease in psychotherapy such as CBT. As outlined in detail in Chap. 2, cognitive impairment is evident across all stages of CKD, is independent of age-related changes, and exists for both lower-order and higher-order cognitive abilities that increase between stages of CKD [30]. Common early cognitive difficulties include impaired attention, information processing speed, short-term memory, mental set shifting, and language processes. As renal disease progresses, impairments in more basic aspects of cognition typically give way to more significant impairments in higher-order executive functioning, worsening memory processes, and more global cognitive impairment.

Psychotherapists working with CKD patients are encouraged to familiarize themselves with common cognitive difficulties and validated screening methods (reviewed in Chap. 2) to be informed as to the specific cognitive difficulties that may be present in their patient and to screen for changes in cognition over the course of longer-term psychotherapy. There is an extreme paucity in the published literature regarding adaptation of standard evidence-based psychotherapies, such as CBT, for patients with cognitive impairment. However, a handful of publications address modifying psychotherapy for older adults with mild cognitive impairment (e.g., [31]), and the CBT for psychosis literature, including published treatment manuals (e.g., [32]), have been developed purposefully for populations who typically exhibit cognitive impairments similar to those of advanced stage CKD patients (i.e., attention, memory, executive function impairments) and are helpful to consider when approaching other cognitively impaired groups.

7.6.1 Strategies for Addressing Cognitive Impairments in Psychotherapy

Following is a review of strategies for addressing and compensating for cognitive impairments when providing psychotherapy to patients with CKD based on the clinical experience of the authors who are experienced clinical neuropsychologists and health psychologists accustomed to modifying psychotherapies for various medical, geriatric, and/or psychiatric populations with cognitive impairments ranging from subtle to significant.

Psychoeducation Once cognition has been screened, one of the most helpful psychotherapeutic strategies is to provide the patient, and when possible a supporting family member, with psychoeducation regarding the nature and extent of their cognitive difficulties [31]. This feedback should be combined with normalizing explanations regarding the incidence and prevalence of cognitive impairment in CKD (see Chap. 2), and real-world examples (preferably reflecting back the patient's own accounts), of how these cognitive difficulties may be experienced by the patient in their day to day life. For example, a patient struggling to remember the name of their new attending physician could be assured this is not likely due to lack of motivation or interest, or onset of Alzheimer disease, but because difficulties with attention secondary to CKD may interfere with the intake of new information. Often patients with chronic medical conditions that involve changes in cognition catastrophize or misattribute cognitive impairments to something much more sinister, such as the onset of a dementia process such as Alzheimer disease, which can further negatively impact psychological symptoms and interfere with treatment adherence and overall well-being. Being provided accurate information about the nature, causes, and probable progression of cognitive impairments common in CKD, as well as information about lifestyle factors which may help mitigate cognitive declines such as adherence to medical management, diet, and exercise recommendations may reduce the frequency and severity of catastrophic misinterpretations and psychological symptoms (again, see Chap. 2 for further details).

Recommendation

- Before beginning psychotherapy, screen for cognitive impairment and provide patients, and family supports when possible, with psychoeducation about the nature of cognitive difficulties common in CKD.

Clinical Pearl

- Patients who experience cognitive changes will often make catastrophic misinterpretations, which further exacerbate psychological symptoms.

Pacing of Therapy Impairments in attention and information processing speed will interfere with how well patients are able to sustain cognitive engagement in psychotherapy and how quickly they are able to follow information that is provided and formulate responses to questions. Although efforts should be made to ensure a quiet, distraction-free environment for the psychotherapeutic session, often therapy is being provided in a noisy or distracting environment such as chairside during dialysis. Sensitivity to inattention secondary to distraction should be considered. Psychotherapists accustomed to working with non-medically ill and non-cognitively impaired populations may feel that therapy is progressing at a slow pace; however, the psychotherapist is advised to go at the pace of the patient, pause frequently to allow patients extra time to process information, and check in often to ensure patients are keeping up with the pace of discussion. Asking patients to repeat back or paraphrase important content is also recommended to ensure patients have attended to and processed therapeutic content, and this will also assist with the encoding phase of new learning/memory. The importance of setting realistic and achievable goals for psychotherapy should consider the slower pace of psychotherapy secondary to cognitive impairments.

Recommendation

- When delivering psychotherapy, pause frequently and check in with patients to ensure they are keeping up with the pace of delivery.

Repetition Impairments in attention, information processing speed, and short-term memory will interfere with the intake or encoding of new information and the transfer of that new information from immediate or very short-term memory into longer-term memory storage. Repetition of important key concepts both within and between sessions is recommended to compensate for these difficulties and better enable patients to encode and consolidate new information into memory. Strategies that can be helpful include the psychotherapist briefly outlining key concepts, then going over these in more detail, then asking the patient to repeat back or paraphrase what they have taken away. Patients may also benefit from having material covered or goals set at the previous session briefly reviewed or repeated at the outset of the following session to help orient them to where they are at in the psychotherapeutic process as well as aid in enhanced learning of previously presented concepts.

Use of Visuals and Handouts Given the identified difficulties with information processing speed, attention and memory, as well as early difficulties with language processing, CKD patients will benefit from the use of visual aids and handouts summarizing key points. This may be accomplished in session with the use of a white board on which the psychotherapist can draw simple graphics and visuals to ground the patient and help orient them to key concepts and content being discussed. For example, in a CBT session, the psychotherapist may draw a large circle to represent a given situation they are evaluating with the patient and include visuals to represent the patient's thoughts, feelings/emotions, and actions/behaviors in that situation

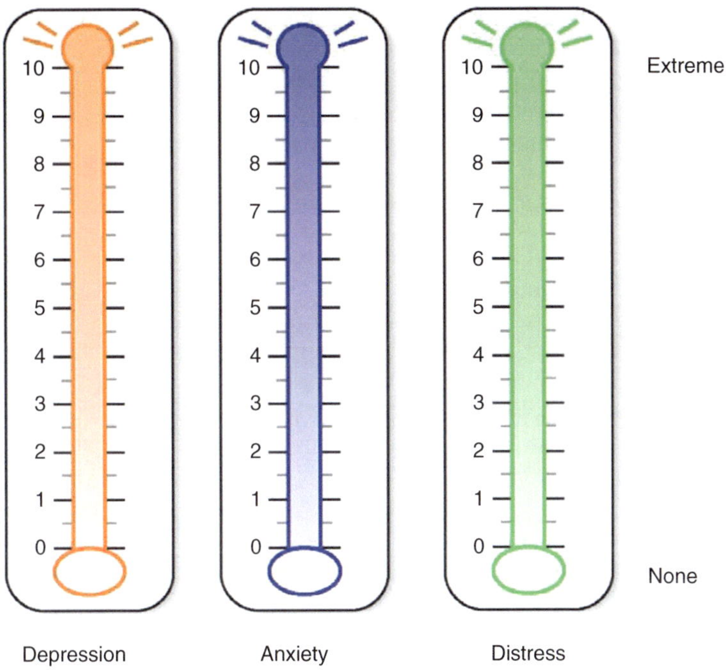

Fig. 7.3 Emotional thermometer

(see Fig. 7.1) in order to decrease working memory load for the patient when engaging in reappraisal of the thoughts and feelings associated with the event. Similarly, an easy way to measure and track level of psychological symptoms each session on a scale from 0 (none) to 10 (extreme) is with the use of a visual "thermometer" (see Fig. 7.3). In addition to this in-session use of visual aids, providing patients with handouts for their use between sessions can also aid engagement and decrease burden on cognitive demands. Handouts can be used to summarize key points for patient review between sessions, as reminders to prompt patients to engage in between session homework activities and even as cue cards to remind patients of coping strategies they have developed for use in certain situations or for managing certain symptoms.

Use of Concrete Examples and Terminology Patients with moderate to severe CKD who are experiencing more prominent executive functioning difficulties such as impairments in mental flexibility, mental set shifting, or abstract reasoning may struggle with abstract terminology or with the cognitive restructuring elements of CBT. Providing these patients with concepts in clear and concise wording with simple, concrete examples is recommended. For example, providing a list or pictorial of common cognitive distortions or a handout with frequently experienced thoughts and feelings associated with particular psychological disorders from which they can circle the ones that apply to them may be more beneficial than asking patients to generate descriptions of their thoughts and feelings, or to generate alternative explanations or interpretations for common cognitive distortions. Among patients with significant global cognitive impairment, greater emphasis on behavioral aspects of CBT is generally recommended; however, this is often challenging to accomplish for advanced CKD patients with significant mobility restrictions.

Recommendation

- Use clear and concise explanations and concrete examples, especially when working with more advanced stage CKD patients who may be experiencing moderate to severe executive cognitive impairment.

Setting Realistic and Achievable Goals and Activity Pacing Working collaboratively with the patient to identify even seemingly small activities that they are able to engage in and setting realistic and achievable goals for behavioral activation or exposure activities is strongly recommended. Celebrating even what appear to be the smallest achievements, such as getting out of bed and showering, can be validating and encouraging to patients with significant cognitive, psychological, and physical challenges. In addition, helping patients to use activity pacing to intersperse reasonably achievable behavioral activity with rest breaks is also an important element unique to providing CBT in a medically compromised patient population. Activity pacing is critical to establish early on so that patients do not "overdo it," experience discomfort or failure, and then avoid further behavioral aspects of treatment. Setting patients up for success with achievable behavioral elements of their treatment will help ensure patients gain a feeling of success and self-efficacy that may further motivate them to remain engaged in psychotherapy and medical management of their condition.

Clinical Pearl

- Setting patients up for success with realistic and achievable goals and behavioral activity or exposures will enhance engagement in psychotherapy.

7.7 Case Vignette Analysis: "One Thing After Another"

Mr. Hastings met with the health psychologist for eight sessions of cognitive behavioral therapy. The first two sessions were spent discussing his goals for therapy and formulating a case conceptualization, which his therapist shared with him, revising as new information came to light. Mr. Hastings learned that his difficulty checking blood sugar had a lot to do with two things: (1) his fear of needles and (2) the anxiety he experienced every time he saw high glucose numbers. These unpleasant emotions led him to avoid checking unless his wife was watching, or he felt very unwell.

He was too embarrassed to tell anyone about this fear and tried his best to hide it. The ongoing difficulty he faced in checking his blood sugar and repeated trips to the emergency department eventually made him feel hopeless about ever being able to manage his diabetes, and the idea of giving up his favorite foods on top of all this was too much to handle.

Over the next few sessions, his psychologist helped him to understand the relationship among his emotions, unhelpful thoughts, and health-related behaviors. They also dedicated several sessions to exposure therapy to reduce his fear of needles. Through newfound problem-solving skills, he set up a meeting with the diabetes nurse educator to learn about other options for monitoring blood sugar and started using a continuous glucose monitoring system that did not require finger sticks and was much easier to use. The team social worker helped him apply for and secure funding for this new monitoring system. With his blood sugar under control and increased sense of self-efficacy, he started making small changes to his diet and began to lose weight. Unfortunately, he needed to start dialysis before losing enough weight for a preemptive living donor transplant. After weighing the pros and cons of peritoneal dialysis versus hemodialysis, he chose automated peritoneal dialysis. This afforded him and his wife the freedom to travel to visit their sons, and he was able to keep his day times entirely free to do whatever he wanted. He was starting to enjoy life again and feeling hopeful that a living donor transplant was in his near future.

7.8 Key Takeaways

- Patients with CKD experience a number of stressors as the disease progresses and new treatments are started.
- Comorbid psychopathology is common in CKD patients and is associated with poorer prognosis.
- Multidisciplinary mental health clinicians working in multidisciplinary settings must ensure that patients have a clear understanding of how patient confidentiality works and how information is shared with other care clinicians.
- Cognitive behavioral therapy (CBT) is an evidence-based nonpharmacological treatment for several psychological disorders, and evidence exists for its efficacy with CKD patients.
- CBT helps patients modify unhelpful thinking patterns, change self-defeating behaviors, and improve overall functioning.
- CBT techniques include cognitive restructuring, behavioral activation, exposure, problem-solving, and relaxation.
- Clinicians should self-educate about CKD symptoms and treatments when working with renal patients by engaging in self-learning or shadowing multidisciplinary colleagues.
- Clinicians should collaboratively identify treatment goals and engage in case conceptualization early in the course of treatment, within the context of a biopsychosocial framework.

- A patient's preferred psychotherapeutic treatment setting may vary based on a number of factors, including their mobility, access to transportation, and dialysis schedule.
- Clinicians should remain flexible when working with renal patients, due to potential changes in health status, treatment plans, and interfering symptoms and side effects.
- Patient progress should be routinely monitored over the course of treatment, and not just at completion of psychotherapy.
- Behavioral interventions should be matched to a patient's current stage of change according to the transtheoretical/stages of change model, and motivational interviewing strategies can be used to increase a patient's motivation for change and decrease ambivalence.
- Cognitive difficulties such as impaired attention, information processing speed, short-term memory, mental set shifting, and language processes are common in patients with CKD and may pose a barrier to psychotherapy.
- Strategies for addressing and compensating for cognitive impairment in psychotherapy include providing psychoeducation about cognitive difficulties, pacing the speed at which therapy proceeds, repeating information, using visual aids and handouts, using concrete examples and terminology, and setting realistic and achievable goals.

References

1. Psychotherapy Act, 2007, S.O. 2007, c. 10, Sched R. https://www.ontario.ca/laws/statute/07p10. Accessed 11 Apr 2021.
2. United States. Department of Health and Human Services. Manage patients with chronic kidney disease: Slow progression & reduce complications [Internet]. Bethesda: National Institute of Diabetes and Digestive and Kidney Diseases [cited 2021 Apr 11]. Available from: https://www.niddk.nih.gov/health-information/professionals/clinical-tools-patient-management/kidney-disease/identify-manage-patients/manage-ckd/slow-progression-reduce-complications.
3. Cukor D, Cohen SD, Peterson RA, Kimmel PL. Psychosocial aspects of chronic disease: ESRD as a paradigmatic illness. J Am Soc Nephrol. 2007;18(12):3042–55.
4. Palmer S, Vecchio M, Craig JC, et al. Prevalence of depression in chronic kidney disease: systematic review and meta-analysis of observational studies. Kidney Int. 2013;84:179–91.
5. Goh ZS, Griva K. Anxiety and depression in patients with end-stage renal disease: impact and management challenges – a narrative review. Int J Nephrol Renovasc Dis. 2018;11:93–102.
6. Liu CH, Yeh MK, Weng SC, et al. Suicide and chronic kidney disease: a case-control study. Nephrol Dial Transplant. 2017;32(9):1524–9.
7. Huang CW, Wee PH, Low LL, et al. Prevalence and risk factors for elevated anxiety symptoms and anxiety disorders in chronic kidney disease: a systematic review and meta-analysis. Gen Hosp Psychiatry. 2021;69:27–40.
8. Engel GL. The clinical application of the biopsychosocial model. Am J Psychiatry. 1980;137:535–44.
9. Shi Y, Xiong J, Chen Y, et al. The effectiveness of multidisciplinary care models for patients with chronic kidney disease: a systematic review and meta-analysis. Int Urol Nephrol. 2018;50:301–12.
10. Seekles ML, Ormandy P, Coyne E. Mapping the UK renal psychosocial workforce: The first comprehensive workforce survey. BMC Nephrol. 2019;20(100)

11. Beck AT. Cognitive therapy: nature and relation to behavior therapy. Behav Ther. 1970;1(2):184–200.
12. Ellis A. Reason and emotion in psychotherapy. New York: Lyle Stuart; 1962.
13. David D, Cristea I, Hofmann SG. Why cognitive behavioral therapy is the current gold standard of psychotherapy. Front Psych. 2018;9(4):1–3.
14. Hofmann SG, Asnaani A, Vonk IJJ, et al. The efficacy of cognitive behavioral therapy: a review of meta-analysis. Cognit Ther Res. 2012;36(5):427–40.
15. Butler AC, Chapman JE, Forman EM, Beck AT. The empirical status of cognitive-behavioral therapy: a review of meta-analyses. Clin Psychol Rev. 2006;26:17–31.
16. Driessen E, Hollon SD. Cognitive behavioral therapy for mood disorders: efficacy, moderators and mediators. Psychiatr Clin North Am. 2010;33(3):537–55.
17. Othman AA, Jaafar WMW, Zainuddin ZN, Yusop YM. Effectiveness of cognitive behaviour therapy on depression among haemodialysis patients: a systematic review of literature. Cogent Psychol. 2020;7(1):1–13.
18. Lerma A, Perez-Grovas H, Bermudez L, et al. Brief cognitive behavioural intervention for depression and anxiety symptoms improves quality of life in chronic haemodialysis patients. Psychol Psychother. 2017;90(1):105–23.
19. Cukor D, Ver Halen N, Rosenthal Asher D, et al. Psychosocial intervention improves depression, quality of life, and fluid adherence in hemodialysis. J Am Soc Nephrol. 2014;25(1):196–206.
20. Duarte PS, Miyazaki MC, Blay SL, Sesso R. Cognitive-behavioral group therapy is an effective treatment for major depression in hemodialysis patients. Kidney Int. 2009;76(4):414–21.
21. Valsaraj BP, Bhat SM, Latha KS. Cognitive behaviour therapy for anxiety and depression among people undergoing haemodialysis: a randomized control trial. J Clin Diagn Res. 2016;10(8):VC06 10.
22. Chan R, Dear BF, Titov N, et al. Examining internet-delivered cognitive behaviour therapy for patients with chronic kidney disease on haemodialysis: a feasibility open trial. J Psychosom Res. 2016;89:78–84.
23. Ng CZ, Tang SC, Chan M, et al. A systematic review and meta-analysis of randomized controlled trials of cognitive behavioral therapy for hemodialysis patients with depression. J Psychosom Res. 2019;126:109834.
24. Safran JD, Segal ZV, Shaw BF, Vallis TM. Patient selection for short-term cognitive therapy. In: Safran JD, Segal ZV, editors. Interpersonal process in cognitive therapy. New York: Basic Books; 1990. p. 226–47.
25. Sage N, Sowden M, Chorlton E, Edeleanu A. CBT for chronic illness and palliative care: a workbook and toolkit. Chichester: Wiley; 2008.
26. Campbell A, Hemsley S. Outcome rating scale and session rating scale in psychological practice: clinical utility of ultra-brief measures. Clin Psychol. 2009;13(1):1–9.
27. Prochaska JO, Velicer WF. The transtheoretical model of health behavior change. Am J Health Promot. 1997;12(1):38–48.
28. Miller W, Rollnick S. Motivational interviewing. 2nd ed. New York: Guilford Press; 2002.
29. Steinberg MP, Miller WR. Motivational interviewing in diabetes care. New York: Guilford Press; 2015.
30. Brodski J, Rossell SL, Castle DJ, Tan EJ. A systematic review of cognitive impairments associated with kidney failure in adults before natural age-related changes. J Int Neuropsychol Soc. 2019;25(1):101–14.
31. Miller MD, Richards V, Zuckoff A, et al. A model for modifying interpersonal psychotherapy (IPT) for depressed elders with cognitive impairment. Clin Gerontol. 2007;30(2):79–101.
32. Wright NP, Turkington D, Kelly OP, et al. Treating psychosis: a clinician's guide to integrating acceptance and commitment therapy, compassion focused therapy, and mindfulness approaches within the cognitive behaviour therapy tradition. Oakland: New Harbinger Publications; 2014.

8 Decisional Capacity Determinations in Psychonephrology

James A. Bourgeois and Calvin H. Hirsch

8.1 Introduction

Among the more common and important aspects of consultation-liaison psychiatry practice with patients with renal disease is the determination of decisional capacity. Beyond the usual circumstances leading to the patient's decisional capacity being questioned by the primary medical teams (e.g., apparent poor understanding of medical condition and intervention options, self-sabotaging behavior leading to questions of "surreptitiously suicidal" behavior, "non-compliance," the patient seen in the immediate aftermath of a medically serious suicide attempt), there are clinical scenarios specific to nephrology practice where decisional capacity is an inherent and critical part of multispecialty care. In this chapter, the authors review general considerations in decisional capacity determinations, review the recent literature for psychiatric and neurologic illness that correlate with impaired decisional capacity, and present a clinical approach to integrate decisional capacity determinations into the comprehensive consultation-liaison psychiatry consultation on the renal disease patient.

J. A. Bourgeois (✉)
Department of Psychiatry, Baylor Scott & White Health, Central Texas Division, Department of Medical Education, College of Medicine, Texas A&M University Health Science Center, Temple, TX, USA
e-mail: james.bourgeois@BSWHealth.org

C. H. Hirsch
Division of General Medicine (Geriatrics), University of California Davis Medical Center, Sacramento, CA, USA
e-mail: chhirsch@ucdavis.edu

A. Hategan et al. (eds.), *Psychonephrology*,
https://doi.org/10.1007/978-3-030-84740-1_8

8.2 Decisional Capacity: Medical Informed Consent

The first consideration in the area of decisional capacity refers to the patient's capacity for a specific medical/surgical decision to accept or reject a proposed intervention versus the patient's capacity for "self-determination" more broadly, beyond a specific intervention. The scenario of assessment of the patient's capacity for a single, discrete, dichotomous medical/surgical decision is more specific and concrete and can be accomplished with a greater degree of certitude "in the moment," while self-determination is inherently future- (not present-)oriented and thus involves a degree of inference and/or speculation on the part of the evaluating physician; thus it is a less precise determination. In many cases, a possibly "impaired" patient may raise questions about both capacity for a discrete decision regarding an intervention *and* eventual self-determination, to the degree that both determinations are to be addressed in a single consultation.

Decisional capacity determinations are, by definition, related to a particular, proposed medical/surgical intervention planned in the near future and are not "global" (e.g., "can the patient make all medical decisions?") or "future" (e.g., "can the patient agree to a surgery when it is scheduled three months from now?"). Decisional capacity for a procedure must be specific to a definable intervention offered for a particular illness. The spirit of decisional capacity, in this vein, fits squarely into the doctrine of informed consent, whereby consent must be informed, voluntary, and not coerced.

A classic paper by Appelbaum and Grisso defines four elements of decisional capacity, with the single proposed intervention defined [1]. By the Appelbaum and Grisso formulation, the patient must be able to demonstrate the following four elements:

(i) He/she must *understand* factual information pertinent to his/her illness and proposed intervention.
(ii) The patient must be able to *appreciate* how the proposed intervention applies to him/her as one with a particular disease and thus must appreciate prognosis of illness versus intervention and be able to weigh the two choices.
(iii) The patient must use a sound, *rational process of reasoning.*
(iv) The patient must *communicate a consistent choice* regarding accepting or rejection the procedure. It is emphasized that the patient may ultimately reject the proposed intervention, as long as a competent and consistent process of decision-making is demonstrated.

Clinical Pearl

Decisional capacity consists of four essential elements:

- Showing an understanding of the illness and proposed procedure.
- Ability to make a binary choice of yes or no for the procedure by appreciating how it specifically will affect them and their prognosis.
- Step 3 must demonstrate intact reasoning consistent with the patient's values.
- Communication of a consistent decision.

An important operational concept in decisional capacity determinations is the "decisional capacity gradient." As various medical procedures are associated with a range of potential benefits versus risks to a particular patient, the decisional capacity rubric used by the physician in the determination of decisional capacity must take this "decisional dimensionality" into account. As a practical matter, one can usually safely infer that clear decisional capacity for a "high on the gradient" intervention can correlate with intact decisional capacity for "low on the gradient" interventions; nonetheless, decisional capacity should be specified for the particular clinical consideration at hand [2].

It is generally considered that research participation requires the highest decisional capacity standard. This is because in addition to the routine clinical considerations of individual risks versus benefits for a given proposed procedure, the patient must further demonstrate validated understanding of the concepts on placebo control, blinding, and random assignment (which varies, depending on the exact research methodology used). The patient must understand that he/she may receive no direct benefit from the trial, that his/her physician nor the subject him/herself will know the treatment condition, and that participation in research may well preclude the receipt of standard clinical care for their illness.

The next highest standard of decisional capacity pertains to the patient's rejection of proposed medical/surgical intervention. Inasmuch as it is presumed that medical and surgical procedures are being offered in a beneficent, "good faith" fashion with the patient's presumed interest at heart, the patient is still allowed to reject the proposed intervention. However, to do so, he/she must demonstrate clear understanding and appreciation of the implications of rejection of the procedure. This is a somewhat "higher" standard than accepting the proposed procedure.

The next decisional capacity standard is to accept the proposed medical surgical procedure. Again, as the patient is acquiescent to the offer of medical/surgical intervention ethically offered in a beneficent framework, the degree of detailed understanding can be somewhat lower than needed to decline the procedure. Nonetheless, the patient needs to demonstrate, by a "what would the typical, reasonable patient do" standard, adequate understanding of risks, benefits, and side effects. The physician is cautioned to not accept the response of "well, I could just die" following a procedure. While this is true, more nuanced understanding of risks requires understanding complications that may occur at a reasonable frequency that do not lead to death. In the example of renal transplantation, these include graft failure, organ rejection, non-function of the graft, bleeding, infection, and the general risks of anesthesia.

Clinical Pearl

Decisional capacity follows a gradient dictated by the amount of understanding and reasoning required to reach an informed decision about participation.

- The highest standard is for informed consent for participation in research based on the assumption that potential harms may outweigh potential benefits, which are not known.
- The second-highest standard is for rejecting a proposed medical or surgical intervention based on the assumption that rejection may subject the patient to a higher risk of an adverse outcome.

- The third-highest standard is for accepting a proposed medical or surgical intervention.
- Lowest standard is appointment of a surrogate decision-maker.

Complex informed consent may have multiple dimensions and branching decision trees. For example, a patient with advanced kidney disease who is expected to require dialysis in the next year may have selected peritoneal dialysis because their rural location is 40 miles from the nearest hemodialysis center. As a result, their nephrologist may be grooming them for peritoneal dialysis. However, in the interim they may be diagnosed with polymyalgia rheumatica (a rheumatological condition characterized by proximal muscle weakness and pain) and require prolonged administration of prednisone. The preliminary informed consent for peritoneal dialysis now becomes complicated by unexpected immunosuppression that increases the risk for peritonitis, changing the risk-benefit calculus. The risk-benefit calculus may change again if the patient's spouse is hospitalized or the patient has a stroke. Changes in the patient's condition require adaptive reasoning and sophisticated planning, with commensurate education and support from involved clinicians.

On the opposite end of the spectrum is informed consent for a minor elective procedure like lancing a boil. The benefits and risks of the procedure are relatively straightforward, and the reasoning behind the decision to accept or forgo the procedure does not require sophistication.

Not all informed consent is solely "in the moment," but can be implicitly about the future. In CKD, much planning revolves around the future choice of peritoneal dialysis versus hemodialysis versus transplant, and assessment of the patient's ability to choose a modality requires that they understand the risks and benefits in the context of their own comorbidities and psychosocial environment, which are dynamic. In hemodialysis, advance planning may be required for placement of permanent venous access, often months before the procedure.

More complex is the determination that a patient is a candidate for peritoneal dialysis or renal transplant as opposed to hemodialysis, and that requires that the patient understands and agrees to the rationale, potential benefits, and potential harms unique to the selection. In effect, the clinician is performing "pre-informed consent" for a particular choice that may be distant in time (months or more) but which places the patient on a path that may lead in a step-wise fashion to additional informed consent for tests or procedures required to qualify for that mode of dialysis. Ultimately, the patient must provide informed consent for the definitive procedure that commits them to a modality.

Because the definitive procedures may be temporally distant, they can at first appear theoretical and amorphous to the patient, increasing the challenge of ensuring that he or she understands the risks and benefits as they crystalize over time with the arrival of new information. In addition, decisional capacity may change due to cognitive decline. Each path the patient embarks upon may lead to new tests and new procedures that ultimately may preclude the originally selected dialysis modality. For example, with the physician's approval, a patient may give "pre-informed consent" for a renal transplant. As a result, the patient may give informed consent

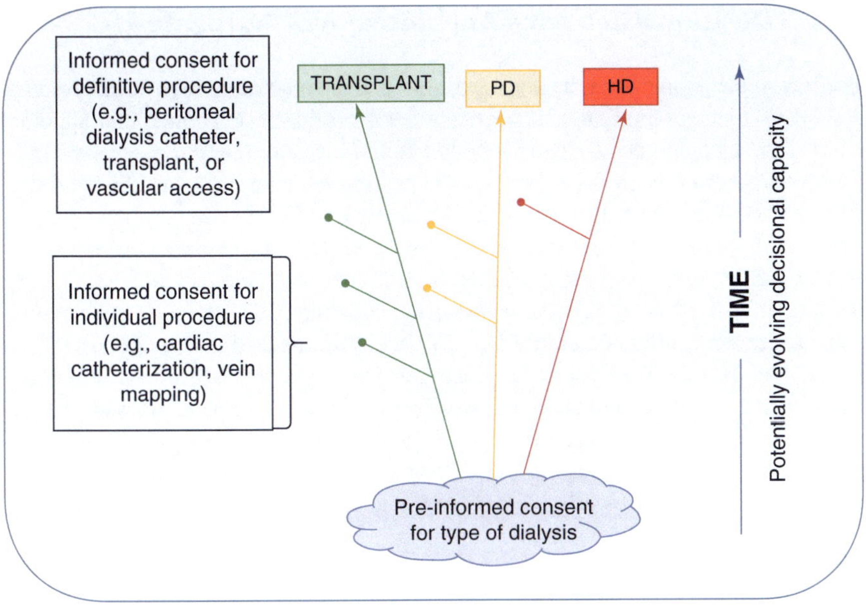

Fig. 8.1 The temporally spaced stages of informed consent for dialysis. The consent process begins with pre-informed consent for a preferred dialysis modality based on the patient's understanding of risks and benefits that are influenced by comorbidities, psychosocial support, and availability of the individual modality. This sets the patient down a preferred path that may require informed consent for specific procedures along the way, culminating in informed consent for the definitive procedure. During the temporal lag between pre-informed consent and consent for the final procedure, the patient's values may change, new comorbidities may arise, and the patient's decisional capacity may evolve due to intercurrent cognitive decline. Thus, informed consent for dialysis is a time-based dynamic process
HD hemodialysis, *PD* peritoneal dialysis

for a cardiac stress test that turns out positive, leading to informed consent for a cardiac catheterization that requires placement of coronary-artery stents, and the patient may then be considered unstable for transplant or prematurely routed to hemodialysis because of catheterization-related acute renal failure (Fig. 8.1).

Recommendation

- Decisional capacity should be assessed at intervals starting early in chronic kidney disease.
- Decision-making capacity extends beyond just informed consent for the invasive procedure to the ability to adhere to medication and lifestyle changes imposed by the CKD.
- Patients must give a "pre-informed consent" for their choice of dialysis well before the definitive procedure so that diagnostic pathways can be mapped out.
- As the pathway is followed for transplant, peritoneal dialysis, or hemodialysis, each may have their own set of procedures requiring informed consent.

8.3 Decisional Capacity: Appointment of Surrogate

The lowest decisional capacity standard, and an issue not routinely assessed systematically, is the appointment of a surrogate decision-maker. Inasmuch that appointment of a surrogate decision-maker (also called a healthcare proxy, or substitute decision-maker in some jurisdictions) is a "procedure" with risks, benefits, and side effects, ascertainment that the patient adequately understands the implications of a surrogate appointment if necessary. The surrogate must be competently identified and appointed, the surrogate will be decisional only when the patient is manifestly impaired, the surrogate may not necessarily act as the patient would have wanted, and the surrogate will at that point have full access to medical information to render a decision. However, surrogate appointment is considered the lowest decisional capacity standard in that the patient, in order to appoint a surrogate, does not necessarily need detailed understanding of his/her own illness and/or proposed procedure(s), only the considerations specific to surrogate appointment. There are many patients who are clearly incapable of medical informed consent, but who can quite capably name a surrogate decision-maker; this should be ascertained as part of the consent process.

8.4 Dispositional Capacity

Despite often being questioned by medical teams at the same time decisional capacity is challenged, disposition capacity is conceptually and fundamentally different and thus must be differentiated from decisional capacity [2]. While decisional capacity determination intuitively and logically fits into the doctrine of informed consent, dispositional capacity is not about informed consent at all. Indeed, a given patient may have only marginal understanding and appreciation about a proposed medical intervention (thus clearly failing a decisional capacity determination) yet be able to demonstrate acceptable self-care skills and an ability to monitor social resources to an adequate degree to be able to care for him−/herself outside of the hospital.

8.5 Neuropsychiatric Illnesses Leading to Impaired Decisional Capacity

While it is reasonable to question decisional and dispositional capacity of patients with psychiatric illnesses (many of which impair cognitive function, reasoning, and reality testing), impaired decisional capacity cannot be assumed a priori based on the clinical presence of *any* psychiatric illness; the determination of decisional capacity is a *separate determination* from that of identifying and managing psychiatric illness(es). Indeed, the presence of a psychiatric commitment order (e.g., following a suicide attempt, or due to disorganized cognitive function) cannot per se be determinative of intact versus impaired decisional capacity. Even in the presence of significant psychiatric illness (which may be the main presenting clinical problem), decisional capacity determination needs to be completed *for the specific proposed intervention* using a comprehensive clinical approach.

Nonetheless, there is an emerging literature on specific psychiatric illnesses and their relative risk of impaired decisional capacity. Put in terms of an "illness gradient," the psychiatric illness group most likely to lead to impaired decisional capacity are *neurocognitive disorders* (major neurocognitive disorder/dementia, delirium) > *psychotic disorders* (schizophrenia, schizoaffective disorder) > *depressive and bipolar disorders* (bipolar I disorder, major depressive disorder) > *anxiety disorders* (generalized anxiety disorder, panic disorder) [3, 4]. While this gradient has good clinical utility, it is only a guide to the evaluation of a given patient.

8.5.1 Neurocognitive Disorders

Of great pertinence to psychonephrology is the fact that renal patients are both at high risk of major neurocognitive disorder/dementia based on systemic comorbidity (e.g., diabetes mellitus, hypertension, systemic lupus erythematosus) and are by definition *delirium-prone* (e.g., with the use of immunosuppressants, corticosteroids, uremia, hepatorenal syndrome). The clinical literature to date clearly establishes that major neurocognitive disorder/dementia and delirium are those psychiatric illnesses most likely to lead to impaired decisional capacity [3, 4]. While this literature does not focus on renal patients per se, the connection between major neurocognitive disorder/dementia and delirium to impaired decisional capacity is unavoidable.

8.5.2 Psychotic and Depressive Disorders

Psychotic disorders (schizophrenia and similar) are likely overrepresented in renal patients, likely due to their greater burden of diabetes mellitus and systemic vascular disease. Regarding depressive disorders, the impact on decisional capacity is dimensional; i.e., mild/moderate depressive disorders do not affect cognitive function, thus decisional capacity, while severe/melancholic/psychotic/catatonic depressive disorder does correlate with impaired decisional capacity.

8.5.3 Specific Decisional Capacity Scenarios in Psychonephrology

Specific to psychonephrology, there are many reasons why renal patients are a high-risk group for needing formal decisional capacity determinations. Renal patients are a high-risk population for impaired decisional capacity due to a high prevalence of cognitive impairment, even in mild-moderate chronic kidney disease (CKD), defined as an estimated glomerular filtration rate (GFR) < 60 mL/minute/1.73 m^2

(see Chap. 12, *Neurocognitive Ramifications of Renal Disease*). The risk of cognitive impairment, and thus impaired decisional capacity, rises as kidney function declines. Compared to persons without CKD, adults with mild kidney disease have a 23% higher odds ratio (OR) of developing cognitive impairment, and this OR increases to 68% among individuals with moderate kidney disease [5]. In studies of CKD, the prevalence of mild cognitive impairment (mild neurocognitive disorder) ranges from 27% to 62%, versus 11% to 26% in matched controls, while the prevalence of major neurocognitive disorder (dementia) approaches 10%. In end-stage renal disease (ESRD), the proportion with major neurocognitive disorder rises to 20–37% of patients [6].

The cognitive impairment in CKD, as in vascular cognitive impairment, is dominated by impairments in executive function, with memory and other domains declining modestly or not at all [7]. Thus, CKD-associated cognitive impairment can be missed by clinicians and even family. In a sample of hemodialysis patients aged 55 and older, 70% had moderate to severe cognitive impairment, but only 3% carried a diagnosis of a neurocognitive disorder [8].

Executive skills are paramount for decisional capacity. A patient must be able to *reason* and apply *judgment* in order to weigh the benefits and harms of an intervention such as dialysis and arrive at a decision. *Organization* and *planning* are more subtle intellectual skills, but are required for adults to act independently and manage their affairs. *Attention* and *speed of mental processing* indirectly impact decisional capacity by affecting the patient's ability to absorb and interpret information that is being presented, increasing the risk of poor or snap decisions that do not reflect the patient's actual enduring preferences.

In addition to their high major neurocognitive disorder/dementia risk, renal patients are a high-risk population for delirium, owing to comorbid systemic illness (e.g., diabetes mellitus, systemic lupus erythematosus) and high-risk medication use (e.g., corticosteroids, immunosuppressants).

Patients who have ESRD and are candidates for renal transplant surgery face specific decisional capacity challenges. Qualification for renal transplant surgery involves an ongoing, iterative, and dynamic determination of candidacy. Beyond the psychological determination of behavioral compliance with the transplant workup and preoperative care and organization of appropriate social resources to the postoperative recovery period, patients must demonstrate a programmatic commitment to postoperative care, lifelong immunosuppressants, and adherence to all medications and clinical monitoring. Beyond these important behavioral and programmatic considerations, renal transplant surgery requires demonstration of decisional capacity for the transplant operation itself.

Patients who have ESRD and who are not appropriate candidates for renal transplant are routinely offered hemodialysis or peritoneal dialysis. In this context, the patient's decisional capacity to accept or forgo dialysis (as a discrete medical procedure with its own risk/benefits/side effects) may need formal determination. This is especially likely to surface with an acutely uremic presentation when the patient is delirious and thus unable to participate in the informed consent process. Acutely delirious presentations are well-known to have widely fluctuating cognitive status and, thus, correspondingly fluctuating decisional capacity at the time of presentation.

An often uncomfortable and existentially dramatic circumstance occurs when an established, ongoing dialysis patient comes to the conclusion that he/she does not want to continue the life-sustaining treatment and, assuming that he/she is not a candidate for renal transplant surgery, accepts death as a predictable consequence of discontinuing dialysis. Assessment for decisional capacity for dialysis refusal and its lethal consequences should be explored in detail and specifically documented, as the patient will promptly become uremic and delirious if dialysis is withheld.

8.6 Clinical Approaches to Decisional Capacity Determinations

While any physician can (and implicitly does, even if often using a more intuitive and less structured clinical methodology) determine decisional capacity, formal decisional capacity determinations are a common practice in consultation-liaison psychiatry consultations. While the clinical focus of a decisional or dispositional capacity consult is ultimately on the capacity decision, it is important for the psychiatrist *not* to "focus solely on the capacity question." This is especially important in that many neuropsychiatric illnesses that may impair decisional capacity (e.g., delirium, psychotic disorders, severe major depressive disorder) are in fact *reversible*, so with appropriate psychiatric treatment, a "capacity impaired" patient may become a "capacity restored" patient.

The first element in responding to a decisional capacity consultation is to determine if the case is one of decisional capacity, dispositional capacity, or both. In the case of *decisional* capacity, the psychiatrist must know what the proposed medical/surgical intervention is and be able to understand the risks/benefits/side effects of the proposed intervention and to understand if the patient's understanding and appreciation are those of a "typical patient." The patient must be able, in common language, to understand both their illness and the proposed intervention, how the intervention applies to their specific illness course, and how the course of illness might be modified by virtue of the proposed intervention, compared to the natural history of the illness without the proposed intervention.

In the case of *dispositional* capacity, the psychiatrist should make routine (if not universal) use of secondary consultants in occupational therapy, physical therapy, and social work to ascertain by standard methodology whether the patient can demonstrate adequate performance at self-care skills (especially the context of their medical illnesses) and whether they can show how they would obtain needed social and supportive resources.

The psychiatric interview should include routine ascertainment of neurocognitive, psychotic, bipolar depressive, anxiety, or other psychiatric illnesses. Thorough workup to elucidate psychiatric illness (e.g., neuroimaging and laboratory studies for delirium and major neurocognitive disorder/dementia) with proposed clinical interventions is essential. Especially in cases where management of an acute psychiatric syndrome that is contemporaneously impairing decisional capacity, the psychiatrist should specify the current decisional capacity status, but propose clinical intervention that, if followed, may reverse impaired decisional capacity to a condition of intact decisional capacity.

It is state of the art for consultation-liaison psychiatric practice to supplement the routine clinical interview with a standardized cognitive assessment, such as the MMSE or MoCA. Though not designed to be solely or specifically determinative of decisional capacity per se, MoCA or MMSE scores < 19 correlate with impaired decisional capacity, while scores > 23 correlate with intact decisional capacity [4, 9]. At the very least, the psychiatrist should be more confident with a determination of "decisional capacity no" with a MoCA score well below 19.

8.7 Bioethical Approaches to Decisional Capacity Determinations in Psychonephrology

Patients with renal disease confront a spectrum of decisions that span a range of complexity, from straightforward decisions about accepting a new medication to a decision to pursue a renal transplant that requires an understanding of the pros and cons of multiple, interrelated, issues like the consequences of immunosuppression, the risk of surgery itself, lifestyle changes, impact on comorbidities like diabetes mellitus, transportation to specialists, and so on. To successfully navigate this web of issues requires sophisticated reasoning and planning, elements of executive function that are commonly impaired as the patient progresses to the advanced stages of CKD. Furthermore, progression of neurocognitive decline does not stop with transplant, peritoneal dialysis, or hemodialysis. One-fifth of renal transplant recipients and one-third of peritoneal dialysis patients develop a major neurocognitive disorder, losing the ability to self-manage their medical problems [6]. This raises ethical questions about offering them a treatment that, in retrospect, may have been inappropriate.

It is unknown what percentage of CKD patients make decisions based on an incomplete understanding of the information presented and instead follow the recommendations of their physicians, family members, or their own misinterpretation of the facts. Current medical ethics are governed by four major principles: autonomy, beneficence, non-maleficence, and social justice [10]. Beneficence (taking a course of action that is most likely to benefit the patient) and non-maleficence (avoiding the probable exposure of the patient to unwanted harm) formerly dominated medical ethics, but are now considered somewhat paternalistic and have been replaced by an emphasis on autonomy – doing what the patient desires as long as it is medically feasible.

If the patient's preferences align with the physician recommendations, it is easy for the physician to assume that the patient has decisional capacity when, in fact, it might be impaired. For example, a nephrologist who wishes to avoid offering hemodialysis because of the patient's rural location may welcome their wish for home peritoneal dialysis and fail to recognize that they do not understand the implications of an overnight dwell time or that they depend on the spouse, who has myelodysplastic syndrome, to hook up the dialysis catheter every night. At some point the patient will be forced to be self-reliant when the spouse is hospitalized or dies, but may not have the requisite executive skills. In this setting, the principle of non-maleficence rises to the top because of the probability that the patient will be unable to correctly perform their own peritoneal dialysis and will become uremic or develop repeated episodes of acute peritonitis. Despite the patient's strong desire for peritoneal dialysis and their willingness to accept the risk of complications, they may not be a suitable candidate.

As advocates for their own patients, clinicians generally should avoid letting societal concerns (social justice) intrude on their ethical decision-making. However, social justice sometimes overlaps with non-maleficence and beneficence. For example, avoidance of a high probability of repeat peritonitis overlaps with a desire to conserve precious health resources consumed by recurrent hospitalizations. Autonomy to make decisions about a course of action or procedure quintessentially demands commensurate executive skills, and it is essential that these be regularly assessed.

Clinical Pearl

- In chronic kidney disease, executive function (organization, planning, judgment, reasoning) may be lost relatively early in the disease before memory, attention, and orientation and will impact the patient's decision-making capacity.

Cognitive assessment, even multi-hour, in-depth neuropsychological evaluation, employs standardized tests with strong psychometric properties that reliably indicate that the test is evaluating a particular cognitive domain. The assumption is that abnormal test results can be extrapolated to the patient's everyday life and ability to make sound healthcare decisions. Clinicians still may be skeptical that a test like the timed Trail Making Test Part B, for which the patient is asked to connect as fast as possible alternating numbers and letters scattered across a page, represents a reliable indicator of broad executive skills. For this reason, multiple tests of a cognitive domain are characteristically administered as confirmation – for example, following the Trails B with a clock-drawing test. Most studies that have evaluated cognitive performance in CKD have used extensive batteries of neurocognitive tests that are impractical for the office setting. Formal neuropsychological testing by a trained neuropsychologist is expensive and not always accessible to the patient.

Common office instruments for mental status evaluation like the Folstein Mini Mental State Examination omit tests of executive function. The Montreal Cognitive Assessment (MoCA) is a time-efficient, office-based cognitive assessment that includes tests of executive function, along with tests of visuospatial skills, memory, language, naming, attention, abstraction, orientation, and delayed recall. Although copyrighted, its use does not require a fee, and it can be downloaded online [11]. In 43 hemodialysis patients and 42 controls, the MoCA showed a sensitivity and specificity of 77% and 79%, respectively, for detecting cognitive impairment when using a cut-off score of $\leq$ 24 out of 30 [12]. Results for the sensitivity and specificity of the MoCA's executive subtests are not available. However, it can be assumed that executive dyscontrol may be missed in a small percentage of patients and that another small percentage may be mislabeled as having executive impairment when they do not. The MoCA also will detect impairment in short-term memory and other domains that may impact self-management of CKD and other comorbidities. It is recommended that the MoCA be repeated at regular intervals, such as annually when CKD is mild to moderate (eGFR 30–59 mL/minute/1,73m^2) and at least semi-annually when severe (eGFR < 30 mL/minute/1.73 m^2).

In balance, using a validated cognitive screen like the MoCA will provide a reasonable assessment of the patient's decisional capacity. The results can be used to balance the ethical principles of autonomy, beneficence, and non-maleficence in making healthcare decisions.

Recommendation

- Evaluate decisional capacity using a time-efficient, validated cognitive screen that assesses executive function in addition to visuospatial skills, memory, language, naming, attention, abstraction, and orientation. An example of such a tool is the Montreal Cognitive Assessment (MoCA).
- Integrate decisional capacity determination into a comprehensive interview, paying attention to neurocognitive disorders.

8.8 Case Vignettes and Analyses

This section presents some patient clinical examples of decisional capacity determination in psychonephrology.

8.8.1 Case Vignette 1: Request for Discharge Against Medical Advice

A patient was a 25-year-old female with chronic systemic lupus erythematosus who presented to the hospital with acute renal failure and delirium. She was confused, irritable, and angry and demanded to leave the hospital "because I know my lupus, it's just a part of me, I am not that sick." A psychiatric consultation was ordered to determine decisional capacity for the patient to leave the hospital against medical advice (dispositional capacity determination). On interview, she had a fluctuating level of consciousness, largely disorganized speech, and a MoCA score of 10/30, and she could not tell the physician how she would take care of herself, as well as denying the seriousness of her illness. An occupational therapy assessment revealed severe impairment in basic activities of daily living skills. She was diagnosed with delirium with impaired decisional capacity to leave the hospital against medical advice.

8.8.2 Case Vignette 2: Request for Changing Treatment to Renal Transplant

The patient was a 45-year-old male with ESRD due to diabetes mellitus who has been on hemodialysis for 2 years. He was variably compliant with hemodialysis and on several occasions has presented with delirium due to acute uremia. He said he wanted to get a renal transplant "so I do not have to do this no more" and that if he got a renal transplant "I will be a normal person again." He could only state that "I could die" regarding possible risks of renal transplant surgery but could not describe graft failure, bleeding, infection, or wound dehiscence as possibilities. On exam, he had a fluctuating level of consciousness and MoCA of 15/30, with poor attention, recall, and orientation. He was diagnosed with delirium due to uremia, rule out vascular dementia due to diabetes mellitus, with impaired decisional capacity for consent for renal transplant.

8.8.3 Case Vignette 3: Request for Hemodialysis Discontinuation

The patient was a 65-year-old male with ESRD on hemodialysis for 5 years. While he initially did well and even somewhat enjoyed the thrice weekly dialysis treatments, attaching well to the dialysis center and becoming friends with other patients, he had done much worse in the previous year. Due to comorbid heart failure, he had had several hospitalizations with increasingly limited functional status. He told his nephrologist that "I appreciate what you have done for me, but, really, I have had enough. I am fatigued and pessimistic and realize that even if I continue dialysis, I know the heart failure will take me pretty soon." On psychiatric interview, he had mild vascular dementia (MoCA of 20/30) and mildly dysphoric affect but was not actively suicidal nor depressed. He was able reasonably to understand how he would die from uremia with hypoactive delirium within a week of discontinuing dialysis and transition to comfort care. He was found to have intact decisional capacity to discontinue dialysis.

8.8.4 Case Vignette 4: Request for Other Organ Transplant

The patient was a 55-year-old female with history of chronic glomerulonephritis. She was admitted to the hospital with delirium from an acetaminophen overdose, requiring N-acetylcysteine to mitigate liver failure. A psychiatric consultation was requested to "see if she is still suicidal" and "to determine decisional capacity if she needs a transplant." On exam, she had a fluctuating level of consciousness, MoCA score of 8/30, and denied memory of the suicide attempt or current suicidal ideation. When told of the seriousness of her condition, she had poor understanding of her illness and could only say "I would consider it" if an orthotopic liver transplantation were to be recommended, and could not understand predictable surgical risks. She was diagnosed with delirium due to liver failure, major depressive disorder, and borderline personality disorder.

8.9 Key Takeaways

- Decisional capacity determinations are an inherent part of the practice of psychonephrology.
- Specific areas in psychonephrology where decisional capacity (including dispositional capacity) determinations are common include:
  - Preoperative decisional capacity for renal transplant surgery.
  - Evaluation of decisional capacity to both accept and discontinue dialysis.
  - Decisional capacity determinations in delirium presentations.
- Dementia is common in renal patients, as is depressive disorder, and these common neuropsychiatric comorbid illnesses may have differential contributions to decisional incapacity.
- Structured decisional capacity determinations are a part of a comprehensive consultation-liaison psychiatry consultation and require formal standardized cognitive assessment.
- In the case of dispositional capacity determinations, the psychiatric interview can be supplemented by in vivo demonstration of adequate activities of daily living and social function with supplemental assessments by occupational therapy, physical therapy, and social work.
- Collaborative approaches between the nephrologist and psychiatrist are recommended for comprehensive assessment and optimal patient care.

References

1. Appelbaum PS, Grisso T. Assessing patients' capacities to consent to treatment. N Engl J Med. 1988;319(25):1635–8.
2. Bourgeois JA, Cohen MA, Erickson JM, Weintraub BR. Decisional and dispositional capacity determinations: the role of neuropsychiatric illness and an integrated clinical paradigm. Psychosomatics. 2017;58:565–73.
3. Boettger S, Bergman M, Jenewein J, Boettger S. Assessment of decisional capacity: prevalence of medical illness and psychiatric comorbidities. Palliat Support Care. 2015;13(5):1275–81.
4. Walaszek A. Clinical ethics issues in geriatric psychiatry. Psychiatr Clin North Am. 2009;32(2):343–59.
5. Etgen T, Chonchol M, Forstl H, Sander D. Chronic kidney disease and cognitive impairment: a systematic review and meta-analysis. Am J Nephrol. 2012;35(5):474–82.
6. Viggiano D, Wagner CA, Martino G, Nedergaard M, Zoccali C, Unwin R, et al. Mechanisms of cognitive dysfunction in CKD. Nat Rev Nephrol. 2020;16(8):452–69.

7. Yaffe K, Ackerson L, Kurella Tamura M, Le Blanc P, Kusek JW, Sehgal AR, et al. Chronic kidney disease and cognitive function in older adults: findings from the chronic renal insufficiency cohort cognitive study. J Am Geriatr Soc. 2010;58(2):338–45.
8. Murray AM, Tupper DE, Knopman DS, Gilbertson DT, Pederson SL, Li S, et al. Cognitive impairment in hemodialysis patients is common. Neurology. 2006;67(2):216–23.
9. Karlawish J. Measuring decision-making capacity in cognitively impaired individuals. Neurosignals. 2008;16(1):91–8. Published online 2007 Dec 5.
10. Gillon R. Defending the four principles approach as a good basis for good medical practice and therefore for good medical ethics. J Med Ethics. 2015;41(1):111–6.
11. Nasreddine Z. MoCA Test Montreal. Québec: MoCA Test, Inc.; 2019. Available from: https://www.mocatest.org
12. Tiffin-Richards FE, Costa AS, Holschbach B, Frank RD, Vassiliadou A, Krüger T, et al. The Montreal cognitive assessment (MoCA) - a sensitive screening instrument for detecting cognitive impairment in chronic hemodialysis patients. PLoS One. 2014;9(10):e106700.

Consultation-Liaison Psychiatry and Collaborative Care Models of the Patient with Renal Disease

9

Briana S. Howarth, James A. Bourgeois, and Nick Kates

9.1 Introduction

Psychiatric illness is common in patients with chronic kidney disease (CKD) [1]. The prevalence of psychiatric illness in a randomly selected group of patients with end-stage renal disease (ESRD) in a hemodialysis unit was investigated [2]. More than 70% of these patients met the criteria for a psychiatric disorder. Depressive disorders were most common (prevalence rate of 29%), followed by anxiety disorders (27%), substance use disorders (19%), and psychotic disorders (10%). CKD with comorbid psychiatric illness often results in higher rates of hospitalization and increased all-cause mortality [3].

Depressive disorders are the most common psychiatric illnesses in CKD, and the impact of depression on quality of life, morbidity, and mortality is profound [4]. Depression that coexists with a chronic medical condition can have a negative

B. S. Howarth (✉)
Geriatric & Consultation Liaison Psychiatry, Halton Healthcare, Oakville, ON, Canada

Department of Psychiatry & Behavioural Neurosciences, McMaster University, Hamilton, ON, Canada
e-mail: bhowarth@haltonhealthcare.com

J. A. Bourgeois
Department of Psychiatry, Baylor Scott & White Health, Central Texas Division, Department of Medical Education, College of Medicine, Texas A&M University Health Science Center, Temple, TX, USA
e-mail: james.bourgeois@BSWHealth.org

N. Kates
Department of Psychiatry and Behavioural Neurosciences, Michael G. DeGroote School of Medicine, McMaster University, Hamilton, ON, Canada
e-mail: nkates@mcmaster.ca

A. Hategan et al. (eds.), *Psychonephrology*,
https://doi.org/10.1007/978-3-030-84740-1_9

impact on patient activation, which is important for self-management, resulting in worse clinical outcomes [5]. In CKD specifically, depression's negative impact has been attributed to alterations in adherence to medications and renal replacement therapy, changes in nutritional status, and an increased risk of self-harm and suicide attempts [6]. This is even more concerning because depression is often under-recognized and undertreated in patients with CKD.

In one sample of patients with ESRD, 80% who identified having comorbid psychotic illness reported receiving psychiatric treatment compared to only 12% of those with comorbid anxiety or depression [2]. This is a multifactorial issue. Depressive symptoms and uremic symptoms overlap, complicating the ability to identify depressive illness. With the recognition that most patients with mild to moderate CKD receive their care within primary care setting, one must also consider the challenges primary care physicians face due to the other demands on their time. Within specialist clinics, care may be fragmented with a focus on CKD management including management of hypertension and diabetes mellitus as the two most prevalent contributors to CKD, but often overlooking for and managing comorbid psychiatric illness. There may also be a misconception on the part of clinicians providing care to patients with CKD that depression and anxiety are simply part of the ESRD experience, rather than discrete comorbid illnesses that need to be fully evaluated and treated.

Clinical Pearl

- Depression is the most common comorbid psychiatric condition in patients with CKD.
- Recognition of comorbid depression can have profound impacts on morbidity and mortality for these patients if recognized and treated.

9.1.1 Case Vignette 1

Mr. S was a 72-year-old male admitted to a medical surgical unit with acute on chronic renal failure. He had ESRD secondary to diabetic nephropathy. He had a history of major depressive disorder with psychotic features and was on a combination of venlafaxine XR 225 mg po daily and aripiprazole 5 mg po daily. Despite correction of acute renal failure, with restoration of baseline renal function and eGFR of 10 mL/min/1.73 m^2, he complained of persistently low energy and nausea, which were negatively impacting his ability to work with the physiotherapy team in the hospital.

Questions to consider are as follows:

- What is your differential diagnosis for Mr. S's complaints of low energy and nausea?
- What is the role of the consultation-liaison psychiatrist in Mr. S's care?

We will return to this case later in this chapter for further analysis.

9.2 The Chronic Care Model

The issues discussed previously underscore the difficulties with managing chronic conditions such as CKD and moving from reactive to proactive care. The focus on acuity and urgency, "putting out fires," is often accompanied by a reduced emphasis on prevention and relapse prevention in between acute episodes nor on self-management, thereby resulting in suboptimal care for patients with CKD. The chronic care model (CCM), as developed by Wagner (2019), provides direction for restructuring models of care for patients living with CKD [7]. The six components of the CCM promote and support clinical interactions between an activated and informed patient and the organized, collaborative, and proactive care team (see Table 9.1). Collaborative care, whereby a mental health professional is part of the care time either on the same site or indirectly, has demonstrated clear benefits in the identification and management of psychiatric illness in patients with comorbid non-psychiatric medical illness in both specialty and primary care practices [8, 9].

The CCM is a framework designed to improve care for patients living with chronic illness like CKD and was born out of concern over inadequate management of patients living with chronic illness, particularly hypertension and diabetes mellitus [10–12]. Research in chronic illness management had identified shortcomings in the management of patients with chronic illness, with delays in the detection of complications or declines in health status. Morbidity in chronic illness was often attributable to failures in self-management, support with inadequate patient education, and

Table 9.1 The main components of the chronic care model

Category		Description
1	Delivery system design	Roles of team members are clearly defined
		Tasks are clearly delegated
		Interventions focus on providing evidence-based care
		Reliance on other health discipline clinicians
2	Self-management support	Promotion of behavioral change and psychosocial support
		Enhancing patients' participation in their care
		Enhancing patients' confidence in their own management
		Patient activation
3	Decision support	Clinical expertise – Collaborative care
		Focus on stepped-care approaches and treatment algorithms
		Care for chronic medical conditions and psychiatric conditions, which is evidence based
		Well-organized and prepared multidisciplinary team
4	Clinical information systems	Supportive information technology
		Patient tracking, proactive scheduling of team meetings, following of evidence-based guidelines and algorithms
5	Health systems	Organization of health care
		Quality of care
6	Community	Nonprofit, governmental, faith-based organizations
		Research and advocacy for better patient outcomes

patient activation [13]. This was mostly due to the healthcare system being structured around acute care management. Patient needs were prioritized based on *urgency* rather than *chronicity/severity* and were reactive rather than proactive, which meant that the nuance of managing patients with chronic illness was often missed.

Recommendation

- When providing psychiatric care to patients with CKD, activating the patient to be an active participant in their psychiatric and nephrology care will have benefits for both their mental and physical health.

The original CCM, as developed by Wagner, identified six categories of intervention, which demonstrated the most benefit for the management of patients with chronic illness, as outlined below [10]:

(i) Delivery system design
(ii) Self-management support
(iii) Decision support
(iv) Clinical information systems
(v) Health systems
(vi) Community

The CCM is extremely applicable in the management of CKD. The prevalence of CKD is steadily increasing due to the aging population and the increasing prevalence of both hypertension and diabetes mellitus. Due to the increasing prevalence and improved identification of patients with mild-moderate CKD in primary care settings, the focus has shifted to developing care models that improve renal, cardiovascular, and psychiatric outcomes. In line with the CCM, many studies have identified that management of CKD has improved outcomes when care between primary care and specialist clinics is better coordinated, including the delegation of tasks to other health professionals, primarily nurses and nurse practitioners, with a focus on patient self-management and clinical decision support [14].

Clinical Pearl

- Patients with CKD have improved outcomes when care between primary care and specialist clinics is coordinated with delegation of tasks to other health professionals.
- These outcomes are further enhanced when a focus is put on patient self-management and patient activation.

Chen et al. conducted an open-label randomized controlled trial to determine the impact of self-management support on the care of patients with CKD [15]. Self-management support consisted of education for patients, delivery of health information, and the availability of support via telephone. The results demonstrated significant improvements in outcomes in terms of increased eGFR and reduced hospital admissions in patients receiving self-management support.

Clinicians can learn from the success of the CCM that can be applied to models of care for patients with CKD when it comes to management of comorbid psychiatric conditions. In patients with CKD, the presence of comorbid psychiatric conditions increases healthcare resource utilization and healthcare costs [16]. Patients with comorbid psychiatric and nonpsychiatric chronic medical conditions are more likely to be of lower socioeconomic status, to have multiple chronic illnesses, and to have an increased risk of overall mortality [16]. We know that in CKD the comorbidity with depressive disorder significantly increases morbidity and mortality, while the increased resource utilization and healthcare costs can largely be attributed to excessive relative reliance on acute care due to reduced access to coordinated care and collaborative mental health care [16]. Collaborative psychiatric care has also been shown to increase the detection and management of psychiatric illness in primary care and specialist practices [8, 9, 17].

9.2.1 Case Vignette 1 (Continued)

Mr. S was later discharged from the hospital. The consultation-liaison psychiatrist was concerned with the dose of venlafaxine XR, given his eGFR, and initiated a gentle down-taper of venlafaxine XR to 150 mg daily. He continued to take aripiprazole 5 mg daily. The low energy and persistent nausea were attributed to uremia. Mr. S was instructed to follow up with his primary care physician, nephrologist, and psychiatrist upon discharge from hospital. When he saw his primary care physician, the nausea had worsened considerably, and he was having passive suicidal ideation.

Question to consider is as follows:

- How could Mr. S's care have been restructured in order to better support the management of both ESRD and major depressive disorder?

We will return to this case later in this chapter for further analysis.

9.3 Collaborative Care and Consultation-Liaison Psychiatry

The definitions outlined in Table 9.2 provide context to the following discussion of collaborative care and consultation-liaison psychiatry [18, 19]. Psychiatric illness is often underdiagnosed and undertreated in patients with comorbid chronic nonpsychiatric medical illness such as CKD. This is further complicated by the fact that patients with depressive disorders can often present with somatic symptoms, especially in older adults, who make up the majority of people with CKD. Out of his work as a consultation-liaison psychiatrist, Katon identified this dilemma and strove to help nonpsychiatric physicians learn to identify psychiatric illness in patients with comorbid chronic nonpsychiatric medical illness [20]. However, simply increasing the rate of accurate diagnosis and initiating treatment for depressive disorders were not sufficient to improve care for patients with depressive disorder in

Table 9.2 Definitions of consultation-liaison psychiatry, shared care, collaborative care, and integrated care

Consultation-liaison psychiatry	Formerly termed "psychosomatic medicine"
	Psychiatrists working at the interface of psychiatry and medicine
	Psychiatry services available to patients admitted to medical/surgical wards as well as some outpatient clinic settings
Shared care	Approach to care which uses skills and knowledge of different clinicians – Usually physicians – To provide better coordinated care to patients with comorbid conditions
Collaborative care	Primary care physician and/or specialist and mental health clinicians share resources, expertise, knowledge, and decision-making wherever they may be working to ensure patients receive effective care from the right clinician in the most convenient location and in a timely and well-coordinated manner
Integrated care	Co-location of primary care physician/specialist and psychiatric clinicians using systematic approach to provide care to a defined population with realigning of distribution, delivery, management, and organization of services to develop comprehensive care

the primary care setting. To achieve this, care needs to be systematic and evidence based, with enhancement of behavioral strategies to involve patients in their own care, which is where collaborative care can play an important role.

9.3.1 Case Vignette 2

Mrs. I was a 73-year-old female with a major depressive episode, precipitated by the sudden death of her husband who had a major neurocognitive disorder and for whom she had been the primary caretaker. Mrs. I had been referred for geriatric psychiatry consultation by the geriatric medicine outpatient clinic. Her medical history was significant for osteoarthritis, non-insulin-dependent diabetes mellitus, hypertension, and CKD. Her medication list included metformin, ramipril, hydrochlorothiazide, and acetaminophen. After diagnosing her with a major depressive episode, the geriatric psychiatrist prescribed sertraline 25 mg po daily for 14 days, to be increased to 50 mg po daily, and asked Mrs. I to follow up in 1 month.

Mrs. I presented to her primary care physician 2 weeks before the scheduled geriatric psychiatry appointment, with progressive worsening of her mood accompanied by low energy, with significant fatigue and lethargy, as well as new signs of cognitive impairment. On assessment, she was alert, though inattentive, and she was oriented to person, but not to place or time. The physician attempted to accomplish an Mini-Mental Status Exam (MMSE) test, but Mrs. I was unable to tolerate the exam. Mrs. I's physician reached out to the geriatric psychiatrist urgently for assistance and asked whether the dose of sertraline should be increased given her worsened mood.

Questions to consider are as follows:

- What is the most likely explanation for Mrs. I's current presentation?
- What investigations must be ordered?

We will return to this case later in this chapter for further analysis.

9.3.2 Collaborative Care

The American Psychiatric Association released a report in 2016, *Dissemination of Integrated Care Within Adult Primary Care Settings* [21]. This report has a useful four-pronged approach as outlined below and is based on Katon's original work [20].

(i) **Collaborative mental health care is *team-based care*.** Teams are often led by primary care clinicians and consist of consultant psychiatrists and care managers.
(ii) **Collaborative mental health care is *population based*.** Collaborative mental health care is not formulaic. It must be adapted to fit the population served by that primary care clinician, thus providing broad applicability, and needs to focus on those not being seen as well as those receiving care.
(iii) **Collaborative mental health care is *measurement-guided care*.** Proactive follow-up with evidence-based tools for determining response to treatment is essential. Integral to this is the concept of treating to target.
(iv) **Collaborative mental health care is *evidence based*.** Drawing on decision support, as outlined by Wagner [10], collaborative mental health care is efficient due to its reliance on evidence-based care, following of guidelines and treatment algorithms, and the use of evidence-based tools for screening and assessing treatment response.

Drawing upon these four principles, several studies have demonstrated that the collaborative care model can improve the detection and treatment of depressive disorders in patients with chronic nonpsychiatric medical illness in both primary care and specialty settings. The Improving Mood-Promoting Access to Collaborative Treatment (IMPACT) study is one of the best-known studies demonstrating this result. The IMPACT study used collaborative care, with a stepped approach to improve the recognition and management of depression in older adults in primary care setting. They demonstrated not only clinically significant symptom improvement but also improved functioning and physical activity, with a reduced risk of myocardial infarction and stroke in the 1 year after completion of the study [9, 22].

Recommendation
- When providing psychiatric care to patients with CKD, utilize appropriate treatment guidelines and a stepped-based care approach to optimize treatment response.

Katon developed another collaborative care program, the Pathways study, for patients with comorbid diabetes mellitus and depressive disorders who were managed in primary care settings [17]. This demonstrated improved outcomes for both depressive disorder and diabetes mellitus, as measured by statistically significant changes in HbA1C over time. Although improvement in depressive symptoms was seen for patients with comorbid depressive disorders and diabetes mellitus, improvement in depressive symptoms alone did not result in improvement in diabetes outcomes. Implementing an active care plan with clear treatment goals for diabetes mellitus and comorbid depressive symptoms is likely to result in improvement in diabetes mellitus, and this is addressed by the collaborative care model.

The collaborative care model will enhance the management of comorbid psychiatric illness and nonpsychiatric medical illnesses like coronary artery disease and CKD, which are common in patients with diabetes mellitus [23]. Through the IMPACT trial, we know that collaborative mental health care is effective when managing psychiatric symptoms in patients with complex comorbid medical conditions but is also effective in managing other aspects of their medical conditions such as blood sugar control and blood pressure management. In complex patients, such as those living with CKD, competing demands and fragmentation of care can have an impact not only on the assessment and management of these comorbid psychiatric conditions but also on the management of comorbid systemic medical conditions such as diabetes mellitus and hypertension. Collaborative care with a team-based, care management approach can address not only comorbid psychiatric conditions but also the management of all chronic conditions, optimizing self-management support around aspects of care such as medication adherence, blood pressure monitoring, and blood sugar monitoring [22]. This approach may have been particularly beneficial for both Mr. S and Mrs. I in case vignettes 1 and 2, respectively, where fragmented care may have contributed to their relatively poorer psychiatric outcomes.

9.3.3 Case Vignette 3

Ms. V was an 83-year-old female with bipolar I disorder. She had been on lithium carbonate for more than 30 years with good control of her manic symptoms. Lithium was discontinued after she developed ESRD with a baseline eGFR of 15 mL/min/1.73 m^2. Discontinuation of lithium precipitated an episode of mania with psychotic features for which she was admitted to an inpatient psychiatry unit. She was started on valproic acid 1500 mg po qhs and olanzapine 20 mg po qhs and discharged. She re-presented to hospital 4 weeks later with a decreased level of consciousness, confusion, and gait ataxia. Bloodwork done in the emergency department showed that the creatinine level had now increased to 436 umol/L (4.93 mg/dL), eGFR was 10 mL/min/1.73 m^2, and serum sodium had increased to 156 mmol/L. Consultation-liaison psychiatry was asked to see Ms. V to rule out delirium.

Questions to consider are as follows:

- What is the differential diagnosis for her presentation of confusion and gait ataxia?
- What is the significance of her elevated serum sodium? What else would you recommend ordering to narrow the differential?

- How might Ms. V's outcomes change if her psychiatric care were co-located with her nephrology care?

We will return to this case later in this chapter for further analysis.

9.3.4 Consultation-Liaison Psychiatry

Consultation-liaison psychiatry is an antecedent of collaborative mental health care. Commonly thought to be the psychiatric care available to inpatients admitted with medical/surgical illness, it in fact encompasses psychiatrists (in both inpatient and outpatient settings) operating at the intersection of medicine and psychiatry. Consultation-liaison psychiatry has formerly been known as "psychosomatic medicine" or "medical psychiatry." But today it is the preferred name as it underscores the critical role consultation-liaison psychiatrists play in integrating psychiatric care into medical-surgical inpatient units and also outpatient medical clinics like nephrology clinics and hemodialysis units [24]. Recognizing this, the Academy of Psychosomatic Medicine changed its name to Academy of Consultation-Liaison Psychiatry in 2017 [25].

With the high prevalence of psychiatric illness in patients with CKD, most nephrology programs are attached to a consultation liaison psychiatry team [24]. There are many roles of the consultation-liaison psychiatrist in these settings (Table 9.3) [19]. The consultation-liaison psychiatrist plays a critical role in helping nephrology teams build their capacity to recognize many psychiatric conditions and their impact on the morbidity of patients with CKD. This includes increasing their knowledge of and ability to recognize common symptoms, simple management strategies, broadening their awareness of community resources and programs, and providing information and resources they can impart to patients to assist them with managing their own condition. This is much easier in a collaborative relationship, where clinicians know they have easy access to support and guidance from mental health professionals and assistance in accessing services.

Table 9.3 Roles of the consultation-liaison psychiatrist to renal patients [19]

Role	Description
Consultation	Assessment and management of psychiatric sequelae to medical conditions
	Diagnosis of psychiatric conditions in the presence of comorbid medical conditions
	Identification and management of drug interactions between psychotropic and non-psychotropic medications
	Psychopharmacological management in comorbid medical conditions
	Effect of non-psychotropic medications on psychiatric conditions
Liaison	Education to nephrology team
	Building capacity with nephrology team to enhance recognition and management of psychiatric conditions
	Advocacy for patients with psychiatric conditions
	Assistance with "difficult" scenarios; e.g., treatment refusal, withdrawal of renal replacement therapy, assessment of decisional capacity

9.4 Collaborative Mental Health Care for CKD Patients

As illustrated throughout this chapter, psychiatric illness is common in patients living with CKD but is under-recognized and undertreated, resulting in increased morbidity and mortality for these patients. Collaborative mental health care has been demonstrated to improve the recognition and management of psychiatric illness in individuals with comorbid medical conditions, and team-based care is a critical component of collaborative mental health care.

The Technology Assisted stepped Collaborative Care Intervention (TACcare) trial [26] is a multicenter randomized controlled trial that is investigating the impact of a short-term collaborative intervention of cognitive behavioral therapy (CBT) and/or psychopharmacology for symptoms of fatigue, depression, and pain in hemodialysis patients. A stepped-care approach, individualizing treatment to patients' needs, implemented and monitored by a care manager was undertaken. Care managers are a critical component of collaborative care as they act as the liaison between patient and other health-care professionals, bridging the activated patient and a well-organized multidisciplinary team.

Recognizing the potential limits of accessing mental health professionals given high demands, collaborative care lends itself well to virtual modes of care. The TACcare trial is unique in that the behavioral component of the intervention is partly delivered by video conference to the hemodialysis unit directly. Primary outcome measures are changes in depression, fatigue, and pain as ascertained by the Beck Depression Inventory-II (BDI-II), Functional Assessment of Chronic Illness Therapy – Fatigue (FACIT-F), and Brief Pain Inventory (BPI) short form. Final results are pending at the time of writing this chapter, but this is an innovative and promising application of collaborative care to improve the management of psychiatric disorders in patients with ESRD. Within the hemodialysis population, other studies have been conducted looking at how collaborative care can improve patient activation, which, as discussed previously, may in turn improve mental health outcomes.

ShareHD is a study in progress investigating the impact of shared hemodialysis care on patient activation and in turn the patient's experience of care, quality of life, and medical outcomes [5]. Patients are educated and activated by the health-care team to be active participants in their hemodialysis. Overall, patients report an improved experience of care, greater independence, and a greater sense of control.

In summary, collaborative care should be an important part of the management of patients with CKD including ESRD. Based upon recent research, its wider implementation will likely result in improved detection and management of comorbid psychiatric illness.

9.5 Case Vignette Analyses

9.5.1 Case Vignette 1

The case of Mr. S demonstrated the broad differential one must take when an individual with CKD presents with depressive symptoms. The differential diagnosis includes major depressive disorder, depressive disorder due to another medical condition (uremia), delirium, and side effects of high-dose venlafaxine XR in the context of reduced eGFR. The consultation-liaison psychiatrist's first role is in the diagnostic assessment of psychiatric illness bearing in mind the contribution of comorbid acute medical processes. Second, psychiatric treatment can be modified bearing in mind acute medical processes (e.g., renal dose adjustment of venlafaxine XR). Third, but likely most important, is the liaison with allied health team to support Mr. S's participation with physiotherapy, for example, creation of a behavioral care plan or direction on how to effectively communicate with Mr. S and how to promote behavioral activation. How could Mr. S's care be restructured in order to better support the management of both ESRD and the major depressive disorder? A collaborative approach that is team based, measurement guided, evidence based, and population focused has been demonstrated to provide earlier recognition of problems and more effective mental health care to patients with comorbid psychiatric and chronic medical conditions. Consultation-liaison psychiatry team embedded in a hemodialysis unit or nephrology clinic can operationalize this and provide opportunities for building capacity within nephrology teams for improved assessment and management of comorbid psychiatric conditions.

9.5.2 Case Vignette 2

Ms. I was presenting with signs suggestive of worsening major depressive episode, but given the relative recency of initiating a selective serotonin reuptake inhibitor (SSRI), hyponatremia secondary to syndrome of inappropriate secretion of antidiuretic hormone (SIADH) must be high on the differential. To further investigate this, the astute psychiatrist should order serum electrolytes and extended electrolytes, blood urea nitrogen, creatinine, serum osmolality, urine electrolytes, and urine osmolality and other routine delirium studies. It is imperative that Ms. I then be seen by her primary care physician acutely or, if needed, directed to the emergency department.

9.5.3 Case Vignette 3

The consultation-liaison psychiatrist must be acutely aware of the differential diagnosis of confusion and gait ataxia in individuals taking antipsychotic medications and mood-stabilizing medications that includes, though is not limited to, neuroleptic malignant syndrome, valproic acid toxicity, hepatic encephalopathy/delirium, uremic encephalopathy/delirium, and stroke. In the case of Ms. V, the elevated serum sodium points to the possibility of diabetes inspidus. Elevated serum sodium with high serum osmolality and low urine osmolality may point toward diabetes insipidus in the context of chronic lithium use. If Ms. V's psychiatric care were co-located with her nephrology care, the comorbid psychiatric condition may have been recognized and managed earlier. Case conferencing can occur more seamlessly; "hallway consultations" may have activated the psychiatry team to detect a change in underlying medical status and facilitated quicker access to specialty nephrology care.

9.6 Key Takeaways

- Psychiatric comorbidities are common in patients living with CKD.
- Depression is often under-detected and undertreated in patients with comorbid CKD, resulting in increased morbidity and mortality and reduced quality of life.
- Psychiatric symptoms in CKD, in particular depression and anxiety, may play a critical role in reducing a patient's ability to manage their own care, thereby lowering patient activation in a condition in which patient activation is already impaired.
- Collaborative care in general can be applied in CKD to enhance patient activation, which may in turn improve comorbid psychiatric illness.
- Collaborative mental health care improves detection and management of psychiatric illness in both primary care and specialist practices in patients with comorbid chronic illness.
- These models need to see building the capacity and expertise of medical and primary care clinicians as one of their key activities.
- Consultation-liaison psychiatry needs to draw upon similar principles and practices to collaborative care models, embedding mental health professionals within primary care and specialist practices to deliver evidence-based mental health care.

References

1. Simoes E, Silva AC, Miranda AS, Rocha NP, Teixeira AL. Neuropsychiatric disorders in chronic kidney disease. Front Pharmacol. 2019;10:932.
2. Cukor D, Coplan J, Brown C, et al. Depression and anxiety in urban hemodialysis patients. Clin J Am Soc Nephrol. 2007;2:484–90.
3. Kimmel PL, Fwu C, Abbott KC, et al. Psychiatric illness and mortality in hospitalized ESKD dialysis patients. Clin J Am Soc Nephrol. 2019;14:1363–71.
4. Kimmel PL, Cukor D, Cohen SD, Peterson RA. Depression in end-stage renal disease patients: a critical review. Adv Chronic Kidney Dis. 2007;14(4):328–34.
5. Wilkie M, Barnes T. Shared hemodialysis care: increasing patient involvement in center-based dialysis. Clin J Am Soc Nephrol. 2019;14(9):1402–4.
6. King-Wing Ma T, Kam-Tao LP. Depression in dialysis patients. Nephrology (Carlton). 2016;21(8):639–46.
7. Llewellyn S. The chronic care model, kidney disease, and primary care: a scoping review. Nephrol Nurs J. 2019;46(3):301–28.
8. Alexopoulos GS, Katz IR, Bruce ML, et al. Remission in depressed geriatric primary care patients: a report from the PROSPECT study. Am J Psychiatry. 2005;162(4):718–24.
9. Unutzer J, Katon W, Callahan CM, et al. Collaborative care management of late-life depression in the primary care setting a randomized control trial. JAMA. 2002;288(22):2836–45.
10. Wagner EH. Organizing care for patients with chronic illness revisited. Milbank Q. 2019;97(3):659–64.
11. Hypertension Detection and Follow-up Program Cooperative Group. Five-year findings of the hypertension detection and follow-up program: I. Reduction in mortality of persons with high blood pressure, including mild hypertension. JAMA. 1979;242(23):2562–71.
12. The Diabetes Control and Complications Trial Research Group. The effect of intensive treatment of diabetes on the development and progression of long-term complications in insulin-dependent diabetes mellitus. N Engl J Med. 1993;329:977–86.

13. Wagner EH, Austin BT, Von Korff M. Organizing care for patient with chronic illness. Milbank Q. 1996;74(4):511–44.
14. Nicholl R, Robertson L, Gemmell E, Sharma P, Black C, Marks A. Models of care for chronic kidney disease: a systematic review. Nephrology. 2018;23:389–96.
15. Chen SH, Tsai Y, Sun C, Wu I, Lee C, Wu M. The impact of self-management support on the progression of chronic kidney disease—a prospective randomized controlled trial. Nephrol Dial Transplant. 2011;26:3560–6.
16. Sporinova B, Manns B, Tonelli M, et al. Association of mental health disorders with health care utilization and costs among adults with chronic disease. JAMA Netw Open. 2019;2(8):e199910.
17. Katon WJ, Von Korff M, Lin EHB, et al. The pathways study – a randomized trial of collaborative care in patients with diabetes and depression. Arch Gen Psychiatry. 2004;61:1042–9.
18. Kates N, Arroll B, Currie E, et al. Improving collaboration between primary care and mental health services. World J Biol Psychiatry. 2019;20(10):748–65.
19. Ali S, Ernst C, Pacheco M, Fricchione G. Consultation-liaison psychiatry: how far have we come? Curr Psychiatry Rep. 2006;8(3):215–22.
20. Davydow DS, Katon JG, Rollman BL, Unützer J. Improving mental and physical health outcomes in general healthcare settings: a Gedenkschrift in honor of Wayne Katon, MD (1950–2015). Gen Hosp Psychiatry. 2015;37(5):375–86.
21. American Psychiatric Association & American Academy of Psychosomatic Medicine Dissemination of integrated care within adult primary care settings. (2016). https://www.psychiatry.org/psychiatrists/practice/professional-interests/integrated-care/learn. Accessed 21 Mar 2021
22. Lin EHB, Von Korff M, Ciechanowski P, et al. Treatment adjustment and medication adherence for complex patients with diabetes, heart Disease, and depression: a randomized controlled trial. Ann Fam Med. 2012;10:6–14.
23. Katon WJ, Lin E, Von Korff M, et al. Collaborative care for patients with depression and chronic illnesses. N Engl J Med. 2010;363(27):2611–20.
24. Rustomjee S, Smith GC. Consultation-liaison psychiatry to renal medicine: work with an inpatient unit. Aust N Z J Psychiatry. 1996;30:229–37.
25. Boland RJ, Rundell J, Epstein S, Gitlin D. Consultation-liaison psychiatry vs. psychosomatic medicine: what's in a name? Psychosomatics. 2018;59:207–10.
26. Roumelioti ME, Steel JK, Yabes J, et al. Rational and design of technology assisted stepped collaborative care intervention to improve patient-centered outcomes in hemodialysis patients (TACcare trial). Contemp Clin Trials. 2018;73:81–91.

Part II

Common Psychiatric Presentations and Their Management in the Patient with Kidney Disease

Common Psychiatric Disorders in the Renal Patient

10

Julia Danielle Kulikowski, Sarah Candace Payne, and Ana Hategan

10.1 Introduction

Chronic kidney disease (CKD) is associated with increased mortality, cardiovascular events, and all-cause hospitalizations. Psychiatric comorbidity further increases these risks when compared to the general population. Globally, the prevalence of end-stage renal disease (ESRD) has increased and is associated with a reduced health-related quality of life and premature death [1–4]. Patients are required to make significant changes to their lifestyle, including diet, activity levels, and general health management. With progression of kidney disease, patients often require renal replacement therapy. These measures act to replace the function of kidney filtration and include hemodialysis, peritoneal dialysis, and kidney transplant. Transplantation is the ultimate form of renal replacement and has been associated with improved quality of life and prolonging of survival.

Psychiatric support to individuals with kidney disease varies among nations and institutions. Growing literature supports interdisciplinary actions among nephrology services and other healthcare teams. This chapter will focus on the importance of psychiatric care in this patient population. CKD and ESRD can be debilitating and are associated with elevated rates of psychiatric comorbidity. Psychiatric disorders are found at higher rates in chronic systemic medical conditions, and CKD and

J. D. Kulikowski (✉) · S. C. Payne
Department of Psychiatry and Behavioural Neurosciences, McMaster University, Hamilton, ON, Canada
e-mail: julia.kulikowski@medportal.ca; sarah.payne@medportal.ca

A. Hategan
Division of Geriatric Psychiatry, Department of Psychiatry & Behavioural Neurosciences, Faculty of Health Sciences, Michael G. DeGroote School of Medicine, McMaster University, Hamilton, ON, Canada
e-mail: julia.kulikowski@medportal.ca; hategan@mcmaster.ca

A. Hategan et al. (eds.), *Psychonephrology*,
https://doi.org/10.1007/978-3-030-84740-1_10

ESRD are of particular areas of concern in this regard. Kidney disease impacts quality of life, and treatment decisions and disease course can destabilize or contribute to comorbid psychiatric disorders, especially if not identified and clinically managed. Societies on renal disease from around the world emphasize the psychological distress that this progressive condition can have on individuals. A comprehensive psychiatric assessment can allow for early connection helping to build therapeutic rapport and familiarity with their care team and allow for psychopharmacologic intervention where appropriate.

10.2 Depressive Disorders

10.2.1 Case Vignette 1: The Depressed Patient

A 62-year-old woman with a prior history of major depressive disorder and CKD presented for follow-up to her nephrologist. Psychiatric consultation was requested for assessment of low mood. Affect had previously been euthymic with the use of the selective serotonin reuptake inhibitor, sertraline 100 mg per day, and nonpharmacological approaches including prior cognitive behavioral therapy for major depressive disorder and behavioral activation. More recently, the patient has been less active with a decline in mood for approximately 3 weeks. Neurovegetative symptoms have emerged with notable poor sleep and early morning awakenings as well as poor concentration, low appetite with 5 lb weight loss, and nihilistic thought content and guilt related to believing that she caused the kidney impairment herself due to poor diet and sedentary lifestyle. She also described passive suicidal ideation. The patient was diagnosed with a recurrent major depressive episode and was connected with the psychiatrist in the nephrology clinic to co-manage her case.

10.2.2 Case Vignette 1 Analysis

In this case, it is important to think about this patient scenario from a biopsychosocial perspective. Biologically, due to the nature of major depressive disorder, there is a predisposition to a recurrent major depressive episode. A history of CKD will also increase this risk for recurrent major depressive episode. Importantly, distress is a common feature in kidney disease and fluctuates with progression of the disease. Psychological and social aspects tie closely into mood stability, and for this reason, patients often benefit from an interdisciplinary team approach with the goal of optimizing patient supports.

10.2.3 Epidemiology and Risk Factors

Depressive disorders in those with kidney impairment have been found at increased rates compared to the general population; in those with CKD or ESRD, depressive disorder occurs at rates three to four times higher than the general population, which is also two to three times more often compared to other chronic systemic diseases

Table 10.1 Mechanisms contributing to depressive disoder in renal patients

Biological	Behavioral
Low heart rate variability Hyperactivity of hypothalamic-pituitary axis	Interpretation of illness Distress Lifestyle factors (smoking, substance use) Sedentary lifestyle Obesity Limited social supports

[1, 4]. Literature shows that the prevalence rate of depressive symptoms and depressive disorder in CKD is 21.4% [4]. Factors associated with depression include younger age, female sex, Black and Hispanic race, lower education and financial income, unemployment, hypertension, smoking, diabetes mellitus, and cardiovascular disease [5, 6]. Similarly, the prevalence rate of depressive symptoms and depressive disorder in ESRD is 22.8% [4]. Factors associated with depression in those with ESRD include younger age, female sex, White race, diabetes mellitus, longer treatment with dialysis, coronary artery disease, cerebrovascular disease, and peripheral vascular disease [7].

Depression and kidney impairment have been theorized to have a bidirectional, reciprocal association [4]. Depression is known to be common with ESRD, in part attributed to psychosocial and biologic changes that accompany renal impairment. Both biological and behavioral factors are discussed as mechanisms contributing to depression in renal impairment (Table 10.1). One such biological influence is that of heart rate variability. Low heart rate variability has been observed in patients with depressive disorder and ischemic heart disease, and this co-occurrence is associated with higher mortality. However, the relation of heart rate variability to renal outcomes is debatable, and studies have indicated that reduced heart rate variability may be a complication of CKD rather than a causal factor [8]. CKD has also been associated with hyperactivity of the hypothalamic-pituitary axis that can lead to depressive disorder as elevated levels of cortisol and norepinephrine lead to inflammation and malnutrition states like cachexia [9]. (For more information on the role of nutrition in CKD, see Chap. 19.)

10.2.4 Diagnosis of Depressive Disorder in Renal Impairment

Diagnosing depressive disorder in the renally impaired patient can be a challenge due to the overlapping physical effects of uremia with the neurovegetative symptoms of clinical depression. Screening for depression through a structured clinical interview remains the gold standard in making a diagnosis; however, depressive disorder can also be assessed through validated rating scales. Such rating scales like the Hamilton Rating Scale for Depression and the Beck Depression Inventory can be helpful means to first identify those with symptoms which should then be further assessed by a structured interview. It is important to distinguish symptoms of uremia versus major depressive disorder (or clinical depression) to best guide treatment and management. Symptoms of uremia (e.g., fatigue, insomnia, poor appetite) can overlap with those of major depressive disorder and be difficult to differentiate.

However, these uremic symptoms can be distinguished from depressive symptoms during a clinical interview. Evidence suggests vascular major neurocognitive disorder (or vascular dementia) to be the most prevalent form of major neurocognitive disorder in the CKD population [10]. Features of vascular dementia overlap with features of major depression and hypoactive delirium. Although neurocognitive disorders are discussed elsewhere, for a review of delirium and neurocognitive disorders of renal disease, please refer to Chap. 12. Because of the overlapping nature of these distinct syndromes, the clinical interview remains the gold standard for diagnosing major depression in renal patients.

10.2.5 Outcomes and Prognostic Considerations

Depressive disorder in CKD is often underrecognized and thus undertreated. Untreated depression is associated with poor medical outcomes including hospitalization, increased length of stay in hospital, cardiovascular events, peritonitis, withdrawal from dialysis, and death from suicide [11, 12]. Compared to the general population, rates of completed suicide are elevated in those on long-term dialysis [12]. Mortality in those with ESRD and major depressive disorder is identified as 1.5 times higher than in those with depressive disorder alone and is correlated with the severity of depression [13]. Due to the nature of the disease, there is a negative impact on the quality of life of individuals with comorbid depressive disorder and CKD or ESRD. Examples of this include limited social support and sexual dysfunction, loss of employment, and less mobility. [3]. Patients with depressive disorder are also less likely to engage in treatment adherence [2]. Cognitive slowing and distorted thinking are common symptoms in depressed patients and may interfere with decision-making abilities at important points in care [14]. (For further review of decisional capacity evaluation, see Chap. 8.)

Kidney disease comes with significant challenges including the psychological interpretation of the illness, physical impairment, the time-consuming nature of treatment, and reliance on dialysis for survival. These issues can cause psychological distress and can cause poor adherence to treatment, smoking, low physical activity, and obesity, which can be perpetuated by lack of social support and poor quality of life.

10.2.6 Treatment of ESRD as It Relates to Depressive Disorder

Peritoneal dialysis is often carried out at home and affords patients greater autonomy versus hemodialysis, which is carried out at a healthcare institution. However, despite increased autonomy, rates of major depressive disorder range from 18.7% to

51% and may be elevated because of the time-intensive nature of this treatment [15]. Hemodialysis can also be financially burdensome [16]. Though time intensive and costly, hemodialysis comes with *greater* social support given the presence of other patients and healthcare workers, which may account for lower rates of depressive syndromes compared to peritoneal dialysis.

Kidney transplant is a more definitive means of renal replacement treatment and can significantly improve the quality of life of patients undergoing dialysis. Rates of major depressive disorder in kidney transplant recipients are higher than the general population and lower than those receiving dialysis [17]. This can be a challenging time in the disease course because transplant often brings initial feelings of hope, which can evolve into feelings of hopelessness, disappointment, anxiety, and disillusionment associated with long waitlists [18]. Challenges following transplant continue with the potential for graft failure, complex medication schedules, medication side effects, and medical complications. Individuals undergoing transplant can have unrealistic expectations of a "normal" life without chronic disease; however, kidney transplantation is often a "progressive" chronic disease that requires ongoing medical management. For this reason, it is important to ensure adequate mental health support throughout the patient's illness and treatment journey.

Clinical Pearl

- A bidirectional connection exists between depression and the pathophysiologic changes seen in kidney impairment.
- Patients should be screened for depressive disorders when starting dialysis and every 6 months thereafter.
- Psychosocial stress, including from managing the kidney disease and nonmedical stressors, can contribute to depressive symptoms and should be monitored at each assessment.

Clinical Pearl

- The link between illness perception and depression is a current area of focus that studies an individual's perception of their illness based on their understanding of the trajectory of illness, chronicity, associated symptoms of the illness, and how the illness is controlled by their own behavior or treatment.

The most common psychotropic medications used to treat depressive disorder are presented in Table 10.2. (See also Chap. 5) Regarding nonpharmacological approaches to treat depressive disorder in renal patients, please refer to Chap. 7.

Table 10.2 Common psychotropic medications used in the general population[a]

Drug class/medication (starting dose/day)[b]		Dose in CKD and ESRD	Main side effects and monitoring
Antidepressants			
SSRIs	Citalopram (10 mg qd) Escitalopram (5 mg qd) Sertraline (25 mg qd)	CKD mild to moderate: no dose adjustment ESRD: use with caution; consider decreasing sertraline maximum dose	Headache, nausea (given with food to decrease GI upset), diarrhea, sweating, insomnia, SIADH/hyponatremia, risk of bleeding, risk of falls/fractures/osteoporosis QTc prolongation at >40 mg dose of citalopram (this is the max recommended dose, 20 mg per day for escitalopram similarly) *First-line treatment* for major depressive and anxiety disorder[c]
SNRIs	Venlafaxine XR (37.5 mg qd)	Normal eGFR: dose 75–225 mg/d eGFR 10–70: consider reducing total daily dose by 25–50% ESRD: reduce total daily dose by 50%	Dry mouth, nausea, constipation, SIADH/hyponatremia, risk of bleeding *First-line treatment* for major depressive disorder, anxiety disorder, OCD, PTSD[c]
	Duloxetine (30 mg qd)	eGFR >30: no dose adjustment eGFR <30: use not recommended	
NaSSA	Mirtazapine (15 mg qhs)	ESRD: consider dose reduction; clearance reduced by 50%	Sedation, weight gain, constipation, mild anticholinergic effects, decreased WBC May be relatively more sedating at lowest doses (<15 mg) and in the first weeks of therapy; in older adults, consider starting at 15 mg to avoid sedation *First-line treatment* for major depressive and anxiety disorder[c]
NDRI	Bupropion XL (150 mg qd)	CKD: consider dose reduction and/or frequency	Dry mouth, agitation, constipation Can lower seizure threshold *First-line treatment* for major depressive disorder; no data to support use in anxiety disorders[c]
Mood stabilizers			
Lithium (150–300 mg qhs)		Severe renal impairment: strong contraindication	GI upset, tremor, benign leukocytosis, hypothyroidism, hyperthyroidism, hyperparathyroidism, interstitial nephropathy, diabetes insipidus, neurotoxicity (with toxicity), cardiac conduction abnormalities, delirium Pre-treatment workup and monitoring tests: CBC, TSH, calcium, eGFR, serum lithium level, ECG *First-line treatment* for acute mania, acute bipolar I depression, maintenance treatment of bipolar disorder[c]

Table 10.2 (continued)

Drug class/medication (starting dose/day)[b]	Dose in CKD and ESRD	Main side effects and monitoring
Valproic acid (valproate) (125–250 mg qd-bid-tid)	CKD: no dose adjustment	GI upset, nausea, vomiting, diarrhea, constipation, hepatotoxicity, pancreatitis, weight gain, tremor, dizziness, ataxia, headache, thrombocytopenia, SIADH/hyponatremia, hyperammonemia; risk of suicidal ideation/behavior Pretreatment workup and monitoring tests: CBC, liver enzymes, serum valproate level; check for serum hyperammonemia when altered mental status *First-line treatment* for acute mania, acute bipolar I depression, maintenance treatment of bipolar disorder[c]
Lamotrigine (12.5–25 mg qd-bid)	ESRD: consider reduced maintenance dosage	Nausea, vomiting, diarrhea, blurred vision, headache, dizziness, ataxia, confusion, Stevens-Johnson syndrome; risk of suicidal ideation/behavior; do not combine with valproate *First-line treatment* for acute bipolar I depression, maintenance treatment of bipolar disorder[c]
Antipsychotics		
Haloperidol (0.25–0.5 mg bid)	CKD: no dose adjustment	EPS: Parkinsonism, akathisia, dyskinesia Avoid use if QTc >500 ms Increased mortality in patients with dementia (major neurocognitive disorder) Gold standard symptomatic treatment for delirium Given IM in ED when other formulations are unavailable
Olanzapine (2.5–5 mg qd)	CKD: no dose adjustment	Anticholinergic, weight gain, hyperglycemia, hypertriglyceridemia Avoid in diabetes mellitus
Risperidone (0.25–0.5 mg qd-bid)	CKD: reduce dose	EPS: Parkinsonism, akathisia, dyskinesia Hyperprolactinemia Pedal edema
Paliperidone (3 mg qd)	CKD: reduce dose ESRD: use not recommended	EPS: Parkinsonism, akathisia, dyskinesia
Quetiapine (12.5–25 mg qd-tid)	CKD: no dose adjustment	QTc prolongation, orthostatic hypotension Anticholinergic, weight gain, hyperglycemia, hypertriglyceridemia
Aripiprazole (2–5 mg qd)	CKD: no dose adjustment	Akathisia, Parkinsonism

(continued)

Table 10.2 (continued)

Drug class/medication (starting dose/day)[b]	Dose in CKD and ESRD	Main side effects and monitoring
Anxiolytics/sedatives		
Lorazepam (0.25–0.5 mg qhs-bid-tid)	CKD mild to moderate: no dose adjustment ESRD: use not recommended	Use with caution in renal impairment Older adults are prone to CNS depression; if used, start at very low dose, depending on patient response, to minimize cognitive impairment and falls Paradoxical reactions: agitation, excitation
Trazodone (12.5–25 mg qhs-bid-tid)	CKD: no dose adjustment; increase carefully	QTc prolongation, orthostasis Priapism
Mirtazapine (7.5–15 mg ghs)	ESRD: consider dose reduction; clearance reduced by 50%	May have sleep-promoting effects at low doses (<15 mg): shortened time to onset of sleep, reduced stage I sleep, increased deep sleep, increased latency of REM sleep, reduced nighttime awakening, improved sleep continuity
Melatonin (1–3 mg qhs)	CKD: no dose adjustment	Drowsiness, dizziness, headache, nausea Used in jet lag, circadian rhythm sleep disorders, delayed phase sleep disorder

Notes: [a]For a more comprehensive review of psychotropic agents along with dosing adjustments in renal impairment, see Stahl SM. Stahl's essential psychopharmacology: Prescriber's guide. 7th ed. New York: Cambridge University Press; 2021

[b]Patients aged >75 (or aged >60 with multiple medication comorbidities) require a lower dose

[c]According to APA and CANMAT guidelines

APA American Psychiatric Association, *CANMAT* Canadian Network for Mood and Anxiety Treatments, *CKD* chronic kidney disease, *EPS* extrapyramidal symptoms, *ESRD* end-stage renal disease, *GAD* generalized anxiety disorder, *GFR* Glomerular Filtration Rate (measured in mL/min/1.73 m^2), *GI* gastrointestinal, *OCD* obsessive-compulsive disorder, *PTSD* posttraumatic stress disorder, *qd* once daily, *qhs* at bedtime, *bid* twice daily, *tid* three time daily, *XL* extended release

10.3 Anxiety Disorders

Anxiety disorders in CKD and ESRD are an area less studied. Existing evidence shows that anxiety symptoms and anxiety disorders are common in patients with CKD and have been associated with poor health-related quality of life and increased hospitalizations and mortality [19]. Poor health-related quality of life is associated with higher risks for ESRD and all-cause mortality in patients with CKD [19]. At this time, there is no known significant difference in the frequency of anxiety-related symptoms among the various stages of CKD. Rates of anxiety symptoms and disorders are approximately two times higher in those with CKD compared to the general population; 12–52% of those with ESRD experience anxiety symptoms and anxiety disorders [20]. High levels of anxiety syndromes are associated with increased hospitalizations and days in hospital, progression to dialysis, and death [16].

Given the chronicity of renal disease, these patients often encounter difficulties in managing life stressors and other psychological stress and illness burden; thus, symptoms of anxiety (and also depression) can fluctuate throughout the disease course. Renal transplant patients can experience feelings of disappointment, depressive symptoms, and psychological loss, which are often unrecognized by healthcare professionals [14]. Comprehensive clinical assessments should include these topics to best understand and connect with patients. Based on the individual and their symptom profile, treatment can include both nonpharmacological and pharmacological approaches. The most common psychotropic medications used to treat anxiety disorders are presented in Table 10.2. For further details regarding psychopharmacology principles in nephrology, please see Chap. 5.

Recommendation
- Stress management, psychological interventions, and screening for symptoms of depressive disorder and anxiety disorders are important for quality of life and treatment outcomes.
- Psychoeducation for healthcare professionals, patients, and family members on depressive and anxiety disorders is an important focus of care.
- The emotional experience is an important aspect of care; identifying and discussing issues of demoralization, death and dying, hopelessness, and existential questions around illness and life is essential.

10.4 Trauma and Stressor-Related Disorders

10.4.1 Case Vignette 2: The Adjustment Disordered Patient

A psychiatric consultation for assessment of depressed mood was requested for a 72-year-old man who was on peritoneal dialysis. He had no prior psychiatric history. Past medical history was relevant for remote myocardial infarction, obstructive sleep apnea, restless legs syndrome, type 2 diabetes mellitus, and dyslipidemia. He also had a history of ESRD. He was a previously active individual who became less active following his myocardial infarction. He was previously described as a "happy and social individual" but became more isolative following initiation of dialysis. Psychiatric assessment revealed low mood for the past month since starting peritoneal dialysis along with anxious thoughts related to anticipated progression of disease and death. These worried thoughts impacted his concentration and impaired sleep with initial and middle insomnia associated with ruminative thoughts about his disease progression. His wife described that he became more anxious particularly about death since he started peritoneal dialysis at home, and she found that his mood was low and often irritable, with difficulty concentrating.

10.4.2 Case Vignette 2 Analysis

Trauma and stressor-related disorders include posttraumatic stress disorder, acute stress reaction, adjustment disorders, and attachment disorders. Within the population of those undergoing kidney replacement therapy, adjustment disorders are seen at increased rates [21]. Stressors can be directly related to the disease and/or the treatment itself such as initiation of dialysis or transplantation and can also result due to other life stressors. In case vignette 2, the patient did not meet the criteria for major depressive disorder, and his presentation was most consistent with an adjustment disorder with mixed anxiety and depressed mood. Psychoeducation around this disorder was provided to the patient and his wife with a focus on strategies to help dampen anxious thoughts and improve sleep. Sleep can be improved by nonpharmacological methods and pharmacological approaches including melatonin. Trazodone or mirtazapine can also be considered to target symptoms of anxiety and mood (see Table 10.2 for dosing information). The nephrology team also provided the patient with education on ESRD and provided support groups and educational groups from their clinic. The patient continued with peritoneal dialysis with added supports and ultimately improved with this enhanced psychosocial approach to care.

Importantly, adjustment disorders have features that overlap with depressive and anxiety disorders and must be carefully assessed as treatment can differ. Adjustment disorder is time limited to stressors within the first 3 months of symptom emergence and can be specified as various types, including with depressed mood, anxious distress, or mixed anxiety and depressed mood [5].

In terms of trauma in patients with ESRD, few studies have looked into the prevalence of this; however, trauma can occur as a direct result of medical intervention and illness. Trauma can occur during or preceding renal care and thus should be included in a diagnostic assessment to best understand each patient. Trauma-related disorder in patients with comorbid ESRD can impair a patient's ability to cope and their ability to maintain adherence to treatment in severe cases.

10.5 Bipolar Disorders

The treatment of bipolar disorder can be complicated in those with systemic medical comorbidities. It is also very common for individuals with bipolar disorder to develop systemic medical comorbidity, occurring in up to 80% of those with this disorder [22]. Bipolar disorder in renal impairment has been less studied despite the significant challenges to providing care. Changes in mental status have the potential to impact treatment decisions and contribute to poor systemic medical outcomes. Depending on the treatment method, dialysis may contribute to fluctuations in drug concentrations, thus making patients potentially susceptible to mania or depressive episodes, each of which can impact adherence and distress [22]. For individuals treated with long-term lithium carbonate, creatinine should be closely monitored during treatment [22]. (For further information on lithium monitoring, see Chap. 6.)

Treatment should be unique to each individual and should focus on a biological and psychosocial approach to best support the patient and caregiver. Care should be interdisciplinary and include all healthcare professionals involved in the various aspects of the patient's care. Close communication between the individual's psychiatrist and nephrologist is often necessary. Pharmacologic approaches are an important topic and will be discussed in Chap. 5. For common psychotropic medications used to treat bipolar disorders, please refer to Table 10.2.

10.6 Psychotic Disorders

10.6.1 Case Vignette 3: The Psychotic Patient

A psychiatric assessment was requested for a 65-year-old man with a history of schizophrenia, who was on hemodialysis. The consult was requested due to recent refusal of hemodialysis and an increase in delusions of persecution. The patient had been on hemodialysis for 1 month with good adherence to care and good rapport with the nephrology team. He was connected with the social worker on one occasion for financial and occupational support. Assessment revealed distress related to the sudden ending of community supports, which left the patient without help for organizing and obtaining his medications. The patient lost track of medications and missed several doses of olanzapine. The psychiatry and nephrology team connected with the family physician and recommended blister packaging to help support the patient with his medication regimen. The social worker working with the nephrology clinic also began meeting with the patient to ensure adequate support in the community. With the changes made to the patient's medication adherence and added community supports, the patient's delusions diminished and the patient returned to hemodialysis with ongoing care from the interdisciplinary team at the dialysis center.

10.6.2 Case Vignette 3 Analysis

As in our case vignette 3, it is important that psychiatry is involved in the care of patients with psychotic disorders early in the course of kidney disease. Building rapport with the patients is an integral step in caring for these patients. As with all psychiatric conditions, disturbances to medication adherence have the potential to impact kidney treatment and can have implications on psychiatric disease. For common antipsychotic medications used to treat psychotic disorders, please refer to Table 10.2.

10.7 Severe Mental Illness

Severe mental illness can be defined as a psychiatric disorder that is chronic, impairs function, and requires ongoing treatment. For the purposes of this review, severe mental illness will include psychotic spectrum disorders, bipolar disorder, and major depressive disorder. Chronic psychotic illnesses are considered a severe mental illness and can often be associated with shorter life expectancies by up to 20 years; systemic medical conditions often account for this shortened life expectancy [23]. Those with severe and persistent mental illnesses also have increased risk factors for diabetes mellitus and cardiovascular disease, which are often not optimally managed [24]. Psychiatric disorders were historically thought to have negative outcomes on transplant due to poor medication adherence, self-injurious behavior, and drug interactions between psychotropics and post-transplant medications [25]. Data has shown that severe mental illness alone is not associated with negative transplant outcomes such as survival rates [26]. Three-year survival rates following kidney transplantation in patients with psychotic disorder have been found to be no different than those without a psychiatric illness [26]. Severe mental illness is not a contraindication to transplant, and in fact, successful transplants do occur in patients with severe mental illness [26]. However, pharmacological treatments used in transplant regimens can interact with psychotropic medications and exacerbate preexisting neuropsychiatric symptoms in those with severe mental illness. For a comprehensive review of toxicity, see Chap. 14. It is important that early intervention and an interdisciplinary approach are used in this patient population as there are biological, psychological, and social issues that can arise which are important to address and think about in caring for these individuals.

Clinical Pearl

- Clinicians must have flexibility in how they provide care to patients. An interdisciplinary approach involves multiple team members to work toward a common goal of supporting and providing inclusive and personalized care for each patient.
- Mental health clinicians should work with nephrology teams and dialysis centers to adopt psychiatrically informed care and models.

10.8 Insomnia and Other Commonly Encountered Sleep Problems

Sleep disorders are common in the general population and are associated with lower quality of life and impairment in the general health of individuals [27]. Sleep disorders become more prevalent in those with chronic illnesses, occurring in up to 80% of those with ESRD [28]. Sleep impairment often goes unrecognized and untreated and can be associated with higher rates of depressive disorder, anxiety disorder, and cognitive impairment [27]. The number of sleep disorders is vast and overlaps with symptoms of other disorders; thus, a clear and comprehensive history and understanding of the progression of sleep disturbance is important for treatment purposes. Common sleep disorders include breathing-related sleep disorders (e.g., obstructive sleep apnea, circadian rhythm sleep-wake disorders) as well as parasomnias (e.g., restless legs syndrome).

Normally, there are decreases in sympathetic activity during sleep with an increased vagal tone [29]; however, the function of the baroreceptor reflex changes in the renal patient and causes hyperactivity of the sympathetic nervous system and decreased vagal tone, making it difficult to fall asleep and stay asleep [29]. Melatonin is an important hormone secreted from the pineal gland that promotes sleep and

Table 10.3 Multifactorial contributors to insomnia

Factors impacting sleep				
Psychological	Lifestyle	Physiologic	Treatment related	Other
Depression Anxiety Mania Distress	Nicotine Alcohol Poor sleep hygiene Caffeine	Changes in melatonin levels/circadian rhythm changes Low iron levels	Timing of dialysis Medication	Comorbid systemic medical conditions Pain Gender/sex Family history

circadian rhythm; melatonin has been shown to be lower in patients with ESRD and does not increase following kidney transplantation [30].

Insomnia is defined as the inability initiating or maintaining sleep and is associated with poor sleep quality and poor quality of life [31]. There are a number of factors that contribute to the development and progression of insomnia (Table 10.3). Factors include older age, female sex, family history, personal history, medical comorbidities, and comorbid psychiatric disorders [27]. Important factors that can worsen or sustain poor sleep include general stress, stress related to stage of renal disease and function, unmanaged pain, progression of systemic medical disease, and method of treatment which can alter circadian rhythm and sleep patterns [30]. Sleep can also be further impaired by physiologic effects of medication or physical discomfort due to nocturnal dialysis.

Restless legs syndrome occurs in 20–30% of individuals with ESRD compared to 3–7% of the general population [32]. Iron deficiency can often be a culprit associated with restless legs syndrome. Low levels of iron leads to the impairment of dopamine production and contributes to restless legs syndrome [32].

There are both pharmacological and nonpharmacological approaches to the treatment of sleep disorders in ESRD. Management will ultimately depend on the underlying etiology, such as the use of continuous positive airway pressure (CPAP) in obstructive sleep apnea, correction of iron deficiency in those with restless legs syndrome, pain management in those with an underlying pain disorder, and treatment of mood in those with comorbid depressive disorder and sleep disturbance. A thorough evaluation of possible contributors to the sleep disorder is essential in order to guide management. Many individuals will benefit from education on sleep hygiene. Cognitive behavioral therapy for insomnia (CBT-I) is a proven treatment for insomnia in the general population and does also have evidence in those with ESRD [33]. Melatonin can be a safe and well-tolerated sleep aid for some individuals with ESRD [33]. When prescription medications are required for the treatment of sleep disorders in those with ESRD, it is important to consider the pharmacokinetic properties of the medication being used as this will impact safe usage and maximum dosage of the drug [34]. In general, there is a higher risk of adverse events associated with the use of benzodiazepines and z-drug (e.g., zopiclone, zolpidem), and agents such as mirtazapine and trazodone may be safer alternatives. (For further details on psychotropic medications with sedative effect, please see Chap. 5.)

Clinical Pearl

- Poor sleep often goes unrecognized and untreated.
- Poor sleep in those with ESRD is multifactorial and can be a result of psychological disorders such as anxiety and depressive disorder, lifestyle factors, ESRD-specific factors, and treatment-related factors.
- Systemic medical illness can also cause sleep impairment and requires review.
- Poor sleep can increase depressive and anxiety-related symptoms, and sleep is commonly impaired in as a result of anxiety and depressive disorders.

10.9 Key Takeaways

- In patients with CKD including ESRD, comorbid psychiatric illness often goes undetected and untreated, and this can have significant impact on various aspects of a patient's health and overall quality of life.
- Patients with CKD and ESRD have increased rates of depressive disorders, anxiety disorders, trauma and stressor-related disorders, and sleep disorders, and the presence of comorbid illness can complicate treatment of renal disease.
- An interdisciplinary approach among members of the healthcare team, including nephrology and psychiatry, is important to address the various biological, psychological, and social factors impacting the patient's psychiatric status and to focus on improving the patient's quality of life.
- Psychoeducation should be provided on the impact of comorbid illness in individuals with chronic disease, which can improve the capacity of knowledge and skills in patients and their families.

References

1. Sonikian M, Metaxaki P, Papavasileiou D. Effects of interleukin-6 on depression risk in dialysis patients. Am J Nephrol. 2010;31:303–8.
2. Cukor D, Rosenthal DS, Jindal RM. Depression is an important contributor to low medication adherence in hemodialyzed patients and transplant recipients. Kidney Int. 2009;75:1223–9.
3. Navaneethan SD, Vecchio M, Johnson DW. Prevalence and correlates of self-reported sexual dysfunction in CKD: a meta-analysis of observational studies. Am J Kidney Dis. 2010;56:670–85.
4. Shirazian S, Grant CD, Aina O, Mattana J, Khorassani F, Ricardo AC. Depression in chronic kidney disease and end-stage renal disease: similarities and differences in diagnosis, epidemiology, and management. Kidney Int Rep. 2016;2(1):94–107.

5. American Psychiatric Association. Diagnostic and statistical manual of mental disorders. 5th ed. Arlington: American Psychiatric Association; 2013.
6. Fischer MJ, Xie D, Jordan N. Factors associated with depressive symptoms and use of antidepressant medications among participants in the Chronic Renal Insufficiency Cohort (CRIC) and Hispanic-CRIC Studies. Am J Kidney Dis. 2012;60:27–38.
7. Lopes AA, Albert JM, Young EW. Screening for depression in hemodialysis patients: associations with diagnosis, treatment, and outcomes in the DOPPS. Kidney Int. 2004;66:2047–53.
8. Thio CHL, van Roon AM, Lefrandt JD, Gansevoort RT, Snieder H. Heart rate variability and its relation to chronic kidney disease: Results From the PREVEND Study. Psychosom Med. 2018;80(3):307–16.
9. Taraz M, Taraz S, Dashti-Khavidaki S. Association between depression and inflammatory/anti-inflammatory cytokines in chronic kidney disease and end-stage renal disease patients: a review of literature. Hemodial Int. 2015;19(1):11–22.
10. Fukunishi I, Kitaoka T, Shirai T, et al. Psychiatric disorders among patients undergoing hemodialysis therapy. Nephron. 2002;91:344–7.
11. Troidle L, Watnick S, Wuerth DB. Depression and its association with peritonitis in long-term peritoneal dialysis patients. Am J Kidney Dis. 2003;42:350–4.
12. Kurella M, Kimmel PL, Young BS. Suicide in the United States end-stage renal disease program. J Am Soc Nephrol. 2005;16:774–81.
13. Farrokhi F, Abedi N, Beyene J. Association between depression and mortality in patients receiving long-term dialysis: a systematic review and meta-analysis. Am J Kidney Dis. 2014;63:623–35.
14. Goh ZS, Griva K. Anxiety and depression in patients with end-stage renal disease: impact and management challenges – a narrative review. Int J Nephrol Renovasc Dis. 2018;11:93–102.
15. Yu ZL, Yeoh LY, Seow YY, Luo XC, Griva K. Evaluation of adherence and depression among patients on peritoneal dialysis. Singap Med J. 2012;53(7):474–80.
16. Loosman WL, Rottier MA, Honig A, Siegert CE. Association of depressive and anxiety symptoms with adverse events in Dutch chronic kidney disease patients: a prospective cohort study. BMC Nephrol. 2015;16:155.
17. Novak M, Molnar MZ, Szeifert L, et al. Depressive symptoms and mortality in patients after kidney transplantation: a prospective prevalent cohort study. Psychosom Med. 2010;72(6):527–34.
18. Tong A, Hanson CS, Chapman JR, et al. 'Suspended in a paradox'-patient attitudes to wait-listing for kidney transplantation: systematic review and thematic synthesis of qualitative studies. Transpl Int. 2015;28(7):771–87.
19. Preljevic VT, Osthus TB, Os I, et al. Anxiety and depressive disorders in dialysis patients: association to health-related quality of life and mortality. Gen Hosp Psychiatry. 2013;35:619–24.
20. Murtagh FE, Addington-Hall J, Higginson IJ. The prevalence of symptoms in end-stage renal disease: a systematic review. Adv Chronic Kidney Dis. 2007;14(1):82–99.
21. De Pasquale C, Veroux M, Indelicato L, et al. Psychopathological aspects of kidney transplantation: Efficacy of a multidisciplinary team. World J Transplant. 2014;4(4):267–75.
22. McLaren KD, Marangell LB. Special considerations in the treatment of patients with bipolar disorder and medical co-morbidities. Ann Gen Hosp Psychiatry. 2004;3(1):7.
23. Chang CK, Hayes RD, Perera G, et al. Life expectancy at birth for people with serious mental illness and other major disorders from a secondary mental health care case register in London. PLoS One. 2011;6(5):e19590.
24. Iwagami M, Mansfield KE, Hayes JF, et al. Severe mental illness and chronic kidney disease: a cross-sectional study in the United Kingdom. Clin Epidemiol. 2018;10:421–9.
25. Zimbrean P, Emre S. Patients with psychotic disorders in solid-organ transplant. Prog Transplant. 2015;25(4):289–96.
26. Evans LD, Stock EM, Zeber JE, et al. Post-transplantation outcomes in veterans with serious mental illness. Transplantation. 2015;99:e57–65.
27. Maung SC, El Sara A, Chapman C, Cohen D, Cukor D. Sleep disorders and chronic kidney disease. World J Nephrol. 2016;5(3):224–32.

28. Hui DS, Wong TY, Ko FW, et al. Prevalence of sleep disturbances in Chinese patients with end-stage renal failure on continuous ambulatory peritoneal dialysis. Am J Kidney Dis. 2000;36:783–8.
29. Neumann J, Ligtenberg G, Klein II, Koomans HA, Blankestijn PJ. Sympathetic hyperactivity in chronic kidney disease: pathogenesis, clinical relevance, and treatment. Kidney Int. 2004;65(5):1568–76.
30. Elder SJ, Pisoni RL, Akizawa T, et al. Sleep quality predicts quality of life and mortality risk in haemodialysis patients: results from the Dialysis Outcomes and Practice Patterns Study (DOPPS). Nephrol Dial Transplant. 2008;23:998–1004.
31. Novak M, Shapiro CM, Mendelssohn D, Mucsi I. Diagnosis and management of insomnia in dialysis patients. Semin Dial. 2006;19(1):25–31.
32. Wijemanne S, Jankovic J. Restless legs syndrome: clinical presentation diagnosis and treatment. Sleep Med. 2015;16:678–90.
33. Maung SC, El Sara A, Chapman C, Cohen D, Cukor D. Sleep disorder and chronic kidney disease. World J Nephrol. 2016;5(3):224–32.
34. Lea-Henry TN, Carland JE, Stocker SL, Sevastos J, Roberst DM. Clinical pharmacokinetics in kidney disease: fundamental principles. Clin J Am Soc Nephrol. 2018;13:1085–95.

Substance Use Disorders and the Kidney 11

Veronica Perez and James A. Bourgeois

11.1 Introduction

Reviewing the diagnostic criteria for substance use disorders is beyond the scope of this chapter; however, the reader can refer to specific sources on this topic, including the *Diagnostic and Statistical Manual of Mental Disorders* – 5th edition (DSM-5). As a general note, the DSM-5 has maintained the term "substance-induced disorders" (encompassing the diagnoses of substance intoxication, substance withdrawal, and specific substance-induced mental disorder) but removed the terms "substance abuse" and "substance dependence" distinction from its diagnostic classification. In their place, the term "substance use disorder" (used synonymously with the term "addiction") was established as a single category. The terms "substance abuse" and "substance dependence" still circulate widely in the literature and among clinicians and are used interchangeably in this chapter as well. Many of the studies on addictive disorders were conducted using the old diagnostic constructs pre-DSM-5. It is important to be familiar with these older diagnostic terms referring to physiological parameters, whereas the newer DSM-5 constructs emphasize the behavioral features of substance use disorders.

V. Perez (✉)
Department of Psychiatry, Baylor Scott & White Health, Central Texas Division, Temple, TX, USA

College of Medicine, Texas A&M University Health Science Center, Temple, TX, USA
e-mail: Veronica.Perez@BSWHealth.org

J. A. Bourgeois
Department of Psychiatry, Baylor Scott & White Health,
Central Texas Division, Department of Medical Education, College of Medicine,
Texas A&M University Health Science Center, Temple, TX, USA
e-mail: james.bourgeois@BSWHealth.org

A. Hategan et al. (eds.), *Psychonephrology*,
https://doi.org/10.1007/978-3-030-84740-1_11

As a clinician caring for patients with licit and illicit substance use, a medical workup may be warranted for acute and long-term management of impairments to renal function linked directly or indirectly to substance use. Nephrological complications of drug use encompass the spectrum of tubular, glomerular, interstitial, and vascular kidney disease, and they contribute to many adverse pathophysiological and metabolic concerns. This chapter focuses on documented and well-established renal complications associated with licit and illicit substances.

Due to the variety of potential etiologies and the array of behavioral risk factors, it can be difficult to ascertain a definite relationship between a specific substance and its relationship to a renal disease. So, although not all substances of abuse have been linked to nephrological impairments, this connection should be considered in the differential diagnosis, along with abstinence as a part of the treatment plan.

As discussed elsewhere in this book, routine measurement of renal function is assessed with serum electrolytes, urinalysis, urine protein excretion, and glomerular filtration rate. Glomerular filtration rate (GFR) is the best measure of kidney function. Knowledge of GFR is important in assessing renal function. The GFR is the number used to determine a patient's stage of renal disease.

Recommendation

- Glomerular filtration rate (GFR) is one of the most important parameters to determine in the clinical evaluation of kidney function since it is generally accepted as the best overall index of kidney function.

Clinical Pearl

- Although patients with systemic medical complications of substance use disorders, including cirrhosis and cachexia, may nonetheless have serum creatinine levels within normal limits, their GFR could be significantly reduced.
- Knowledge of GFR is important in determining medication dose adjustments in patients with impaired renal function.

A mathematical calculation using the patient's age, race, sex, and serum creatinine is used to calculate a GFR. Because of the inaccuracy of using creatinine alone, several formulae have been developed to estimate GFR [1]. The Cockcroft-Gault equation estimates creatinine clearance (CrCl) without adjustment for body surface area [2]:

$$\mathrm{CrCl}\left(\mathrm{mL}/\mathrm{min}\right)=\frac{\left(140-\mathrm{age}\left[\mathrm{years}\right]\right)\mathrm{x}\left(\mathrm{body\ weight}\left[\mathrm{kg}\right]\right)}{72\ \mathrm{x\ serum\ creatinine}\left(\frac{\mathrm{mg}}{\mathrm{dL}}\right)}$$

(Multiply the result by 0.85 for females because of average lower muscle mass.)

Let us begin the discussion of substance use disorders and the kidney by reviewing a case vignette highlighting one of the most common medical conditions associated with substance abuse and kidney injury.

11.2 Case Vignette: "A Rapid Crush"

A 43-year-old Caucasian man presented to the emergency department with chief complaint of myalgias and generalized weakness. He denied any recent injury or trauma. From chart review and prior presentations, he had known history of polysubstance use, including alcohol abuse, but no other significant past medical history. On attempts to interview him, he was agitated and confused and a poor historian. His vital signs were significant for tachycardia and hyperthermia. Laboratory results revealed multiple electrolyte abnormalities and elevated creatinine kinase, which was five times the upper limit of normal. A urine sample was collected for urine drug screening and appeared brownish-red in color. The urine was positive for blood on dipstick testing. However, red blood cells were not visualized on microscopy. Urine drug screening and a blood alcohol level were pending. Continue reading on for clues to the diagnosis. A case analysis is also presented at the end.

11.3 Substance Use and the Kidney

11.3.1 Alcohols

There are many adverse health effects of acute alcohol intoxication and chronic, heavy consumption of alcohol. It is typical for patients with heavy alcohol consumption to present with a myriad of fluid and electrolyte abnormalities. Most of the time, these abnormalities arise in the context of gastrointestinal fluid and electrolyte losses, in addition to underlying malnutrition. Common renal issues related to alcohol (ethanol and other alcohol) consumption are described below.

- **Alcoholic ketoacidosis** is a metabolic complication attributed to the combined effects of ethanol (also called ethyl alcohol, grain alcohol, or alcohol) and poor dietary intake on glucose metabolism. This syndrome is characterized by clinical history of alcohol ingestion, hyperketonemia, and anion gap metabolic acidosis, usually without significant hyperglycemia.
  - Diagnosis of alcohol use contributing to anion gap acidosis is made by obtaining a thorough history, validation of ketoacidosis in the absence of significant hyperglycemia, and exclusion of other disorders.
  - Urine test results can be weakly positive or negative for ketones in this scenario. For many patients, beta-hydroxybutyrate comprises most of the ketonuria. However, standard tablets or dipsticks use the nitroprusside reaction that is positive when acetone or acetoacetate is present but is negative with beta-

hydroxybutyrate. Therefore, a specific serum beta-hydroxybutyrate level can be requested if requiring confirmation.

Clinical Pearl

- Even if ethanol (alcohol) is no longer detectable on laboratory assessment, severe anion gap acidosis following a binge drinking episode can be present. According to the National Institute on Alcohol Abuse and Alcoholism (NIAAA), the definition of binge drinking is a pattern of drinking ethanol (alcohol) that brings blood alcohol concentration to 0.08%, which corresponds to five or more drinks for men and four or more drinks for women within a 2-hour period.

- **Non-anion gap acidosis** secondary to diarrhea is another common finding in this patient population.
- **Hypokalemia** is often seen in connection with gastrointestinal losses and secondary hyperaldosteronism (through reduced renal flow, which stimulates the renin-angiotensin mechanism with resultant hypersecretion of aldosterone). Certain diuretics given without a potassium-sparing agent can exacerbate low potassium levels. Without correction, hypokalemia can accelerate or worsen delirium due to hepatic encephalopathy, in part through ammoniagenesis. Hypokalemia (along with hypophosphatemia) increases the risk for subsequent rhabdomyolysis.
- **Hypomagnesemia** is another frequent electrolyte abnormality among individuals with alcohol use disorder. Magnesium depletion results from poor nutritional intake plus impaired renal preservation of magnesium or poor gastrointestinal absorption. The correction of hypomagnesemia is also critical to allow repair of any renal potassium wasting.

Recommendation

- Severe hypomagnesemia should be treated with intravenous infusion, whereas oral replacement can be used for milder forms of hypomagnesemia.

- **Hypophosphatemia** in patients with heavy, chronic alcohol consumption can occur and can lead to delirium due to hepatic encephalopathy and rhabdomyolysis or even be life-threatening. Similar to hypomagnesemia, hypophosphatemia is attributed to gastrointestinal losses, as well as increased renal excretion.
  - Malnourished patients with alcohol use disorder and resultant hypophosphatemia are more susceptible to ischemic muscular injury because potassium release at the level of the microcirculation is an important mechanism for vasodilatation that sustains muscle perfusion during physical activity.
  - Patients with chronic renal disease (especially those undergoing dialysis) often take phosphate binders with meals to reduce dietary absorption of phos-

phate. Prolonged use of these binders can contribute to hypophosphatemia especially if combined with alcohol use disorder and malnutrition. Treatment involves the aggressive repletion of phosphate for at-risk individuals. Since phosphate is one of the body's major intracellular anions, severe deficits of phosphate and other electrolytes place individuals at risk of a potentially life-threatening condition known as refeeding syndrome following the reintroduction of nutritional support.

- **Renal tubular acidosis** is a disease that occurs when the kidneys have impaired ability to excrete acids into the urine, resulting in high acidity in the blood. The finding of a reduced serum bicarbonate can represent compensation for respiratory alkalosis. Diagnosis of renal tubular acidosis is based on characteristic changes in urine pH and electrolytes. Treatment includes correcting these abnormalities.
- **Hepatorenal syndrome** is a type of progressive and life-threatening renal failure in patients with advanced liver disease. Chronic heavy alcohol consumption can lead to hepatorenal syndrome in the setting of fulminant liver failure or cirrhosis. There are no specific tests for hepatorenal syndrome, and it is diagnosed by excluding other causes of renal failure (such as severe volume depletion, nephrotoxic agents, and oliguric acute renal failure). This syndrome is thought to reflect a state of profound renal vasoconstriction and splanchnic vasodilatation associated with severely impaired liver function. Renal transplantation is the definitive treatment. Treatment options for those who are ineligible or awaiting transplant include combinations of albumin, vasoconstrictor sympathomimetic agents, and a somatostatin analog to inhibit endogenous vasodilators. Dialysis may also be crucial to help take over the function of the impaired kidney while awaiting transplantation.

Clinical Pearl

– A gradual rise in serum creatinine accompanied by oliguria (low urine output) and low urinary sodium concentration are characteristic laboratory findings in hepatorenal syndrome.

- **Toxic alcohol consumption** must be included within the discussion of alcohol consumption since these alcohols (methanol, ethylene glycol, and isopropyl alcohol) are sometimes substituted for ethanol. Methanol, ethylene glycol, and isopropyl alcohol make up the most common ingested toxic alcohols. Treatments for methanol or ethylene glycol poisoning include ethanol or fomepizole (which is more effective and safer), which both act to inhibit the production of the metabolic products of these alcohols. As long as kidney function is maintained, alcohol will be removed by renal excretion. If severe intoxication is present, hemodialysis may be necessary to remove the alcohol and the toxic products as well as treat concurrent metabolic acidosis.
  – *Methanol* is found in solutions used for deicing and in some paint products, such as varnish or shellac. Methanol toxicity can lead to blindness

secondary to its metabolites formic acid and formaldehyde, which damage the optic nerve. The metabolic products of these alcohols (facilitated by the enzyme alcohol dehydrogenase) are severely toxic and produce organ damage and anion gap acidosis from the nonvolatile organic acids produced.

- *Ethylene glycol* is found in antifreeze. Ethylene glycol poisoning is a medical emergency because it is rapidly absorbed and reaches peak serum levels within hours after oral ingestion. Generally, it is eliminated via exhaled carbon dioxide and through the kidneys. However, at higher doses, the kidneys become the predominant pathway for the excretion of ethylene glycol, glycolic acid, and oxalic acid. Of note, metabolic abnormalities may not be present early on, and the laboratory measurement of ethylene glycol is not readily available in most medical centers; therefore, diagnosis requires a high index of suspicion. Osmolar gap (measured minus calculated osmolality) is a representative, early laboratory finding. Then anion gap metabolic acidosis evolves, as ethylene glycol undergoes metabolism to its acidic derivatives.

Clinical Pearl

- The presence of "tent-shaped" (octahedral) or needle-shaped oxalate crystals in the urine can support a diagnosis of ethylene glycol intoxication. However, their absence does not rule out ethylene glycol poisoning.

- *Isopropyl alcohol* is another common toxic alcohol of ingestion and can be found in rubbing alcohol and other solvents. Unlike the two previous alcohols discussed, isopropyl alcohol *itself* is toxic. Isopropyl alcohol is metabolized to acetone and excreted by the kidneys and the lung. There is no production of organic acids, and therefore, there is no anion gap acidosis (unless another medical condition is contributing). Clinical presentation resembles ethanol intoxication but without the characteristic odor of ethanol metabolism. Additional accompanying features may include gastritis, ketonuria, and a high osmolar gap.

Clinical Pearl

- An anion gap metabolic acidosis usually is the first clue in toxic alcohol ingestions; however, ethanol-related and starvation ketoacidosis are far more common etiologies.

In summary, Table 11.1 summarizes the common physical problems associated with ingestion of alcohols. Table 11.2 briefly illustrates the pharmacological management for alcohol use disorder [3].

Table 11.1 Common physical issues associated with ingestion of alcohols

Ethyl alcohol (ethanol)	Toxic alcohol
Alcoholic ketoacidosis	*Methanol:* blindness, organ damage, anion gap acidosis
Non-anion gap acidosis	*Ethylene glycol:* anion gap acidosis
Hypokalemia	*Isopropyl alcohol:* gastritis, ketonuria, high osmolar gap; it resembles ethanol intoxication without the odor of ethanol metabolism
Hypomagnesemia	
Hypophosphatemia	
Renal tubular acidosis	
Hepatorenal syndrome	

Table 11.2 Medications for alcohol (ethanol) use disorder [3]

Medication	Indication	Typical dosing	Renal dosing	Notes
Acamprosate	Alcohol dependence	666 mg PO tid	333 mg PO tid	Contraindicated with CrCl <30 ml/min
Disulfiram[a]	Alcohol dependence	250–500 mg PO daily	Not defined	Half-life is unknown; slow elimination could lead to accumulation
Naltrexone	Alcohol dependence	50 mg PO daily; 380 mg IM q 4 weeks	Not defined	Mechanism of action is opioid antagonist so wait to start at least 7–10 days after last opioid use to initiate naltrexone to prevent induction of opioid withdrawal

[a]Disulfiram is no longer manufactured in Canada and is only accessible through compounding pharmacies. However, it is still used in the USA and Europe

11.3.2 Anabolic Androgenic Steroids

Anabolic androgenic steroids are a family of naturally occurring and synthetic-derived hormones, which have potential for abuse by athletes or others seeking to increase their muscle mass. The mechanism of injury due to anabolic androgenic steroid abuse is not well established and is likely multifactorial. Chronic renal disease may result from excessive androgen, likely occurring over a span of many years. This may be confounded in the context of polysubstance abuse, especially opioids used for pain management for intense body building or athletic endeavors.

11.3.3 Cannabis

Cannabis, also referred to as marijuana, comes from the genus flowering plants in the family of *Cannabaceae*. It contains chemicals called cannabinoids that have effects on the central nervous system (CNS) and is used recreationally for this purpose. There are two well-known cannabinoid receptors: cannabinoid type 1 receptor (CB1), located mostly at the CNS level, and cannabinoid type 2 (CB2) receptor, located mostly in the immune system tissue. Activation of CB1 is responsible for the psychoactive effects of cannabis. Cannabinoid receptors have been found to be expressed in the podocytes of the glomeruli, with potential benefits of reducing proteinuria and protection against fibrosis [4].

11.3.4 Dissociatives

Dissociatives, also known as dissociative hallucinogens, are a class of substances that generate distorted auditory and visual perceptions and feelings of dissociation or detachment. The main difference between dissociatives and classical hallucinogens is the additional experience of depersonalization. Most notable substances in this class include phencyclidine, ketamine, dextromethorphan, and Salvinorin A.

- **Phencyclidine (PCP)** works primarily as an N-methyl-D-aspartate (NMDA) receptor antagonist, initially marketed as an anesthetic. However, due to high risk of many adverse side effects, its medical indication was short-lived. PCP use can produce many mind-altering effects including but not limited to hallucinations, distorted perceptions, and severe aggressive behavior. Medical complications from use may result in unsteady gait, seizures, and coma, to name a few. These unfavorable but common side effects are precursors for the development of rhabdomyolysis as previously described.
- **Ketamine** is also an NMDA receptor antagonist. It was discovered around the introduction of phencyclidine and determined to be better tolerated than the anesthetic. Ketamine is still widely used in medicine for indications including anesthesia, for pain management, as an anticonvulsant, and for the treatment of refractory major depressive disorder. Common side effects can include agitation, confusion, elevated blood pressure, and tremors. The development of rhabdomyolysis is a potential concern in the unfortunate settings. Additionally, a 2011 literature review helped bring to light ketamine-induced vesicopathy, which is ultimately a pattern of lower urinary tract symptoms connected to ketamine use [5]. Although the pathogenesis of ketamine induced bladder symptoms is unclear, potential pyelonephritis, acute renal failure, or other kidney problems may ensue.
- **Dextromethorphan** is typically known as an over-the-counter cough suppressant. However, it has become a popular substance of abuse primarily due to its accessibility, as well as its sedative (although it possesses psychostimulant properties at lower doses) and dissociative properties. It has multiple mechanisms of action including NMDA receptor antagonism and nonselective serotonin reup-

take inhibition. Rhabdomyolysis and subsequent renal injury may be produced secondary to complications of dextromethorphan abuse including autonomic instability, diarrhea, sedation, and respiratory depression.

- **Salvinorin A** is the main psychoactive component of the plant *Salvia divinorum*. Little is known about its toxicology, adverse effects, or long-term safety at this time.

11.3.5 Hallucinogens

Hallucinogens are a group of heterogeneous, psychoactive substances used for the purposes of altering one's perceptions, thoughts, and mood. These specific substances have a long history of medicinal and religious ceremonial use. In fact, some are still sanctioned for certain religious ceremonies and traditions. Hallucinogens are a diverse group of compounds, including lysergic acid diethylamide (LSD), psilocybin, 3,4-methylenedioxymethamphetamine (MDMA), N,N-dimethyltryptamine (DMT), and mescaline. Hallucinogens as a class are not characteristically known for long-term abuse or addiction, but rather intermittent use and brief experimentation. Therefore, more research is needed on the long-term physiological and psychiatric effects of these substances. Due to the nature of illicit substance use, complications from autonomic instability, altered perception with potential for trauma or injury, and poor dietary practices could theoretically contribute to renal impairments. That being said, MDMA is one hallucinogen with documented negative impacts on the kidney, as described below.

- **3,4-Methylenedioxymethamphetamine (MDMA),** also known as "ecstasy," is a synthetic drug of abuse with stimulant and hallucinogenic properties. It is metabolized by the liver and excreted by the kidney. MDMA induces its effect by releasing and inhibiting uptake of serotonin, dopamine, and norepinephrine in the CNS. Its toxic effects can include hyperthermia, hyponatremia, rhabdomyolysis (with consequential acute kidney injury), and cardiac or neurologic damage. Hypotonic hyponatremia following MDMA use is a consequence of arginine vasopressin release. Similar to cocaine, accelerated hypertension and acute kidney injury due to marked sympathomimetic effects can be other complications of MDMA use.

11.3.6 Inhalants

Inhalants are a group of substances that are inhaled for their psychoactive properties. Inhalants comprise solvents, aerosols, gases, and nitrites. Although the intoxication or "high" that inhalants produce usually last only a few minutes, people may attempt to prolong these effects by repeated inhalation, thus risking toxic reactions or even death. There are several well-established long-term effects of inhalants, including kidney damage. Toluene, a solvent used in many industrial products, is perhaps the most notable nephrotoxic inhalant. Metabolic acidosis, hypokalemia, hepatorenal injury, distal renal tubular acidosis, and rhabdomyolysis are potential consequences of toluene intoxication. Hippuric acid (hippurate) is derived from toluene metabolism and the principal mechanism leading to a normal anion gap metabolic acidosis. In the distal nephron, hippurate also increases the excretion of sodium and potassium. Diagnosis of toluene intoxication can be very difficult due to patients being reticent to report its use, in addition to clinicians not asking about this particular substance of abuse.

Clinical Pearl

- Urinalysis may be helpful in the diagnosis of toluene intoxication as hippuric acid crystals (derived from toluene metabolism) can be detected with microscopy.

11.3.7 Novel Psychoactive Substances

Novel psychoactive substances are a group of synthetic compounds made for the purposes of mimicking traditional substances of abuse. They may entice potential users with affordability and the ability to circumvent detention by routine drug screening.

- **Synthetic cannabinoids** are a group of human-made compounds with chemical effects similar to that of delta-9-tetrahydrocannabinol (THC), the psychoactive component of cannabis. They are popular among young individuals and those who want to deceive mandated or random urine drug testing. The chemical composition of many of these synthetic products is unknown and can differ dramatically from each product, making it difficult to detect by routine urine drug screening. Potential direct nephrotoxic effects of synthetic cannabinoids have been supported by some studies [6].
- **Synthetic cathinones**, also known as "bath salts," are "designer" drugs with active ingredients similar to the psychostimulants but may also have hallucinogenic properties. These man-made agents are chemically related to cathinone, a substance found in the shrub *Catha edulis* (also known as khat). The composition of bath salts tends to be variable and includes alpha-pyrrolidinopentiophenone, mephedrone, methylone, or methylenedioxypyrovalerone. Due to their psychostimulant properties, vasoconstriction can occur, producing renal hypoperfusion or ischemia, as well as renal tubular necrosis. Rhabdomyolysis is another potential complication which could lead to acute kidney injury.
- **Gamma-hydroxybutyric acid (GHB)** is a naturally occurring neurotransmitter and also a psychoactive substance with potential for abuse. Due to its incapacitating and amnestic properties, it is regrettably used as a date rape drug. In settings where alcohol is co-ingested, respiratory arrest has been reported, likely due to GHB's ability to reduce the elimination rate of alcohol. Renal complications are possible in the context of autonomic instability, sedation, respiratory depression, and trauma or injury.

- **Krokodil**, an illicitly produced desomorphine with significant impurities, is a novel substance of abuse with sedative and pain-relieving properties. It gets its name from the severe skin damage following injection use. Because of the severity of tissue damage, bacterial infections and sepsis can occur and contribute to renal dysfunction. Additionally, injection drug use is associated with many other potential complications, which is elaborated on later in this chapter in Sect. 11.4, *Persons Who Inject Drugs*.

11.3.8 Opioids

"Opiate" and "opioid" are often used interchangeably to describe a class of pain-relieving drugs that bind to opioid receptors. Traditionally, opiates include morphine, thebaine, and codeine, which are natural derivatives of the opium poppy plant, *Papaver somniferum*. Opioids, on the other hand, tends to refer to semisynthetic and synthetic drugs in this class. And although the development of substance use disorders is multifactorial, both opiates and opioids have high addictive and abuse potential. Potential renal complications are discussed below. Of note, fentanyl (a highly potent synthetic opioid) and kratom (*Mitragyna speciosa*, a tropical evergreen with psychostimulant-like properties at low doses and opioid-like properties at higher doses) are more novel substances of abuse but are included in the discussion of opioid-related renal injury as a whole. Physical problems associated with the use of opioids are discussed below (see also Table 11.3).

- **Rhabdomyolysis** is a common cause of acute renal failure associated with the use of multiple substances, including opioids. Clinical presentations may include a history of tonic-clonic seizures but classically a markedly elevated serum creatine kinase level. Opioid misuse can lead to respiratory depression and even death due to overdose. Subsequent stupor and immobilization can lead to pressure-induced muscle damage and then rhabdomyolysis. The presence of volume depletion, hypotension, acidosis, and hypoxemia further increases the likelihood of acute tubular necrosis and rhabdomyolysis. Treatment depends on the phase of the disease at the time of presentation. If severe renal failure is not present, an attempt at aggressive intravascular volume resuscitation is the preferred management. However, if severe electrolyte abnormalities or other comorbid medical conditions are present, then acute dialysis may be indicated.
- **Drug-induced thrombotic microangiopathy** has been documented in cases of intravenous use of oral extended-release opioids, including oxymorphone and oxycodone. The reason for developing this syndrome is not clear, but postula-

Table 11.3 Common physical problems associated with the use of opioids

Rhabdomyolysis
Drug-induced thrombotic microangiopathy
Urinary retention
HIV-associated nephropathy (HIVAN) (see Sect. 11.4)
Heroin-associated nephropathy (HAN)

Table 11.4 Medications for opioid use disorder [3]

Medication	Indication	Typical dosing	Renal dosing	Notes
Buprenorphine	Opioid dependence	2–24 mg SL daily	None	Also comes in a combined product with naloxone
Methadone	Opioid dependence	Variable	If CrCl <10 mL/min or on HD/PD, then decrease dose by 25–50% and titrate slowly	Max of 30 mg initial dose; no supplementation needed after dialysis
Naloxone	Opioid overdose	0.4–2 mg SC/IM/IV q 2–3 min PRN; 1 mg each nostril for intranasal q 3–5 min PRN	None	Should be prescribed to anyone on chronic opioids (especially in combination with sedatives, alcohol, or other illicit drug use) and/or opioid use disorder
Naltrexone	Opioid dependence	50 mg PO daily; 380 mg IM q 4 weeks	Not defined	Recommended to wait 7–10 days after last opioid use to start naltrexone to prevent induction of opioid withdrawal; may have to wait longer if starting after methadone use

Note: HD hemodialysis, *PD* peritoneal dialysis

tions include attributions to the opioid medication itself, the chemicals used to formulate the pills for intravenous use, or potentially the polyethylene oxide coating of the tablets. The clinical presentation resembles that of cocaine-induced thrombotic microangiopathy.

- **Urinary retention** due to opioid use is well-established and attributed to mu-opioid receptor agonism. Acute urinary retention is usually painful and becomes life-threatening, requiring emergent catheterization for management.
- **Heroin-associated nephropathy (HAN)** is a nephrotic syndrome, described back in the 1970s. The pathogenesis remains unclear; however, it has been suggested that injected heroin and/or adulterants produce an immune response and subsequent renal deposition of immune complexes within the kidney. Some animal studies have shown that morphine (the active metabolite of heroin) may have a direct effect on the glomerulus, causing proliferation of fibroblasts and a decrease in degradation of renal glomerular type IV collagen [7].

Table 11.4 illustrates the pharmacological approaches for opioid use disorder [3]

Clinical Pearl

- Buprenorphine is often prescribed as a combination with naloxone. Naloxone is inactive if taken sublingually. However, it becomes active if injected and can induce withdrawal, therefore helping prevent diversion (abuse of buprenorphine).

11.3.9 Sedative-Hypnotics

Sedative-hypnotics are a group of substances that induced depression of the central nervous system. Aside from sedation, sedatives have a range of therapeutic benefit including anxiolytic, anticonvulsant, and muscle relaxation properties. Due to these desired effects, this class of medication is commonly abuse and has high addictive potential. Similar to opioids, sedative misuse can lead to respiratory depression and possibly overdose. Muscle damage from injury or prolonged immobilization can lead to rhabdomyolysis, a contributor to subsequent kidney injury.

Recommendation

- Special caution should be taken with prescription of sedatives in the geriatric and medically compromised populations, since accidental or intentional misuse can increase risk of falls, injury, confusion, and delirium.

11.3.10 Psychostimulants

Psychostimulants is an umbrella term to describe many substances, both licit and illicit, which are activating within the body and central nervous system. Prescribed psychostimulants have a wide range of medical indications including the treatment of attention deficit hyperactivity disorders, narcolepsy, obesity, asthma, and sinus congestion. However, psychostimulants also unfortunately have a high potential of abuse and addiction due to their desired acute effects including increased alertness and focus, elevated mood, and weight loss. Chronic effects can present a challenge to clinicians, as discussed below.

- **Amphetamines** are central nervous psychostimulants used to treat attention deficit hyperactivity disorder and narcolepsy. Common among the psychostimulants as a whole, the marked sympathomimetic effects of amphetamine use can lead to acute kidney injury in the context of volume depletion, rhabdomyolysis, and accelerated hypertension. Of note, polyarteritis nodosa is a rare multisystem disorder characterized by diffuse inflammation and damage to small and medium-sized arteries of multiple organ systems, including the kidneys. It is thought to be an autoimmune disease; however, the exact pathogenesis is unclear. No predisposing causes have been found, but this disorder has been observed in drug users (particularly with amphetamines), as well as individuals with hepatitis B.
- **Cocaine** is an alkaloid extracted from *Erythroxylum coca*, a shrub plant indigenous to the Andes Mountains of South America. It is a highly addictive psychostimulant drug that can be used through absorption, inhalation, and injection. It has a relatively short half-life, with the majority of cocaine metabolized and the remainder excreted unchanged in the urine. A broad range of renal complications can occur with acute and chronic cocaine use. Renal complications are generally due to renovascular or renal tubular injury; however, glomerular damage is also possible. Cocaine acts to stimulate the sympathetic nervous system by inhibiting

catecholamine reuptake at the sympathetic nerve terminals. Cocaine-induced central sympathetic stimulation and direct cardiac effects may lead to tachycardia, hypertension, and vasoconstriction.

- **Chest pain and cardiac concerns (e.g., myocardial infarction)** succeeding cocaine use are common reasons for users to present to the emergency room. A cardiac workup is routine; however, renal function should also be assessed to rule out acute kidney injury from acute hypertension and vasoconstriction. Kidney infarction is associated with cocaine use due to the vasoconstrictive effects of cocaine. Renal arteriosclerosis, which is associated with end-stage renal disease, can also occur secondary to cocaine use.
- **Rhabdomyolysis** is a common cause of acute renal failure linked to cocaine. The mechanism of renal injury is multifactorial. Muscle ischemia caused through prolonged cocaine-induced vasoconstriction of intramuscular arteries or direct myofibrillar damage is the proposed mechanism of cocaine-induced rhabdomyolysis. Additionally, contaminating agents such as arsenic and strychnine can contribute to the development of rhabdomyolysis [8]. Furthermore, stress from hyperactivity, crush injury secondary to a drug-induced stupor or coma, and immobilization for prolonged periods can result in rhabdomyolysis.
- There have been few case reports of **acute interstitial nephritis** associated with cocaine use and proven by biopsy [9].
- **Cocaine-related vasculitis** is a vasculitic syndrome largely attributed to the use of cocaine contaminated with levamisole. Approximately 70% of illicit cocaine consumed in the United States was contaminated with levamisole [10]. Levamisole is most notable as an anthelmintic agent in veterinary medicine. In addition to use as a bulking agent, it can be added to cocaine to potentiate the stimulant effects by inhibiting both monoamine oxidase and catechol-O-methyltransferase activity and consequently prolonging the action of catecholamines in the neuronal synapse and accentuating the cocaine reuptake inhibition effect. Levamisole metabolites are also known to have a psychostimulatory effect. Levamisole-induced syndrome has a characteristic clinical presentation including history of cocaine use and distinctive vasculopathic purpura skin lesions (typically involving ears, nose, cheeks, and extremities). Hematuria, proteinuria, and worsening renal function may also be present, but renal manifestation is not very common. Treatment is usually supportive, and the lesions can resolve spontaneously within few weeks especially upon the cessation of cocaine use.

Clinical Pearl

- Clinicians should be aware that cocaine-related vasculitis is a vasculitic syndrome largely attributed to the use of cocaine contaminated with levamisole.

   - **Thrombotic microangiopathy** is a rare complication of cocaine use, specifically in the setting of malignant hypertension. Thrombotic microangiopathy is a clinical syndrome characterized by the presence of hemolytic anemia, thrombocytopenia, and organ damage secondary to the formation of microscopic blood clots in the capillaries and small arteries, with the kidney being frequently affected. The exact pathogenesis is unknown. Treatment with plasmapheresis and fresh frozen plasma can help minimize serious bleeding complications and long-term chronic renal failure.
- **Methamphetamines** are another member of the psychostimulant class. Originally developed as nasal decongestants and bronchial inhalers, methamphetamines are highly addictive and now widely misused recreationally. Although chemically related to amphetamine, a slight difference (i.e., the double methyl group) in methamphetamine allows it to cross the blood-brain barrier faster and makes it more potent. Methamphetamine use can result in renal injury and/or failure with mechanisms similar to other stimulants.

11.3.11 Tobacco

Most remarkable for its deleterious effects on the respiratory system, tobacco use can also have harmful effects on renal function. Increased blood pressure, reduced blood flow, narrowing of blood vessels, damage to arterioles, and arteriosclerosis all contribute to accelerated loss of renal function. Accelerated atherosclerotic vascular disease can progress to ischemic nephropathy in the context of impaired perfusion of the kidneys. This can be further exacerbated with comorbid diabetes mellitus and hypertension, both common in individuals with substance use disorders. Cigarette smoking has also been correlated to proteinuria. Consequent ischemic manifestations in other organs (cerebral vascular accidents, myocardial infarctions, and lower extremity peripheral arterial disease) can occur. Idiopathic nodular glomerulosclerosis, a progressive vasculopathic lesion and diagnosis of exclusion, is linked to hypertension and cigarette smoking. Table 11.5 briefly illustrates the pharmacological management for tobacco use disorder [3].

Recommendation

- Combination therapy for smoking cessation has been shown to be the most effective approach. This may include various combinations of medications (e.g., varenicline, bupropion), nicotine replacement therapy (i.e., nicotine patch, gum, lozenge, inhaler), and a smoking cessation program.

Table 11.5 Medications for tobacco use disorder [3]

Medication	Indication	Typical dosing	Renal dosing	Notes
Bupropion	Nicotine dependence	150–450 mg ER PO daily	Consider decreased dose or use of IR form	Helpful for comorbid depressive disorder
Varenicline	Nicotine dependence	Taper up to 2 mg/day	Start 0.5 mg PO daily and max of 0.5 mg PO bid if CrCl <30 mL/min	Offered in a starter pack with taper instructions; usual course of treatment is for 12 weeks
Nicotine inhaled	Nicotine replacement therapy	6–16 cartridges inhaled per day (4 mg per cartridge)	Not defined	Varenicline or bupropion, along with NRT, and a smoking cessation program is usually the most effective plan for smoking cessation
Nicotine nasal	Nicotine replacement therapy	1 spray per nostril 1–5 times per hour over 8 weeks, then taper	Not defined	
Nicotine transdermal	Nicotine replacement therapy	7–21 mg patch q 24 h	Not defined	
Nicotine transmucosal	Nicotine replacement therapy	2–4 mg lozenge or gum q 1–2 h PRN	Not defined	

Note: ER extended release, *IR* immediate release, *NRT* nicotine replacement therapy

Clinical Pearl

– The EAGLES (Evaluating Adverse Events in a Global Smoking Cessation Study) trial was a large, multi-site global trial that looked at individuals with and without psychiatric illness and the risk of neuropsychiatric adverse events attributable to varenicline or bupropion relative to nicotine patch or placebo. From this trial, bupropion and varenicline did not show an increase in adverse psychiatric events compared to nicotine patch or placebo, and varenicline was shown to be most effective for smoking cessation overall [11]. Therefore, in 2016, the FDA removed the black box warning about varenicline use, which alerted patients about possible risk for serious neuropsychiatric events like depression and suicidality.

11.4 Persons Who Inject Drugs

Persons who inject drugs include individuals who use substances through intravenous, intramuscular, and subcutaneous ("skin popping") routes of administration. Infections and illnesses are spread through the use and sharing of contaminated drug paraphernalia, unhygienic environments, and poor adherence with medical recommendations, including vaccinations. There is a high rate of viral, bacterial, and fungal contamination associated with injection and subcutaneous drug use. Heroin, cocaine, and methamphetamine are the most notable illicit substances with highest risk infections. HIV, hepatitis B and C viruses, and staphylococcal or streptococcal bacteria tend to be the most common pathogens, but this is not all inclusive. The spectrum of effects on the kidney secondary to injection or subcutaneous substance use ranges from nephrotic syndromes, nephritic syndromes, or combination of both. Below are some of the more common complications related to injection drug use.

- **Hepatitis B and C virus-associated nephrotic syndromes** are a set of renal disorders associated with illicit substance use, especially the substances that are injected. Hepatitis B virus-associated nephrotic syndrome should be differentiated from other causes of membranous nephropathy, as immunosuppressive treatment is contradicted due to potential for exacerbating hepatitis B viral replication. Hepatitis C virus-associated nephrotic syndrome is usually a combination of nephritic and nephrotic syndromes.

Recommendation

– All patients presenting with nephrotic syndrome of unknown etiology should be tested for hepatitis B and C virus infection.

- **Amyloidosis** is a rare disease that occurs as a result of amyloid, an abnormal protein, that build ups within various organs, including the kidneys. Primary amyloid deposition in the kidneys is well known to produce nephrotic syndrome. However, secondary amyloidosis due to substance use can also affect the kidneys in the same manner. Secondary amyloidosis is caused by chronic infection or inflammatory disease, which is a known complication of injection or subcutaneous drug use. Clinical presentations include nephrotic-range proteinuria, renal insufficiency, and normal or enlarged kidneys.

Recommendation

– A renal biopsy may be indicated to confirm the presence of amyloidosis.

- **Hepatitis C virus (HCV)-related glomerulonephritis.** True to its namesake, hepatitis C is a cause of viral infection in the liver. However, chronic hepatitis C infection can lead to renal diseases. Essential mixed cryoglobulinemia and membranoproliferative glomerulonephritis (MPGN) with or without cryoglobulinemia are included in potential renal disorders from HCV infection. In addition to urine renal laboratory findings, patterns of serum complement can prove to be helpful in the diagnosis of mixed cryoglobulinemia. Renal biopsy features of mixed cryoglobulinemia include intraluminal thrombi in glomerular capillaries and a substructure of curvilinear fibrils in the subendothelial space on electron microscopy. Treatment is usually comprised of antiviral therapy, angiotensin antagonism, and immunosuppressants in severe disease.

- **HIV-associated nephropathy (HIVAN)** is a kidney disease associated with infection by the human immunodeficiency virus. The pathogenesis of HIVAN is not completely understood. However, the fact that this disease disproportionately affects persons of African descent implies there is likely genetic predisposition. HIVAN is characterized by significant proteinuria and rapidly progressive end-stage renal disease. Its distinct histology represents a form of focal and segmental glomerular sclerosis with collapse of the glomerular tufts (also referred to as collapsing focal and segmental glomerulosclerosis) [12]. Treatment includes aggressive treatment of HIV, dialysis, and ultimately renal transplantation.
- **Postinfectious glomerulonephritis.** Due to the nature of injection drug use, bacterial infections, abscesses, sepsis, and endocarditis are unfortunate but routine conditions associated with injection drug use. Postinfectious glomerulonephritis is a disease that can occur in the kidneys, following infection from bacteria introduced at the injection site. Postinfectious glomerulonephritis is characterized by the presence of proteinuria, hematuria, and red blood cell casts within the urinary sediment. *Staphylococcus aureus* is a typical bacterium found in the skin flora and is also a common pathogen. Other pathogens may include the *Streptococcus*, gram-negative, or *Candida* species. Poststreptococcal glomerulonephritis is a syndrome specific to infection with the streptococcus species.

Clinical Pearl

- If renal failure develops within days to weeks after onset of antibiotic therapy toward endocarditis or abscess, the acute allergic interstitial nephritis should become higher on the differential.

Recommendation

- In the absence of injection drug use, intranasal transmission of viral infections should be considered since contaminated drug-sniffing devices are also potential sources of viral transmission.

11.5 Substance Use Disorders and Renal Transplant

Patients with end-stage renal disease and comorbid substance abuse (as well as comorbid psychiatric illness) are less likely to be placed on a waiting list for kidney transplant and also less likely to receive a transplant once placed on the list [13]. There are many speculations about why this may be including poor adherence with treatment recommendations and potential inferior outcomes after transplantation. Some programs require a period of abstinence prior to being eligible to be placed on the transplantation waiting list. However, there have not been any studies that are able to determine exactly how long the period of abstinence should be in order to improve outcomes. Nevertheless, a period of abstinence cannot predict lifelong recovery following transplantation, just as substance use prior to renal transplantation does not condemn an individual to lifelong substance use after transplant. It has been difficult to predict which patients with substance use disorders will do well and abstain from substance use after transplantation. The consensus seems to be those with motivation toward abstinence, willingness to change, engagement in recovery services, treatment of comorbid psychiatric illness, and ample social support are more likely to be successful following transplantation.

11.6 Substance-Induced Versus Other Comorbid Psychiatric Illness

Substance-related and addictive disorders and other comorbid psychiatric illness are conditions with common risk factors including heritability, brain variances, and environmental influences. Therefore, it is not uncommon for individuals to experience both conditions simultaneously. Comorbid addiction and other psychiatric illness can complicate diagnosis and treatment, especially difficulties in determining if each condition is preexisting or substance induced, not to mention that the clinical presentations of acute intoxication to post-withdrawal symptoms can mimic other primary psychiatric etiologies. In order to improve outcomes in patients with dual diagnosis, both comorbid psychiatric illness and substance use disorders must be addressed concurrently. Dual diagnosis treatment usually entails addressing acute safety concerns, stabilization of mood, psychosis, and other psychiatric symptoms and developing an ongoing treatment plan toward recovery from substance abuse.

Recommendation
- Screening for and treatment of comorbid psychiatric disorders should always be performed in patients with substance use disorders.

11.7 Recovery Programs and Interventions

Treatments for patients with substance use disorders are typically unique to the patient and evolve to reflect the patient's desire, motivation, and actions toward recovery. A safe and monitored detoxification ("detox") from substance use is desired; however, some patients will detox on their own. Following detox, subsequent residential treatment facility ("rehab") should be advocated early on in a patient's plan for abstinence, since this allows them to focus on their goals and well-being with limited access to their external psychosocial stressors and triggers. However, rehab is not feasible for everyone due to financial and time constraints, as well as work and family obligations. In this instance or following rehab, an outpatient treatment program should be pursued. Since substance use disorders and other psychiatric illness tend to be co-occurring, patients with substance use disorders should be referred to a psychiatrist, or an addiction specialist if available, for psychopharmacological management.

Since there are very limited approved medications and only for a few substances, patient participation in psychotherapy should be strongly emphasized and encouraged. Appropriate psychotherapy modalities should be suggested to fit the needs of the patient, as well as their ability to engage in therapy. Therapies shown to be helpful with substance use disorders include cognitive behavioral therapy (CBT), motivational enhancement therapy (MET), motivational interviewing (MI), and twelve-step facilitation. Recovery specific programs such as Alcoholics or Narcotics Anonymous, Celebrate Recovery, and Smart Recovery, to name a few, are free, widely available, and shown to be highly effective in a motivated and committed individual. For more structured outpatient programing, partial hospitalization programs and intensive outpatient programs could be considered. Although none of the above recommendations are specific to patients with renal disease, this patient population will benefit with these recommendations, along with close collaboration with their medical providers. Nephrology social workers should be utilized if possible to address more specific psychosocial needs of patients with renal disease, including those patients undergoing dialysis and awaiting renal transplantation.

Recommendation

- It is helpful to assess the readiness of your patient to work toward treating their substance use disorder in order to determine the best treatment option for him/her at any given time. The Transtheoretical Model (also referred to as the stages of change) lists six stages of change to help with assessments [14]. See Table 11.6 for a brief description of the six stages of change [14].

Table 11.6 The six stages of behavior change according to transtheoretical model [14]

	Stage of change	Description of stage
1	Precontemplation	Individual does not intend to make changes or may not be aware that they have a behavior that needs changing
2	Contemplation	Individual is considering change and possibly weighing the pros and cons; however, ambivalence about change may persist
3	Preparation	Individual is ready to change his/her behavior and taking small steps toward change
4	Action	Individual has changed his/her problematic behavior and building new healthier habits
5	Maintenance	Individual is sustaining his/her behavior change, is in recovery, and is working to prevent relapse
6	Termination (or relapse)	The ultimate goal is termination, meaning the individual is no longer at risk or returning to his/her problematic behavior. However, since addiction is a chronic medical illness, relapse is commonly part of the cycle and should not be viewed as failure

Clinical Pearl

– Individuals do not necessarily follow the *stages of change* in any consecutive order. In fact, it is normal for individuals to move back and forth between stages or even jump around various stages.

11.8 Case Vignette Analysis: "A Rapid Crush"

Based on the patient's clinical presentation and medical workup described in the vignette, the most likely diagnosis is rhabdomyolysis. Although no substance was directly identified in the vignette, it would be reasonable to keep rhabdomyolysis secondary to substance use high on the differential, especially given the patient's history of polysubstance abuse. As you have read in this chapter, multiple substances could contribute to a similar presentation. The most common drugs associated with rhabdomyolysis include cocaine, phencyclidine, methamphetamines, MDMA, heroin, and alcohol. Early identification and aggressive treatment with fluid replacement can help reduce the risk of kidney injury. When able, this patient should be engaged in conversation about his substance use and mental well-being and referred for appropriate recovery programs and interventions. Figure 11.1 summarizes the key points of the differential diagnosis of rhabdomyolysis in patients with substance use.

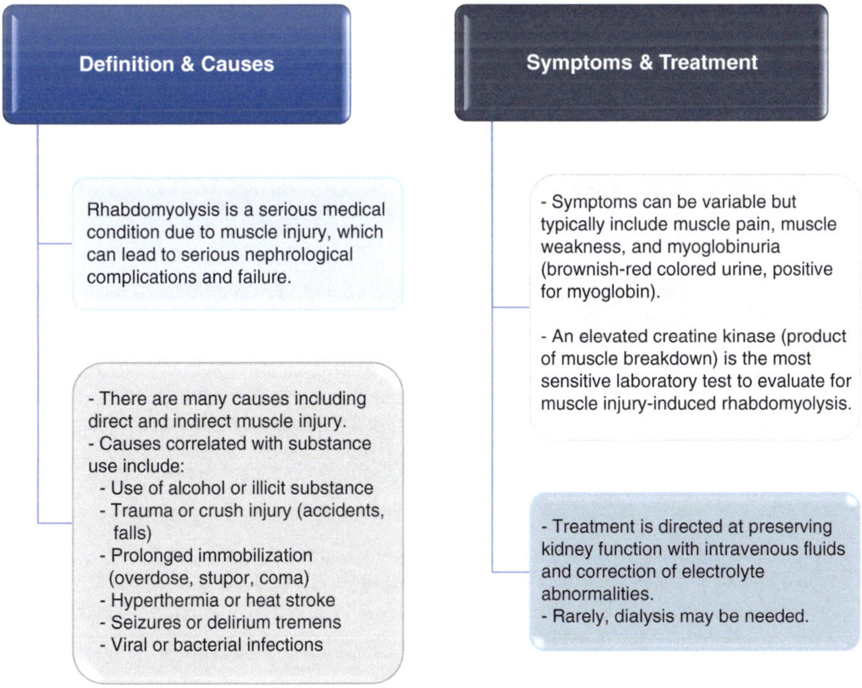

Fig. 11.1 Rhabdomyolysis: causes, clinical presentation, and treatment

11.9 Key Takeaways

- Routine measurement of renal function is assessed with serum electrolytes, urinalysis, urine protein excretion, and glomerular filtration rate (GFR).
- Glomerular filtration rate is one of the most important parameters to determine in the clinical evaluation of kidney function since it is generally accepted as the best overall index of kidney function.
- It is typical for patients with heavy alcohol consumption to present with a myriad of fluid and electrolyte abnormalities. Most of the time, these abnormalities arise in the context of gastrointestinal fluid and electrolyte losses, in addition to underlying malnutrition.
- In toxic alcohol ingestions, an anion gap metabolic acidosis usually is the first clue. However, ethanol-related and starvation ketoacidosis are considerably more prevalent etiologies.
- Rhabdomyolysis is a common cause of acute renal failure associated with the use of multiple substances. Classically, a markedly elevated serum creatine kinase (CK) level and characteristic urine findings (brownish-red color, positive for blood on dipstick but negative on microscopy) are present.
- Cocaine-related vasculitis is a vasculitic syndrome largely attributed to the use of cocaine contaminated with levamisole.
- Comorbid psychiatric illness should always be evaluated for and addressed or treated as appropriate in patients with substance abuse or use disorders.

References

1. Hojs R, Bevc S, Ekart R, Gorenjak M, Puklavec L. Kidney function estimating equations in patients with chronic kidney disease. Int J Clin Pract. 2011;65(4):458–64.
2. Cockcroft DW, Gault MH. Prediction of creatinine clearance from serum creatinine. Nephron. 1976;16(1):31–41.
3. Puzantian T, Carlat DJ, editors. Medication fact book for psychiatric practice. 4th ed. Newburyport: Carlat Publishing; 2018.
4. Nam DH, Lee MH, Kim JE, et al. Blockade of cannabinoid receptor 1 improves insulin resistance, lipid metabolism, and diabetic nephropathy in db/db mice. Endocrinology. 2012;153(3):1387–96.
5. Middela S, Pearce I. Ketamine-induced vesicopathy: a literature review. Int J Clin Pract. 2011;65(1):27–30.
6. Pendergraft WF 3rd, Herlitz LC, Thornley-Brown D, Rosner M, Niles JL. Nephrotoxic effects of common and emerging drugs of abuse. Clin J Am Soc Nephrol. 2014;9(11):1996–2005.
7. Jaffe JA, Kimmel PL. Chronic nephropathies of cocaine and heroin abuse: a critical review. Clin J Am Soc Nephrol. 2006;1(4):655–67.
8. Crowe AV, Howse M, Bell GM, Henry JA. Substance abuse and the kidney. QJM. 2000;93(3):147–52.
9. Alfaro R, Vasavada N, Paueksakon P, Hernandez GT, Aronoff GR. Cocaine-induced acute interstitial nephritis: a case report and review of the literature. J Nephropathol. 2013;2(3):204–9.
10. McGrath MM, Isakova T, Rennke HG, Mottola AM, Laliberte KA, Niles JL. Contaminated cocaine and antineutrophil cytoplasmic antibody-associated disease. Clin J Am Soc Nephrol. 2011;6(12):2799–805.

11. Anthenelli RM, Benowitz NL, West R, et al. Neuropsychiatric safety and efficacy of varenicline, bupropion, and nicotine patch in smokers with and without psychiatric disorders (EAGLES): a double-blind, randomised, placebo-controlled clinical trial. Lancet. 2016;387(10037):2507–20.
12. Izzedine H, Deray G. The nephrologist in the HAART era. AIDS. 2007;21(4):409–21.
13. Sandhu GS, Khattak M, Woodward RS, et al. Impact of substance abuse on access to renal transplantation. Transplantation. 2011;91(1):86–93.
14. Prochaska JO, Velicer WF. The transtheoretical model of health behavior change. Am J Health Promot. 1997;12(1):38–48.

12 Neurocognitive Ramifications of Renal Disease

Calvin H. Hirsch

12.1 Introduction and Epidemiology

Chronic kidney disease (CKD) is a major risk factor for cognitive decline, which affects 10–40% of adults with CKD [1] when defined as clinically significant albuminuria or a glomerular filtration rate (GFR) of <60 mL/min/1.73 m^2. (In this chapter, CKD is defined as a GFR <60 mL/min/1.73 m^2 unless otherwise specified.) Eight percent of the US population met these criteria in 2010, with over 571,000 under treatment for end-stage renal disease (ESRD) [2]. In the REGARDS study of 24,505 adults with a mean age of 65, cognitive status was assessed using the Six-Item Screener (SIS) [3]. After adjustment for age and demographic factors, cardiovascular disease prevalence, and risk factors for cardiovascular disease, the authors found that among participants with CKD, each 10 mL/min/1.73 m^2 decrement in GFR was associated with an 11% increase in the prevalence of cognitive impairment. Persons with CKD were 23% more likely to have cognitive impairment than individuals without CKD (95% CI 1.06–1.43), after adjustment for confounders [3].

In patients with ESRD on hemodialysis, the prevalence of cognitive impairment has been found to range from 30% to 80% [4, 5]. In a cross-sectional analysis of 4686 Japanese adults, mean age 71.5 years, performance on tests of executive function and processing speed remained significantly lower in the subgroup with CKD after controlling for age, sex, education, and multiple cardiovascular risk factors [6]. Cross-sectional analysis of data from the SPRINT-MIND study (Systolic Blood Pressure Intervention Trial-Memory and Cognition in Decreased Hypertension)

C. H. Hirsch (✉)
Division of General Medicine (Geriatrics), University of California Davis Medical Center, Sacramento, CA, USA
e-mail: chhirsch@ucdavis.edu

A. Hategan et al. (eds.), *Psychonephrology*,
https://doi.org/10.1007/978-3-030-84740-1_12

showed that CKD was independently associated with worse cognitive performance [7]. In unadjusted analyses, global cognitive performance, executive function, attention, and memory declined progressively as the urine albumin-creatinine ratio (ACR), a measure of proteinuria, increased. After adjustment for confounders, executive function remained significantly but inversely associated with the ACR ($p = 0.002$), while tests for attention and global cognitive function showed only a weakly significant association, given the multiple comparisons ($p = 0.03$ and 0.04, respectively). In multivariable modeling, only executive function among the individual cognitive domains showed a robust association with the estimated glomerular filtration rate (eGFR) beginning at <60 mL/min/1.73 m^2 ($p < 0.001$); the association with global cognitive function was only weakly significant ($p = 0.02$) [7].

Clinical Pearl

- 6% to 40% of patients with CKD have cognitive impairment.
- In patients needing hemodialysis, the prevalence of cognitive impairment ranges from 30% to 80%.
- CKD affects executive function (organization, judgment, planning, reasoning, processing speed) more than memory.

In a combined cohort comprising 28,384 participants of the ONTARGET and TRANSCEND studies (mean age 67 years), 4555 had microalbuminuria (≤300 mg albumin/g creatinine) or macroalbuminuria (>300 mg albumin/g creatinine). After extensive adjustment for confounders, including risk factors for and prevalent cardiovascular disease and baseline GFR, microalbuminuria significantly predicted cognitive decline over 5 years of follow-up as defined by a three-point drop or more in the Mini-Mental State Examination (MMSE) score. Notably, incident microalbuminuria and macroalbuminuria during follow-up significantly predicted 30% and 77% increased odds of cognitive decline, respectively [8]. These results suggest that albuminuria has a graded, independent association with cognitive impairment.

Etgen et al. performed a meta-analysis of studies assessing the relationship between CKD and cognitive impairment [9]. Seven cross-sectional studies compared patients with mild (GFR = 45–60 mL/min per 1.73 m^2) and moderate (<45 mL/min/1.73 m^2) renal impairment to those with no kidney disease. Those with mild CKD were 32% more likely to have cognitive impairment, and the probability of cognitive impairment rose to 68% in patients with moderate CKD. The ten longitudinal studies that were analyzed also demonstrated that CKD predicts cognitive decline, with average odds ratios that were only slightly smaller than those seen in the cross-sectional studies [9].

The prevalence of both mild neurocognitive disorder (or mild cognitive impairment (MCI)) and major neurocognitive disorder (or dementia) is increased in CKD patients compared to age- and sex-matched controls. The terms "mild neurocognitive disorder" and "MCI," as well as major neurocognitive disorder and

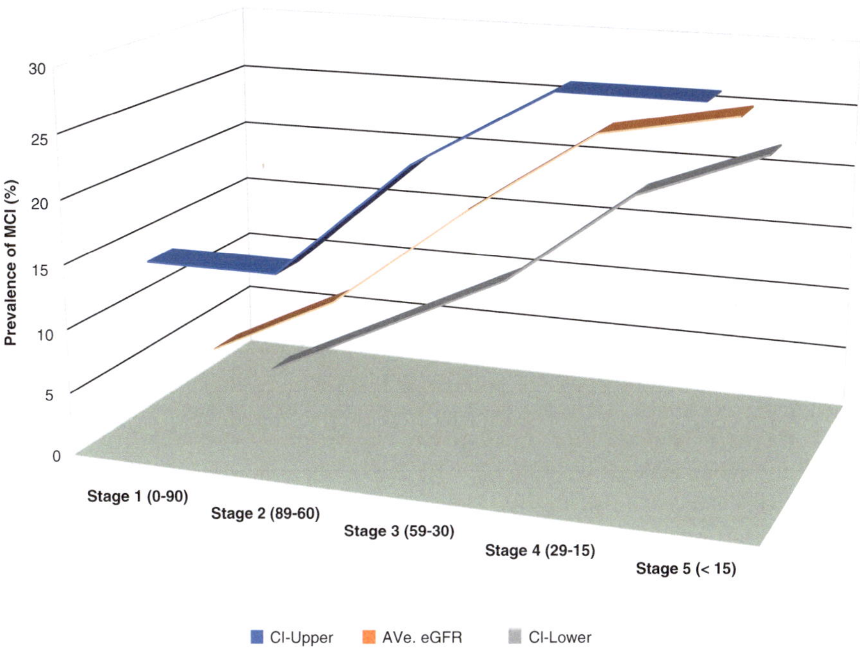

Fig. 12.1 Association of mild cognitive impairment with worsening renal function in patients aged 50–70. CI-Upper: Upper boundary of 95% confidence interval. CI-Lower: Lower boundary of 95% confidence interval. Ave. eGFR: Average estimated glomerular filtration rate. Stages refer to the five stages of chronic kidney disease. Numbers in parentheses refer to the eGFR in mL/minute/1.73 m^2. (Data abstracted from Viggiano et al. [10])

dementia, are used interchangeably in this chapter. Compared to controls without CKD, the prevalence of MCI in all stages of CKD ranges from 27% to 62%, compared to 11% to 26% in matched controls (Fig. 12.1). In a 2020 review, the age-adjusted prevalence of dementia reached as high as 20% in renal transplant recipients, 33% in peritoneal dialysis patients, and 37% among patients on hemodialysis [10].

Clinical Pearl

- At all stages of CKD, mild and major neurocognitive disorders occur more frequently than in patients without CKD:
  - Mild neurocognitive disorder has a prevalence ranging from 27% to 62%.
  - Major neurocognitive disorder is frequent among dialysis patients:
    - Up to 37% prevalence in hemodialysis
    - Up to 33% prevalence in peritoneal dialysis
  - Major neurocognitive disorder is frequent in renal transplant patients, up to 20% prevalence.

12.2 Anatomic and Cognitive Correlates of CKD

12.2.1 Magnetic Resonance Imaging (MRI) Findings

CKD has an independent and adverse impact on brain architecture. Among patients undergoing brain MRI, patients on hemodialysis had significantly more cerebral and hippocampal atrophy and a greater prevalence and severity of deep white matter disease than controls, after adjusting for demographic factors and risk factors for vascular disease. In the hemodialysis group, "silent" (asymptomatic) infarcts were common, with nearly 20% having small-vessel infarcts and nearly 8% showing large-vessel infarcts [11]. White matter lesions on MRI, believed to represent small-vessel ischemic disease, can be found in up to 70% of CKD patients [4] and are prominent in the prefrontal cortex [10], which plays a key role in executive function. CKD increased the odds of progressive white matter disease by over 40% during a 5-year follow-up (OR, 1.43; 95% CI 1.19–3.07), after adjusting for age, sex, and cardiovascular disease risk factors. However, the albumin-creatinine ratio (ACR) may be a stronger predictor of MRI changes than the eGFR. Based on the BRINK (Brain IN Kidney disease) study of 240 brain MRI scans of patients with varying stages of CKD, eGFR was not significantly associated with cortical thickness or brain volume when adjusted for demographic and cardiovascular disease risk factors, whereas the ACR maintained a significant, graded association with the extent of cortical atrophy. The magnitude of the ACR also independently predicted white matter volume, although declining eGFR still showed a borderline-significant trend ($p = 0.09$) [12]. The pattern of involvement on MRI resembles that seen in advanced small-vessel cerebrovascular disease [13], consistent with a predominantly vascular etiology.

12.2.2 Patterns of Cognitive Impairment in CKD

In a sample of 338 patients aged 55 and older requiring hemodialysis, 14% had mild cognitive impairment and over 70% had moderate to severe cognitive impairment, leaving just 13% with normal cognition compared to a control group. However, only 3% of the hemodialysis patients had previously been diagnosed with cognitive impairment [5] (see Chap. 8). This failure to recognize cognitive impairment may result from the pattern of affected domains.

Figure 12.2 illustrates the average odds ratios for the presence of impaired cognition in a sample of 4686 older Japanese patients with mild (eGFR 45–59 mL/min/1.73 m^2) and moderate to severe CKD (eGFR <45 mL/min/1.73 m^2) on three cognitive screens: the Trail Making Test-A (TMT-A), the Digit-Symbol Substitution Test (DSST), and the Story Memory Test [6]. The TMT-A and DSST primarily evaluate information-processing speed and attention and are considered tests of executive function; the Story Memory Test assesses immediate recall of a minute-long recorded story [14]. Cognitive impairment was defined as a test score more than 1.5 standard deviations below the age-specific norm. Subjects with mild to

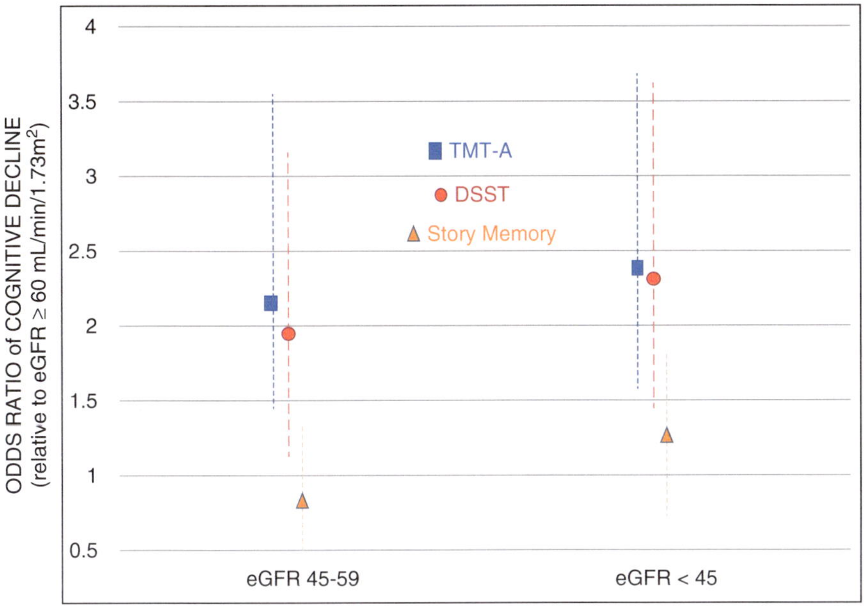

Fig. 12.2 **Association of cognitive decline with CKD stages 3 and 4**, adjusted for potential confounders, including demographic variables, BMI, diabetes mellitus, diagnosed hypertension, heart disease, and functional status. The study population consisted of 4686 Japanese elders ≥age 65 (mean age 72.2 years). TMT A = Trail Making Test Part A, DSST = Digit Symbol Substitution Test – both tests of processing speed and executive function. eGFR in mL/min/1.73 m^2. All tests utilized standardized thresholds for cognitive decline, defined as a score < 1.5 standard deviations below the age-specific mean. Vertical lines denote 95% confidence intervals; those passing below 1 indicate lack of statistical significance. (Data abstracted from Lee et al. [6])

moderate CKD did not have an increased likelihood of memory impairment, whereas they were at least twice as likely to have impaired executive function, even when CKD was mild. Data from the Chronic Renal Insufficiency Cohort (CRIC), a cohort study of 825 adults aged 55 and older with CKD, extend these findings to tests of global cognitive function. Subjects were classified into normal, mild, moderate, and severe CKD (Fig. 12.3). The timed TMT-A and the TMT-B (Trail Making Test-B, a more rigorous test of executive function) significantly worsened as the eGFR declined. Although the Modified Mini-Mental State Examination score (3MS; based on a 100-point scale) significantly declined with worsening eGFR, the average score never went below the cut-off for mild cognitive impairment (MCI) [15]. These results suggest that patients with even mild CKD can have reductions in executive skills, which affect organization, planning, reasoning, judgment, and speed of mental processing, even while they may appear cognitively intact during clinical encounters.

Cognitive impairment in CKD thus resembles that seen in patients with cerebrovascular disease. The multicenter Aging Brain Project performed autopsies on 92 patients who had previously undergone extensive neuropsychiatric testing. In this

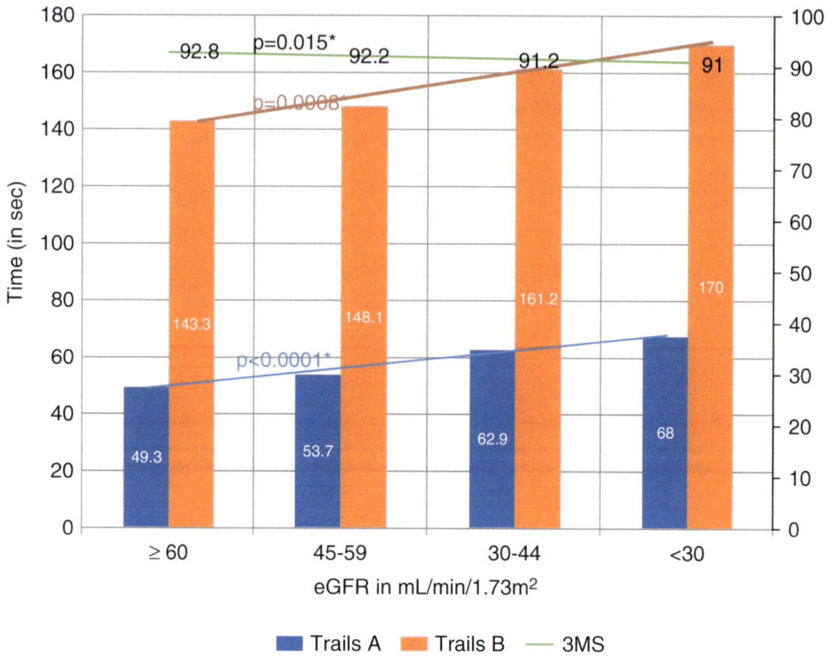

Fig. 12.3 **eGFR and performance on neuropsychiatric screening tests.** Trails A refers to the Trail Making Test-Part A (blue bars), Trails B refers to the Trail Making Test-Part B (orange bars), and 3MS refers to the 100-point Modified Mini Mental State Exam (green). The p-values refer to the statistical significance of the trend lines shown for each measure. (Data abstracted from Yaffe et al. [14])

cohort, patients with autopsy-proven cerebrovascular disease showed a higher prevalence of low executive function (45%) than memory loss (18%), compared to a 10% prevalence of low executive function and a 71% prevalence of memory loss in those with Alzheimer-related pathology on autopsy [13].

12.3 Pathophysiology of Cognitive Impairment in CKD

12.3.1 Delirium

As CKD reaches the advanced stages without the intervention of dialysis, accumulated uremic toxins that would normally be excreted by the kidney injure the blood-brain barrier, induce neuroinflammation, and lead to neurotoxicity. Other sequelae of the uremic syndrome, such as hyperphosphatemia and hypocalcemia, can contribute to the encephalopathy [16]. By definition, this uremic delirium is potentially reversible with dialysis but may be superimposed on more permanent cognitive deficits. The delirium may manifest as fluctuations in memory, poor concentration, poor executive function, depression, and apathy. More severe uremic delirium may cause disorientation, slurred speech, psychosis, and ultimately a reduced level of consciousness [16].

12.3.1.1 Medication Toxicity Causing Delirium

Age-related changes in pharmacokinetics (drug metabolism) and pharmacodynamics (drug action) increase the risk for adverse drug reactions. CKD adds to this risk by affecting the clearance of many drugs, necessitating dose adjustments. Inadequate dose adjustments or failure to substitute (where possible) drugs that are less dependent on renal clearance can result in iatrogenic neurotoxicity and delirium. In patients who received intraoperative opioids during surgery, those with CKD were 60% more likely to experience delirium compared to those without CKD after multivariable adjustment (OR, 1.6; 95% CI 1.2–2.1) [17].

Polypharmacy (≥5 prescription medications) becomes more prevalent with age and with CKD as a result of multimorbidity, increasing the potential for adverse drug reactions and harmful drug-drug interactions even in an academic medical setting. In a study of 200 German patients with CKD (eGFR <60 mL/min/1.73 m^2; mean age 78 years) who were receiving care in a teaching hospital, 37% met the criteria for polypharmacy [18]. In that cohort, 41.5% were prescribed drugs with inadequate renal dosing or relatively contraindicated due to the CKD [18].

Delirium may also be a nonspecific manifestation of infection, other acute illnesses, and metabolic stress. The risk for delirium is increased by underlying cognitive impairment, which affects up to 40% of patients with CKD [1].

Clinical Pearl

- Delirium may be caused by uremic toxins in inadequately treated advanced CKD.
- In CKD, delirium may result from the toxic effects of renally cleared medications.
- The risk of neurotoxicity is increased by polypharmacy (≥5 prescription medications).
- The risk of delirium is increased when there is preexisting CKD-related cognitive decline.

Recommendation

- In CKD, renally dose all drugs.
- Minimize the use of potentially inappropriate medications, especially drugs with known central nervous system side effects.
- Watch for potential drug-drug interactions that could result in medication toxicity.

12.3.2 Cerebrovascular Disease and Stroke

Cerebrovascular disease is believed to be the predominant etiology of neurocognitive decline in CKD. This is not surprising, insofar as atherosclerotic cardiovascular disease is associated with a large proportion of cerebrovascular disease, and traditional risk factors for atherosclerotic cardiovascular disease like hypertension, diabetes mellitus, and hyperlipidemia disproportionately affect persons who develop CKD. Strokes can occur in a large-vessel distribution, but at least 25% are related to small-vessel disease, which heightens risk for symptomatic and asymptomatic ("silent") brain infarcts as well as cerebral microbleeds in these patients. A stroke doubles the risk of a major neurocognitive disorder (dementia) in both CKD and non-CKD patients [4], but prior to the onset of major neurocognitive disorder, ischemic lacunar infarcts and cerebral microbleeds may cause subtle decrements in executive function.

CKD independently confers an increased risk of all stroke subtypes [19]. In adults aged 65 and older, CKD roughly doubles the risk of atrial fibrillation, compared to those without CKD (12–18% vs. 7–8%) [20], causing a commensurate rise in the risk of thromboembolic stroke. The increased incidence of strokes stems, in part, from the complex relationship between CKD and hemostasis. In mild to moderate CKD, platelets become hyperreactive, resulting in an increased risk of thrombosis in vessels that may be damaged by atherosclerosis, contributing to non-embolic infarcts. However, more advanced CKD reduces platelet adhesion and aggregation, resulting in a pro-hemorrhagic state [20]. As a consequence, the volume of the intracerebral hematoma in hemorrhagic strokes may be up to three times greater than in patients without CKD [19], and CKD has been independently associated with cerebral microbleeds, which often are clinically silent [21].

Over an average of 6 years of follow-up among 3257 non-demented participants of the Rotterdam Study (mean age 59.6 years), four or more cerebral microbleeds predicted declines in executive function, information processing, and memory as well as new-onset dementia, after adjustment for demographic factors and a propensity score for cardiovascular risk [22]. In longitudinal analysis, worsening GFR predicted the appearance of new cerebral microbleeds on MRI [23]. Lacunar infarcts, a manifestation of small-vessel disease, increased in cross-sectional prevalence as the GFR declined [24]. Their number and volume have been associated with worse information processing speed and executive function [25].

Subcortical white matter lesions seen on computed tomography (CT) and MRI brain scans have been attributed to ischemic small-vessel disease and increase in prevalence and number as CKD worsens [23]. The severity of white matter lesions has not shown a statistically significant relationship with executive function [26], suggesting that white matter lesions themselves may not be pathogenic of cognitive decline but may serve as a marker for small-vessel dysfunction.

12.3.3 Other Pathophysiologic Mechanisms

12.3.3.1 Uremia

Traditional stroke risk factors like diabetes mellitus, hypertension, and hyperlipidemia do not fully explain the extent of cognitive dysfunction in CKD. The cerebral microvasculature plays an essential role in many core cerebral processes such as cerebrovascular autoregulation and blood-brain barrier permeability [27], which can be affected by so-called uremic toxins. These refer broadly to the accumulation of metabolic toxins resulting from increased production and reduced renal excretion. At least seven can cause cognitive impairment or have other adverse neurological effects, with variable penetrance across the blood-brain barrier. Those that are water-soluble can be removed by dialysis, but larger and protein-bound molecules remain [10], contributing to the progression of cognitive impairment even after the initiation of renal replacement therapy. The accumulation of uremic substances, notably guanidino compounds derived from the metabolism of arginine, can be directly neurotoxic. Guanidino compounds accumulate in various brain regions and induce the production of cytokines, resulting in neuroinflammation and oxidative stress that cause injury and apoptosis of brain astrocytes and neurons, contributing to cognitive decline.

Uremic toxins can induce endothelial dysfunction and disrupt the blood brain barrier, which can lead to the influx of uremic and other metabolites, inflammatory mediators, and potentially toxic medications into the central nervous system [16, 28]. Uremic toxins that have entered the brain through disruption of the blood-brain barrier normally would be cleared by the glymphatic system, an astrocyte-mediated brain fluid transport system that removes metabolic waste from the extracellular space of the brain and is most active during sleep [29]. However, aging, neuroinflammation, and vascular dementia contribute to glymphatic dysfunction and may reduce clearance of uremic neurotoxins [10, 30].

12.3.3.2 Endothelial Dysfunction

A hallmark of CKD, endothelial dysfunction is exemplified by micro- and macroalbuminuria, but it occurs throughout the body. Brain markers of endothelial dysfunction include MRI evidence of small-vessel disease as evidenced by lacunar infarcts, cerebral microbleeds, and white matter lesions. It can be assessed directly by measuring retinal arteriolar and venular dilation in response to flickering light and through plasma biomarkers such as soluble E-selectin and soluble vascular cell adhesion molecule-1. The cerebral microvasculature serves a variety of functions, including regional regulation of cerebral blood flow in response to perfusion pressure (autoregulation), microregulation of perfusion in response to neuronal activity (neuronal coupling), the production of new neurons from neural stem cells (neurogenesis), and regulation of blood-brain barrier permeability. Disruption of any of these functions may cause ischemia, brain injury, and neuronal dysfunction, potentially contributing to cognitive impairment [28].

Using data from the Maastricht Study of 3011 subjects aged 40–75, Rensma and colleagues constructed a composite measure of endothelial dysfunction and evaluated its association with cognitive domains [27]. After adjustment for demographic and cardiovascular risk factors as well as depression and biomarkers of inflammation, their composite measure of endothelial dysfunction was significantly and negatively associated with processing speed and memory ($p < 0.05$), with a trend toward a negative impact on executive function [27].

12.3.3.3 Neuroinflammation

Inflammatory cytokines, such as interleukin (IL)-6, IL-1β, and tumor necrosis factor (TNF) α, increase as renal function worsens [31]. The disruption of the blood-brain barrier caused by the uremic state allows inflammatory cytokines to enter the central nervous system. In the mouse model, CKD results in activation of pro-inflammatory molecules and signs of oxidative stress within the brain and causes disruption of endothelial tight junctions, thus impairing the blood-brain barrier [32].

In the multicenter Chronic Renal Insufficiency Cohort (CRIC), biomarkers of inflammation showed a complex relationship with measures of cognitive performance. At baseline, compared to subjects in the lowest tertile of IL-1β, IL-6, and TNF-α, subjects in the second and third tertiles had significantly worse performance on global performance (assessed by the 3MS), attention and processing speed (assessed by the Trail Making Test (TMT)-A), executive function (assessed by the TMT-B), and verbal memory (assessed by the Buschke Selective Reminding Test) after adjustment for age. However, the magnitude of reduced performance was least for verbal memory. Over 6.2 years of follow-up, absolute changes in cognitive measures were small. After multivariable adjustment, participants in the highest tertile of high-sensitivity C-reactive protein remained more than twice as likely to have a significant decline in attention and processing speed as subjects in the lowest tertile (HR, 2.27; 95% CI 1.26–4.06). However, participants in the highest tertile of TNF-α were half as likely to show a reduction in executive function (HR, 0.47; 95% CI 0.27–0.84) [33]. This paradoxical effect may reflect the opposing roles that TNF plays, depending on its concentration. At physiological levels, it helps maintain normal synaptic function, but at increased levels, it can impair synapses and contribute to memory loss [10]. It should be noted that the investigators measured systemic concentrations, which might not reflect concentrations found within the central nervous system.

12.3.3.4 Miscellaneous Factors

Hyperhomocysteinemia

Elevated levels of homocysteine (hyperhomocysteinemia) increase the risk of cardiovascular events by promoting atherosclerosis, and patients with CKD show elevated levels of homocysteine because of complex metabolic reactions that remain incompletely understood. Homocysteine is formed by the metabolism of the amino acid, methionine. To prevent the accumulation of homocysteine, the enzymatic cofactors folate and vitamin B_{12} promote the regeneration of methionine from homocysteine. Deficiencies in either folate or B_{12} thus can lead to hyperhomocysteinemia. In CKD, uremia disrupts the metabolism of folate and impairs tissue uptake of transcobalamin, the biologically active form of B_{12}, despite adequate stores. Prior to the onset of anuria in CKD-5, uremia also creates a state of functional B_{12} deficiency by decreasing absorption of transcobalamin in the proximal tubule and causing increased loss in the urine [34].

The high prevalence of hyperhomocysteinemia in CKD and its contribution to cerebrovascular disease suggest that hyperhomocysteinemia may be a modifiable risk factor for cognitive decline. The multicenter Homocysteine Study (HOST) evaluated initial and 1-year change in cognitive performance in 659 US veterans with advanced kidney disease (eGFR <30 mL/min/1.73 m^2) using the Telephone Interview of Cognitive Status (modified) supplemented by tests of attention, executive function, and working memory. In this 5-year prospective trial, half of participants received high-dose folate, pyridoxine, and vitamin B_{12}, while the other half received placebo. Although the high-dose B vitamins significantly reduced homocysteine levels, cognitive function was similar in both groups (with a similar prevalence of cognitive impairment), and both groups showed statistically similar rates of change after 1 year, confirming the negative results of earlier clinical trials [35]. However, only approximately one-third of the treatment group achieved normalization of homocysteine levels, underscoring the complexities of metabolism of homocysteine, B_{12}, and folate in CKD.

Alterations in the Gut Microbiome

The healthy intestinal tract contains over 100 trillion bacteria, of which roughly 90% are from the Firmicutes and Bacteroidetes phyla. The gut microbiome has a commensal relationship with the host, being the principal means of degrading ingested plant polysaccharides, degrading oxalate, regulating the immune system, and synthesizing short-chain fatty acids like butyrate, propionate, and acetate, which maintain the integrity of the gut epithelial layer.

As renal insufficiency progresses, rising concentrations of urea correspond to a qualitative and quantitative change in the gut microbiota related in part to selection of gut bacteria that secrete uricase and gut-derived uremic toxins like *p*-cresyl sulfate and indoxyl sulfate, which have been linked to cardiovascular events, mortality, and vascular disease [36, 37]. Ammonia derived from urea leads to a breakdown in the gut epithelial barrier causing a leakage of microbial toxins that in turn contribute to the systemic inflammation seen in CKD [36].

The few studies available suggest that prebiotics (nondigestible carbohydrates that beneficially modify the gut microbiome) show promise in reducing gut-derived uremic toxins. Small trials of probiotics in CKD have produced preliminary evidence that they may reduce levels of pro-inflammatory cytokines and lower the levels of the uremic toxin, indoxyl sulfate [37]. It is unknown whether either of these interventions can slow the incidence and progression of cognitive impairment in CKD, nor are there data on the role of healthy-donor fecal transplants.

The Effect of Anemia in CKD

Lower levels of kidney-derived erythropoietin and chronic inflammation result in a high prevalence of anemia in patients with CKD. Lower levels of hemoglobin reduce blood viscosity and oxygen delivery to the brain despite an increased cerebral blood flow [38], and this reduced oxygen delivery occurs in neuronal tissue already compromised by small-vessel atherosclerosis, dysfunctional vascular autoregulation and neuronal coupling, neuroinflammation, and uremic toxins. Reduced as well as elevated hemoglobin levels have shown a statistically significant, quadratic association with the risk of developing Alzheimer disease and the rate of change in global cognition [39]. However, a similar relationship was not demonstrated in 762 adults aged 55 and older in the Chronic Renal Insufficiency Cohort (CRIC). In models adjusting for demographic and extensive clinical factors, anemia as defined by the World Health Organization (hemoglobin <13 mg/dL in men, <12 mg/dL in women) showed no statistically significant association with cognitive function (global, verbal fluency, delayed recall, naming, attention, and executive function) or change in any of these measures over a median of 2.9 years [40]. However, because anemia was measured as a categorical variable, it is not known whether there are patient-specific threshold levels of hemoglobin below which neurocognitive effects can be recognized.

Sleep Disturbances

Patients with CKD experience a variety of sleep disturbances, including reduced total sleep time, insomnia, disturbances in circadian rhythm, restless legs syndrome, and sleep-disordered breathing, the latter defined as episodes of apnea or hypopnea during sleep resulting in transient hypoxemia [10]. Sleep-disordered breathing affects approximately 17% of men and 9% of women aged 50–70, separate from the presence of CKD [41]. About 25% of sleep apnea in CKD is centrally mediated, i.e., a reduction in respiratory drive from neuronal dysfunction [10]. Results from a meta-analysis suggest that patients with sleep apnea perform worse on tests of executive function but not necessarily memory [41]. Data also suggest that renal replacement therapy can lead to improvements in sleep quality [10], and nocturnal hemodialysis has been shown to significantly reduce the incidence of sleep apnea without continuous positive airway pressure [42]. However, the choice of renal replacement therapy may have other effects on cognitive function, as outlined in the next section.

12.4 Transition to Renal Replacement Therapy and Effects on Cognitive Function

As CKD progresses, there is reduction in tissue oxygen delivery from anemia and small-vessel disease with physiologic compensation through increased cerebral blood flow. This compensation is partially offset by impairments to cerebral autoregulation and increased concentrations of cerebral osmolytes causing alterations in osmotic pressure. In-center hemodialysis remains the most common method of providing maintenance dialysis. Intermittent hemodialysis removes excess fluid and cerebral osmolytes at a high rate, subjecting the patient to intradialytic hypotension. Cerebral blood flow may decrease up to 22% during hemodialysis, further impairing oxygen delivery to neural tissue [38, 43]. The removal of extra fluid by ultrafiltration can further reduce cerebral blood flow [38]. This intradialytic reduction in cerebral oxygen delivery has been referred to as "cerebral stunning," leading to reversible and irreversible cognitive loss.

Among 212 participants in the Chronic Renal Insufficiency Cohort (CRIC) with a GFR of $\leq$20 mL/min/1.73 m^2, 89 transitioned to dialysis prior to their follow-up cognitive assessment. Compared to subjects who remained off dialysis, those who transitioned demonstrated significantly worse executive function without significant changes in memory or global cognition, after adjustment for demographic factors [44], but it is unclear whether executive function worsened prior to or after initiation of dialysis. Hemodialysis patients (mean age 67 years) performed significantly worse on a cognitive battery during hemodialysis compared to the day before or day after [45]. Murthy and Shukia assessed executive function (using the Trail Making Test-B and the Frontal Assessment Battery) before and after hemodialysis. Although all scores were significantly worse than in healthy subjects, the authors observed a significant improvement after dialysis [46]. A prospective cohort of 97 hemodialysis patients also demonstrated the relationship between reduced cerebral blood flow and cognitive function by showing that cerebral arterial mean flow velocity and cognitive function both declined significantly during hemodialysis [47]. Taken together, these studies confirm that intradialytic cognitive worsening occurs in hemodialysis and support the concept of cerebral stunning. These studies also suggest that the effects of cerebral stunning are reversible in the short term but that over time patients requiring hemodialysis develop worse cognitive function compared to ESRD patients not on dialysis.

It is unknown if slower and more frequent hemodialysis (e.g., nocturnal hemodialysis), by reducing the rate of fluid and osmotic shifts, slows cognitive decline compared to conventional hemodialysis. Peritoneal dialysis has a similar benefit of avoiding rapid fluid and osmotic shifts, but this advantage may be offset by exposure to a high glucose load. Studies have suggested better cognitive function in peritoneal dialysis versus hemodialysis patients, but the methodological quality of these studies has been questioned [43]. Kidney transplant eliminates osmotic and fluid shifts seen in hemodialysis and peritoneal dialysis, removes uremic toxins, restores calcium-phosphate homeostasis, and reduces inflammatory mediators [43], although the latter may result from immunosuppressive therapy.

However, the cerebrovascular disease characterizing CKD persists and may result in further cognitive decline. Inconclusive data suggest that in unadjusted analyses, transplant recipients may perform better on tests of attention and auditory verbal learning compared to hemodialysis patients [48]. These differences may reflect selection bias, as the transplant patients were healthier, with significantly less diabetes mellitus and heart disease.

12.4.1 Delirium Induced by Hemodialysis

Rapid dialysis time can lead to *dialysis disequilibrium syndrome* (DDS) that can present in milder forms as fatigue, nausea, headaches, and restlessness near the end of hemodialysis. In its more severe form, the patient may experience seizures, increased intracranial pressure, delirium, and even coma [16]. DDS results from an imbalance in osmotic concentration in the brain resulting from rapid removal of urea from plasma while urea is cleared from the brain more slowly, causing acute brain edema. Using slower, shorter, but more frequent hemodialysis may prevent DDS from occurring [16]. DDS is due exclusively to hemodialysis and does not occur in peritoneal dialysis or following transplant.

12.5 Cognitive Assessment in CKD

As the foregoing discussion emphasized, cognitive changes in CKD, as in vascular cognitive impairment, initially affect attention, processing speed, and executive function before progressing to clinically meaningful changes in memory, language, praxis, and orientation. Executive skills involving organization, judgment, decision-making, reasoning, and planning are essential for coping with the multiple, often complex requirements of managing the metabolic derangements of moderate to severe CKD, as well as the comorbidities that co-occur. Patients are asked to adhere to an increasingly complex pharmacopoeia to prevent hyperphosphatemia and hyperkalemia as well as manage comorbid conditions. They are encouraged to follow dietary restrictions and reduce fluid and salt intake while balancing these demands against personal preferences and cultural norms.

Patients with CKD also need to be able to take a proactive role in making important choices about future renal replacement therapy so that planning can begin about which type of dialysis to consider (peritoneal versus hemodialysis), how to meet qualifications for home peritoneal or hemodialysis versus in-center dialysis, and how to cope with lifestyle and career changes that will be necessary to accommodate the chosen modality of dialysis. In patients receiving hemodialysis, the prevalence of severe cognitive impairment approaches 40%, while recognition of the neurocognitive disorder in community samples ranges from 3% to 15% [5, 49].

Clinical management of CKD consequently requires routine neuropsychiatric screening to evaluate the patient's ability to adhere to difficult treatment regimens and to assess their capacity to consent for medical interventions. Changes in executive function and memory can be subtle and may go unrecognized by family members. Patients with declining cognitive abilities may still insist on taking responsibility for their medications, driving, and making important decisions that affect their finances and social situation. Cognitive assessment helps family and caregivers to become aware of the patient's cognitive deficits and provides an opportunity to counsel them about taking a larger role in the patient's medical management and personal affairs.

Most studies of the impact of CKD on cognitive performance have used extensive batteries of validated neurocognitive tests that are not feasible in clinical practice. Time-efficient, office-based tests of global cognitive function that omit the executive domain, like the Mini Mental State Examination, will miss early signs of executive dyscontrol.

The Montreal Cognitive Assessment (MoCA) includes tests of executive and visuospatial skills, naming, memory, language, attention, abstraction, delayed recall, and orientation and requires less than 15 min to administer. It has been validated in multiple languages and versions, reducing the risk of artificially inflating performance on future tests due to learning. The MoCA was evaluated in 43 hemodialysis patients and 42 healthy controls. Using a cut-off of ≤24 out of 30 for the diagnosis of cognitive impairment, the MoCA showed a sensitivity and specificity of 76.7% and 78.6%, respectively, and correlated well with a formal neuropsychiatric inventory [50]. The MoCA is copyrighted but can be accessed and downloaded without a fee [51].

Recommendation

- Perform regular office-based neurocognitive screening when the eGFR drops below 60 mL/min/1.73 m^2.
- Use a validated instrument that assesses executive skills as well as memory, language, praxis, and orientation.
  - An example is the Montreal Cognitive Assessment.

12.6 Case Vignette

Alfrédo was a 64-year-old man with CKD. After emigrating from Mexico as a child, he was raised in Los Angeles and completed 2 years of junior college before going to work at a large rural winery, where he advanced to supervisor of operations. He did not seek regular health care. When he was 47, he went to a clinic complaining of excessive thirst and urination and was diagnosed with type 2 diabetes mellitus. At the visit, his blood pressure was elevated at 160/96 mm Hg. He received prescriptions for glimepiride and lisinopril, which he took sporadically. At age 62, he was hospitalized for intermittent chest pressure, chronic fatigue, and peripheral edema and was diagnosed with coronary heart disease, heart failure, and renal insufficiency, with a serum creatinine of 2.6 mg/dL (230 μmol/L). His echocardiogram showed an enlarged heart and a reduced ejection fraction of 45%. His cardiac catheterization revealed significant coronary stenosis, for which he received two drug-eluting stents. His hemoglobin A_1C was markedly elevated at 11.7% (0.117), and his fasting blood sugar averaged 220 mg/dL (12.2 mmol/L). He also had an elevated total cholesterol and low-density lipoprotein. He was discharged on a low-dose aspirin, clopidogrel, atorvastatin, amlodipine, short and long-acting insulin, metoprolol, losartan, furosemide, and nitroglycerin.

On examination in your office currently, he was an obese, pleasant, neatly dressed man with a slight Spanish accent. His medications have now increased to 12 with the addition of tamsulosin for enlarged prostate and empagliflozin for diabetes mellitus. His wife, Rosalie, was present for the history and asks the doctor to tell her husband to "take it easy." She worried that Alfrédo was getting too frustrated trying to operate his laptop and also bringing more of his work home. He spent hours most evenings assembling the next day's work schedule for his crew. On examination, his blood pressure was 140/77 mm Hg. He had a normal heart and lung exam, 1+ edema to the mid-shin, and a normal neurological exam. His creatinine was 3.7 mg/dL (283 μmol/L), and his finger-stick random blood sugar was 210 mg/dL (11.66 mmol/L). His urinalysis was remarkable for significant (4+) proteinuria. He met the criteria for advanced CKD (CKD stage 4) with evidence of significant progression over 2 years. The need for dialysis was anticipated in about a year. He had expressed interest in peritoneal dialysis during the night so that he could continue working at the winery and proudly described how he was preparing for the bottling of last year's vintage.

12.7 Case Vignette Analysis

Alfrédo had the classic risk factors for atherosclerotic cardiovascular disease and likely has cerebrovascular disease. Up to 40% of patients with CKD have evidence of cognitive impairment [1], but the cognitive changes may be subtle and unrecognized in the clinical setting because of the predominance of executive dysfunction. He did not complain of cognitive problems, was pleasant and articulate, and was able to rattle off details about his winery's operations. His nephrotic-range proteinuria independently predicted significant cognitive decline over 5 years [8], and his wife's comments to the doctor raised concern that he already was experiencing problems with executive function.

Because of concern about cognitive impairment, the doctor subsequently administered the Montreal Cognitive Assessment as a neurocognitive screen and found that Alfrédo struggled with the clock drawing test and the Mini-Trails B, both tests of executive function. He made two mistakes subtracting serial 7 s from 100. His response to the simile questions was overly concrete. However, he was able to recall four of five items at 5 min and correctly answered all the orientation questions. His total score was 24 out of 30. His doctor was also concerned about Alfrédo's polypharmacy and the potential for adverse drug reactions. The empagliflozin was presently contraindicated with an eGFR <30 in his case. She ordered a homocysteine level with plans to recommend high-dose vitamin B_{12} and folate if very high, which was predicted due to the advanced CKD [34]. She also recommended a probiotic supplement due to predicted changes in his gut microbiome that may be contributing to neuroinflammation [36]. Because of Alfrédo's cognitive decline, the doctor worried about his ability to adhere to the complexities of safe home peritoneal dialysis. She also was concerned about his polypharmacy and planned to recommend a pill box. She would reappoint him within a month to discuss her concerns about his cognition and to learn if his wife would be willing and able to assume more responsibility for the administration of the peritoneal dialysis and dispensing his medication.

12.8 Key Takeaways

- Atherosclerotic cardiovascular disease is both a contributor to chronic kidney disease (CKD) and a risk factor for stroke and small-vessel cerebrovascular disease that are responsible for a large proportion of the cognitive impairment seen in CKD.
- Small-vessel disease can lead to "silent" cerebral microbleeds and lacunar infarcts that gradually erode cognitive function.
- In mild-moderate CKD, cognitive decline can be subtle, impacting executive function more than memory, language, praxis, and orientation, allowing CKD neurocognitive disorder to progress unrecognized until late in its course.
- Patients on peritoneal dialysis and those who have undergone renal transplantation have slightly less cognitive impairment than hemodialysis patients, but these comparisons are biased by the selection of healthier candidates for peritoneal dialysis and transplant.
- Many of the pathophysiological processes that lead to small-vessel disease and neuroinflammation remain, regardless of the mode of dialysis, resulting in a high residual risk of cognitive impairment.
- CKD is independently associated with an increased risk of developing atrial fibrillation, which can result in thromboembolic strokes.
- CKD is responsible for the accumulation of uremic toxins and endothelial dysfunction, which lead to inflammation within the central nervous system that compounds the damage done by cerebrovascular disease.
- CKD also causes an increase in homocysteine levels, which adds to risk of atherosclerotic cardiovascular disease and thus worse small-vessel disease.
- CKD adversely affects the gut microbiome, causing changes in microflora and the creation of gut-derived toxins that leak through the epithelial layer whose integrity is damaged by the loss of protective short-chain fatty acids.
- Through uremic toxins and as-yet unidentified mechanisms, CKD can induce hypopnea and apnea, some of it centrally mediated, contributing to cerebral hypoxia and impaired cognition.
- In ESRD, hemodialysis has been shown to cause a rapid, measurable impairment in executive function that corresponds to dialysis-induced reductions in cerebral blood flow. Although cognitive function improves after hemodialysis, patients

Table 12.1 Clinical measures to slow or prevent neurocognitive decline in chronic kidney disease

Preventive measures	Strength of evidence	Comments
Control risk factors for atherosclerosis (e.g., hypertension, diabetes mellitus, hyperlipidemia, obesity, smoking)	+++	Evidence strong for preventing stroke, uncertain for preventing neurocognitive decline
Anticoagulation for atrial fibrillation per accepted guidelines	++++	Strong evidence-based efficacy for reducing thromboembolic stroke risk
Check homocysteine level		
Consider high-dose vitamin B_{12} and folate if level high homocysteine	+	Theoretical benefit not proven in clinical trials. Low risk to patient
Prebiotics or probiotics to improve gut microbiome	++	Modest evidence for reduction of inflammatory mediators arising from dysbiosis, no evidence for preventing neurocognitive decline
Sleep study to assess for apnea and hypopnea	+++	Strong evidence for reduction of sleep disordered breathing with positive airway pressure, patient may be more alert and attentive. No evidence for preventing neurocognitive decline
Cognitive screening with Montreal Cognitive Assessment (MoCA) at least yearly when eGFR is <60 mL/min/1.73 m^2	+++	Solid evidence for recognizing impairment in executive function as well as memory and other cognitive domains
Neuropsychological testing	++++	Gold standard for detecting cognitive dysfunction and useful when early cognitive impairment is suspected but not detected on MoCA. However, it is expensive, requires referral, is time-consuming, and is not always accessible to the patient
In patients with ESRD requiring dialysis, consider alternatives to hemodialysis, if feasible (e.g., peritoneal dialysis, home nocturnal hemodialysis, renal transplant)	++	Moderate evidence that hemodialysis may promote cognitive dysfunction. Peritoneal dialysis, home hemodialysis, and renal transplantation all have significant associated risks and do not eliminate risk for neurocognitive decline

with ESRD who undergo maintenance hemodialysis have worse cognitive function than ESRD patients who can be managed without it.

- The risk of cognitive impairment independently conferred by CKD cannot fully be eliminated, but thoughtful clinical management can reduce that risk (Table 12.1). Patients with CKD should be screened at regular intervals (e.g., annually) with a validated, office-friendly instrument that includes an evaluation of executive function, such as the Montreal Cognitive Assessment (MoCA). Whenever possible, the family should be educated about significant cognitive deficits that may affect the patient's daily activities, such as medication management. By CKD stage 4, patients should be educated

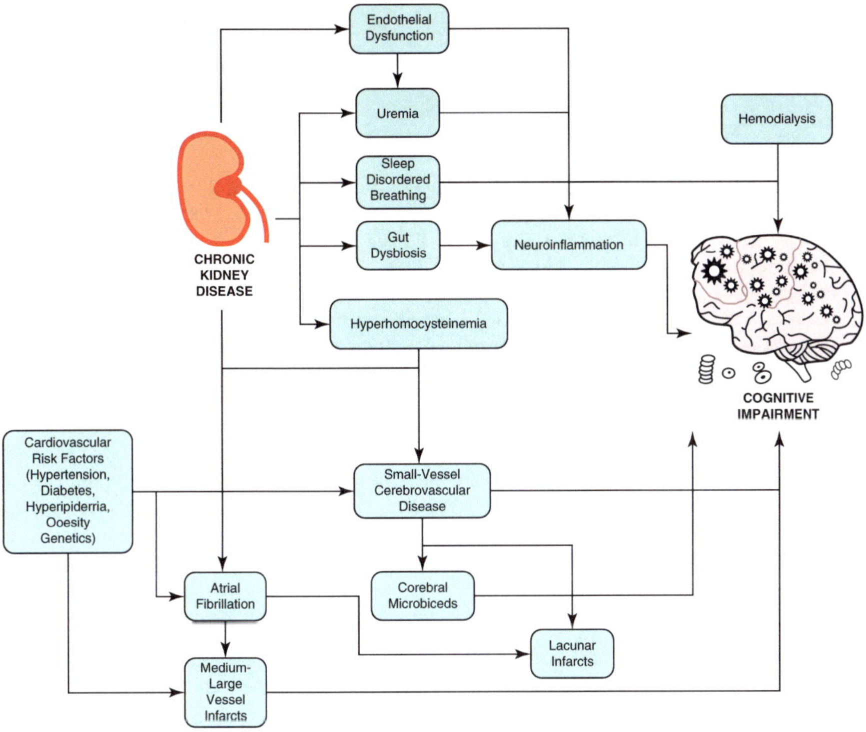

Fig. 12.4 Pathophysiology of cognitive impairment in chronic kidney disease. This paradigm illustrates how chronic kidney disease causes multiple pathophysiologic processes that culminate in cognitive impairment

about the different modalities of renal replacement therapy for which they are candidates, and screening for cognitive impairment that could guide planning for dialysis should be increased to more frequent intervals (e.g., every 6 months).

- The above mechanisms are summarized in Fig. 12.4.

Clinical Pearl

- Cerebrovascular disease, particularly of small vessels, is the major cause of neurocognitive decline in CKD.
- Other contributors to cognitive decline in CKD include:
  - Uremic toxins
  - Endothelial dysfunction
  - Neuroinflammation
  - Hyperhomocysteinemia
  - Alterations in the gut microbiome
  - Hemodialysis

References

1. Drew DA, Weiner DE, Sarnak MJ. Cognitive impairment in CKD: pathophysiology, management, and prevention. Am J Kidney Dis. 2019;74(6):782–90.
2. Webster AC, Nagler EV, Morton RL, Masson P. Chronic kidney disease. Lancet. 2017;389(10075):1238–52.
3. Kurella Tamura M, Wadley V, Yaffe K, McClure LA, Howard G, Go R, et al. Kidney function and cognitive impairment in US adults: the reasons for geographic and racial differences in stroke (REGARDS) study. Am J Kidney Dis. 2008;52(2):227–34.
4. Bugnicourt JM, Godefroy O, Chillon JM, Choukroun G, Massy ZA. Cognitive disorders and dementia in CKD: the neglected kidney-brain axis. J Am Soc Nephrol. 2013;24(3):353–63.
5. Murray AM, Tupper DE, Knopman DS, Gilbertson DT, Pederson SL, Li S, et al. Cognitive impairment in hemodialysis patients is common. Neurology. 2006;67(2):216–23.
6. Lee S, Shimada H, Park H, Makizako H, Lee S, Doi T, et al. The association between kidney function and cognitive decline in community-dwelling, elderly Japanese people. J Am Med Dir Assoc. 2015;16(4):349.e1-5.
7. Weiner DE, Gaussoin SA, Nord J, Auchus AP, Chelune GJ, Chonchol M, et al. Cognitive function and kidney disease: baseline data from the systolic blood pressure intervention trial (SPRINT). Am J Kidney Dis. 2017;70(3):357–67.
8. Barzilay JI, Gao P, O'Donnell M, Mann JF, Anderson C, Fagard R, et al. Albuminuria and decline in cognitive function: the ONTARGET/TRANSCEND studies. Arch Intern Med. 2011;171(2):142–50.
9. Etgen T, Chonchol M, Forstl H, Sander D. Chronic kidney disease and cognitive impairment: a systematic review and meta-analysis. Am J Nephrol. 2012;35(5):474–82.
10. Viggiano D, Wagner CA, Martino G, Nedergaard M, Zoccali C, Unwin R, et al. Mechanisms of cognitive dysfunction in CKD. Nat Rev Nephrol. 2020;16(8):452–69.
11. Drew DA, Bhadelia R, Tighiouart H, Novak V, Scott TM, Lou KV, et al. Anatomic brain disease in hemodialysis patients: a cross-sectional study. Am J Kidney Dis. 2013;61(2):271–8.
12. Vemuri P, Knopman DS, Jack CR Jr, Lundt ES, Weigand SD, Zuk SM, et al. Association of kidney function biomarkers with brain MRI findings: the BRINK study. J Alzheimers Dis. 2017;55(3):1069–82.
13. Reed BR, Mungas DM, Kramer JH, Ellis W, Vinters HV, Zarow C, et al. Profiles of neuropsychological impairment in autopsy-defined Alzheimer's disease and cerebrovascular disease. Brain. 2007;130(Pt 3):731–9.
14. Makizako H, Shimada H, Park H, Doi T, Yoshida D, Uemura K, et al. Evaluation of multidimensional neurocognitive function using a tablet personal computer: test-retest reliability and validity in community-dwelling older adults. Geriatr Gerontol Int. 2013;13(4):860–6.
15. Yaffe K, Ackerson L, Kurella Tamura M, Le Blanc P, Kusek JW, Sehgal AR, et al. Chronic kidney disease and cognitive function in older adults: findings from the chronic renal insufficiency cohort cognitive study. J Am Geriatr Soc. 2010;58(2):338–45.
16. Hamed SA. Neurologic conditions and disorders of uremic syndrome of chronic kidney disease: presentations, causes, and treatment strategies. Expert Rev Clin Pharmacol. 2019;12(1):61–90.
17. Davani AB, Snyder SH, Oh ES, Mears SC, Crews DC, Wang NY, et al. Kidney function modifies the effect of intraoperative opioid dosage on postoperative delirium. J Am Geriatr Soc. 2020;
18. Sommer J, Seeling A, Rupprecht H. Adverse drug events in patients with chronic kidney disease associated with multiple drug interactions and polypharmacy. Drugs Aging. 2020;37(5):359–72.
19. Ghoshal S, Freedman BI. Mechanisms of stroke in patients with chronic kidney disease. Am J Nephrol. 2019;50(4):229–39.
20. Aursulesei V, Costache II. Anticoagulation in chronic kidney disease: from guidelines to clinical practice. Clin Cardiol. 2019;42(8):774–82.
21. Lau WL, Nunes ACF, Vasilevko V, Floriolli D, Lertpanit L, Savoj J, et al. Chronic kidney disease increases cerebral microbleeds in mouse and man. Transl Stroke Res. 2020;11(1):122–34.

22. Akoudad S, Wolters FJ, Viswanathan A, de Bruijn RF, van der Lugt A, Hofman A, et al. Association of cerebral microbleeds with cognitive decline and dementia. JAMA Neurol. 2016;73(8):934–43.
23. Yao T, Song G, Li Y, Wang D. Chronic kidney disease correlates with MRI findings of cerebral small vessel disease. Ren Fail. 2021;43(1):255–63.
24. Ikram MA, Vernooij MW, Hofman A, Niessen WJ, van der Lugt A, Breteler MM. Kidney function is related to cerebral small vessel disease. Stroke. 2008;39(1):55–61.
25. Benjamin P, Lawrence AJ, Lambert C, Patel B, Chung AW, MacKinnon AD, et al. Strategic lacunes and their relationship to cognitive impairment in cerebral small vessel disease. Neuroimage Clin. 2014;4:828–37.
26. Richards E, Bayer A, Hanley C, Norris JE, Tree JJ, Tales A. Reaction time and visible white matter lesions in subcortical ischemic vascular cognitive impairment. J Alzheimers Dis. 2019;72(3):859–65.
27. Rensma SP, van Sloten TT, Houben A, Köhler S, van Boxtel MPJ, Berendschot T, et al. Microvascular dysfunction is associated with worse cognitive performance: the Maastricht study. Hypertension. 2020;75(1):237–45.
28. Assem M, Lando M, Grissi M, Kamel S, Massy ZA, Chillon JM, et al. The impact of uremic toxins on cerebrovascular and cognitive disorders. Toxins (Basel). 2018;10(7):303.
29. Mestre H, Mori Y, Nedergaard M. The brain's glymphatic system: current controversies. Trends Neurosci. 2020;43(7):458–66.
30. Rasmussen MK, Mestre H, Nedergaard M. The glymphatic pathway in neurological disorders. Lancet Neurol. 2018;17(11):1016–24.
31. Gupta J, Mitra N, Kanetsky PA, Devaney J, Wing MR, Reilly M, et al. Association between albuminuria, kidney function, and inflammatory biomarker profile in CKD in CRIC. Clin J Am Soc Nephrol. 2012;7(12):1938–46.
32. Jing W, Jabbari B, Vaziri ND. Uremia induces upregulation of cerebral tissue oxidative/inflammatory cascade, down-regulation of Nrf2 pathway and disruption of blood brain barrier. Am J Transl Res. 2018;10(7):2137–47.
33. Kurella Tamura M, Tam K, Vittinghoff E, Raj D, Sozio SM, Rosas SE, et al. Inflammatory markers and risk for cognitive decline in chronic kidney disease: the CRIC study. Kidney Int Rep. 2017;2(2):192–200.
34. Capelli I, Cianciolo G, Gasperoni L, Zappulo F, Tondolo F, Cappuccilli M, et al. Folic acid and vitamin B12 administration in CKD, why not? Nutrients. 2019;11(2):383.
35. Brady CB, Gaziano JM, Cxypoliski RA, Guarino PD, Kaufman JS, Warren SR, et al. Homocysteine lowering and cognition in CKD: the veterans affairs homocysteine study. Am J Kidney Dis. 2009;54(3):440–9.
36. Hobby GP, Karaduta O, Dusio GF, Singh M, Zybailov BL, Arthur JM. Chronic kidney disease and the gut microbiome. Am J Physiol Renal Physiol. 2019;316(6):F1211–7.
37. Velasquez MT, Centron P, Barrows I, Dwivedi R, Raj DS. Gut microbiota and cardiovascular uremic toxicities. Toxins (Basel). 2018;10(7):287.
38. Sprick JD, Nocera JR, Hajjar I, O'Neill WC, Bailey J, Park J. Cerebral blood flow regulation in end-stage kidney disease. Am J Physiol Renal Physiol. 2020;319(5):F782–91.
39. Shah RC, Buchman AS, Wilson RS, Leurgans SE, Bennett DA. Hemoglobin level in older persons and incident Alzheimer disease: prospective cohort analysis. Neurology. 2011;77(3):219–26.
40. Kurella Tamura M, Vittinghoff E, Yang J, Go AS, Seliger SL, Kusek JW, et al. Anemia and risk for cognitive decline in chronic kidney disease. BMC Nephrol. 2016;17:13.
41. Yaffe K, Falvey CM, Hoang T. Connections between sleep and cognition in older adults. Lancet Neurol. 2014;13(10):1017–28.
42. Seifter JL, Samuels MA. Uremic encephalopathy and other brain disorders associated with renal failure. Semin Neurol. 2011;31(2):139–43.
43. Van Sandwijk MS, Ten Berge IJ, Majoie CB, Caan MW, De Sonneville LM, Van Gool WA, et al. Cognitive changes in chronic kidney disease and after transplantation. Transplantation. 2016;100(4):734–42.

44. Kurella Tamura M, Vittinghoff E, Hsu CY, Tam K, Seliger SL, Sozio S, et al. Loss of executive function after dialysis initiation in adults with chronic kidney disease. Kidney Int. 2017;91(4):948–53.
45. Murray AM, Pederson SL, Tupper DE, Hochhalter AK, Miller WA, Li Q, et al. Acute variation in cognitive function in hemodialysis patients: a cohort study with repeated measures. Am J Kidney Dis. 2007;50(2):270–8.
46. Murthy VS, Shukla VS. A study of executive function in patients with chronic kidney disease before and after a single session of hemodialysis. J Neurosci Rural Pract. 2020;11(2):250–5.
47. Kelly D, Rothwell PM. Disentangling the multiple links between renal dysfunction and cerebrovascular disease. J Neurol Neurosurg Psychiatry. 2020;91(1):88–97.
48. Griva K, Hansraj S, Thompson D, Jayasena D, Davenport A, Harrison M, et al. Neuropsychological performance after kidney transplantation: a comparison between transplant types and in relation to dialysis and normative data. Nephrol Dial Transplant. 2004;19(7):1866–74.
49. Murray AM. Cognitive impairment in the aging dialysis and chronic kidney disease populations: an occult burden. Adv Chronic Kidney Dis. 2008;15(2):123–32.
50. Tiffin-Richards FE, Costa AS, Holschbach B, Frank RD, Vassiliadou A, Krüger T, et al. The Montreal Cognitive Assessment (MoCA) – a sensitive screening instrument for detecting cognitive impairment in chronic hemodialysis patients. PLoS One. 2014;9(10):e106700.
51. Nasreddine Z. MoCA test montreal. Québec: MoCA Test, Inc; 2019. Available from: https://www.mocatest.org

Sexuality and Sexual Dysfunction in the Renal Patient

13

Sehrish Ali, Vishnu P. Parvathareddy, and Natasha N. Dave

13.1 Introduction

Sexual dysfunction has a linear relationship to kidney disease, whereas progression of kidney disease is associated with malfunction and is associated with impaired quality of life, poor self-esteem, depression, and adverse cardiovascular outcomes. It is defined as the inability to carry out or enjoy a sexual activity with another individual. Sexual dysfunction is unfortunately prevalent in both women and men with kidney disease, yet it remains under-recognized and undertreated. The prevalence of sexual dysfunction in pre-dialysis patients is approximately 50%, irrespective of gender [1]. Roughly 80% of men on dialysis have erectile dysfunction, which increases with age [2]. Despite this prevalence, sexual dysfunction is likely underdiagnosed due to both patient/physician discomfort in discussing sexual health and overall lack of studies in patients with kidney disease.

While the exact mechanisms of sexual dysfunction are still being uncovered, it is postulated that this is often due to the lack of pulsatile or cyclic release of hypothalamic and pituitary hormones [3]. In addition to hormonal imbalances, several

S. Ali
Section of Nephrology, Department of Medicine, Baylor College of Medicine, Houston, TX, USA

Section of Nephrology, Michael E. DeBakey Veterans Affairs Medical Center, Houston, TX, USA

V. P. Parvathareddy
Section of Nephrology, Department of Medicine, Baylor College of Medicine, Houston, TX, USA

N. N. Dave (✉)
Strive Health, Denver, CO, USA

A. Hategan et al. (eds.), *Psychonephrology*,
https://doi.org/10.1007/978-3-030-84740-1_13

psychosocial and contributing conditions associated with kidney disease can promote dysfunction, including depressive disorders, poor self-image, neuropathy, mineral bone disease, diabetes mellitus, hypertension, and anemia [1, 4, 5]. Successful identification and treatment of sexual dysfunction must be inclusive of gender identity and sexual orientation. A comprehensive assessment should include review of clinical symptoms, thorough physical examination, degree of dysfunction via screening tools, additional laboratory testing, and/or specialist referral.

13.2 Case Vignette

A 40-year-old G3P3 (gravida 3, para 3) woman with a past medical history of lupus nephritis, hypertension, end-stage kidney disease (ESKD) on home hemodialysis for 3 years being dialyzed via an arteriovenous fistula, secondary hyperparathyroidism, and anemia was seen in clinic for a follow-up visit. She endorsed symptoms of decreased sexual desire, vaginal dryness, dyspareunia, hot flashes, sleep disturbances, and irregular periods for the past 1 year with worsening vasomotor symptoms in the previous 4–6 months. Her surgical history was notable for hysterectomy following the birth of her third child. Her blood pressure was stable on three medications, and her laboratory values including hemoglobin, iron studies, phosphorus, calcium, and parathyroid hormone were within the normal range. Her Kt/V (a parameter of the efficacy of hemodialysis treatment) was adequate with no recent changes to her dialysis prescription. She denied any issues with fluid shifts in the previous 6 months. She asked if these symptoms were menopause related and what treatment options were available as her symptoms were disrupting her quality of life.

13.3 Sexuality and Kidney Disease

13.3.1 Gender and Sexual Orientation

Gender expression and identity may not align with an individual's biological attributes. Individuals may identify with different gender or genders, which is communicated based on societal factors such as cultural constructs or perceptions. Transgender and gender nonconforming individuals, persons whose gender identity differs from their primary sexual organs, are considered gender minorities. Sexual orientation refers to the sexual attraction an individual feels to another person [6]. Nonheterosexual orientations are classified as sexual minorities (often identified as lesbian, gay, or bisexual) that include homosexuality or bisexuality. Sexual and gender minorities experience significant health-care disparities. Recognizing and understanding the unique needs of gender and sexual minorities (lesbian, gay, bisexual, transgender, queer LGBTQ+) is an important aspect when evaluating general and sexual health [7]. There is a considerable absence of kidney research in transgender/gender nonconforming individuals [8, 9]. For example, the effects of gender-affirming hormone use and sexual reassignment surgery on kidney function has not yet been studied [7].

Clinical Pearl
- Significant health-care disparities exist in chronic kidney disease rates and outcomes among sexual and gender minorities.

Recommendation
- When evaluating general and sexual health, recognizing and understanding the unique needs of gender and sexual minorities is an important aspect.
- Multidisciplinary efforts to eliminate health disparities affecting LGBTQ+ people are recommended.

13.4 Sexual Dysfunction in Women with Chronic Kidney Disease

- **Pathophysiology in Women**

  The pathophysiology of sexual dysfunction in women with kidney disease is due to hormonal disturbances that occur among all levels of the hypothalamic-pituitary-ovarian axis [10]. To understand these derangements, it is necessary to review normal reproductive physiology.

  Reproductive Physiology: The gonadotropin-releasing hormone (GnRH) is secreted from the hypothalamus, which conjures the anterior pituitary gland to release luteinizing hormone (LH) and follicle-stimulating hormone (FSH) in a pulsatile fashion. LH triggers ovulation and helps the corpus luteum mature, whereas FSH assists in the growth of the ovarian follicle. Both hormones induce ovarian synthesis of progesterone and estradiol that in turn provides negative feedback for this axis. Progesterone inhibits GnRH, FSH, and LH, while estradiol inhibits GnRH and FSH. For ovulation to occur, elevated estradiol levels are required for mid-cycle LH surge. After ovulation, progesterone is secreted from the corpus luteum to prepare the uterus for embryo implantation. If implantation does not occur, the corpus luteum degenerates causing diminished levels of progesterone leading to menstruation [11].

  Reproductive Pathophysiology in Women with Kidney Disease: The precise processes of hormone disruption in women with kidney disease are poorly understood. Women with kidney disease have demonstrated preserved basal levels of GnRH, LH, and FSH but are unable to secrete GnRH in a pulsatile manner that is required for ovulation [3, 10]. The downstream effects of this include lack of LH/FSH rise consequently blunting estradiol synthesis and secretion. With low levels of estradiol, women are unable to mount a mid-cycle LH peak, which leads to anovulation. The etiology of GnRH inhibition remains ill-defined but is likely multifactorial from reduced clearance of leptin, prolactin, endorphins, and gonadotropins [12–14].

- **Clinical Features in Women**

  The clinical manifestations in women with sexual dysfunction are variable and can range from organ-specific symptoms such as vaginal dryness or dyspareunia to a constellation of systemic symptoms due hypogonadism (see Table 13.1). Understanding the clinical features can help clinicians better characterize and ultimately treat sexual dysfunction.

  1. **General/Systemic Symptoms**

     Hypogonadism: The development of hypogonadism has been outlined in the above section (Reproductive Pathophysiology in Women with Kidney

Table 13.1 Clinical manifestations of sexual dysfunction in women and men

	Women	Men
General	*Hypogonadism:* General: Short term: skin aging, depression, sleep disturbances, urinary incontinence, hot flashes Long term: cognitive decline, cardiovascular and mineral bone disease Specific to sexual function: loss of libido, hypoactive sexual desire disorder, difficulty in arousal and/or orgasm *Hyperprolactinemia:* Galactorrhea	*Hypogonadism/low testosterone:* General: Fatigue, decreased energy, sleep disturbances, negative mood, depression, lack of secondary sexual characteristics, such as facial, axillary, and pubic hair, decreased muscle strength, diminished bone mass. Specific to sexual function: loss of libido, impotence, the presence of small soft testicles, reduced spermatogenesis causing decreased sperm count and poor semen quality and decreased fertility. *Hyperprolactinemia:* Gynecomastia, infertility, loss of libido
Sex organ specific	Atrophic vaginitis: vaginal dryness, decreased pubic hair, pruritus, dyspareunia Decrease vaginal lubrication Dyspareunia	*Erectile dysfunction/impotence:* Neurologic cause: other signs of neuropathy or neurogenic bladder Vascular cause: signs of impaired lower extremity blood flow Both neurologic and vascular causes are likely to be associated with normal sized testicles *Testicular damage:* damage to seminiferous tubules, atrophy of Sertoli cells, interstitial fibrosis and calcification
Fertility considerations	Amenorrhea or irregular cycles Dysfunctional uterine bleeding Early menopause Infertility	Impaired spermatogenesis, decreased volume of ejaculate, either low or complete azoospermia, low percentage of motility Infertility

Disease) [15]. A constellation of short- and long-term findings can be seen in Table 13.1.

Specific to sexual function, loss of sexual desire and satisfaction leads to interpersonal conflict and poor self-esteem. Women with kidney disease can report a myriad of issues in this realm, which can span to include difficulty in arousal or achieving orgasm [16]. The context of these symptoms may shed light on the underlying cause. For example, women with ESKD have reported difficulty participating in sexual intercourse with a dialysis catheter. Therefore, it is important to consider dialysis access and fluid shifts as a potential factor in the development of these symptoms [17].

Hyperprolactinemia: Elevated prolactin levels in kidney disease are believed to be multifactorial due to irregular inhibition of dopaminergic activity, increased secretion due to secondary hyperparathyroidism, and reduced clearance [12, 18].

2. **Vaginal Complications**

   Low estradiol levels lead to atrophic vaginitis characterized by vaginal itching, discharge, dyspareunia, decreased lubrication, and pubic hair. Estrogen deficiency also increases the vaginal pH level predisposing these patients to urinary tract infections [19].

3. **Menstruation**

   Menstrual abnormalities are common in women with kidney disease and can consist of irregular menstrual cycles, dysfunctional uterine bleeding, amenorrhea, and anovulation [20]. These women are also at risk of developing menopause on average 4.5 years earlier than healthy women; therefore, it is crucial to map out menstrual patterns and development of other symptoms [15].

4. **Fertility Considerations**

   The inability to conceive in this population can be a result of deranged hormonal interplay leading to anovulation or early ovarian failure as well as declining sexual interest leading to decreased frequency of intercourse. Although rare, some women with kidney disease have successfully conceived but face significant risks including worsening estimated glomerular filtration rate (eGFR), proteinuria, hypertension, pregnancy complications, and poor fetal outcomes [21–23]. All women of child-bearing age with kidney disease should receive counseling on these risks [22, 23].

- **Evaluation of Sexual Dysfunction in Women**

  Female Sexual Functioning Index (FSFI) is a validated tool used for addressing six domains of female sexual function including desire, lubrication, arousal, orgasm, pain, and satisfaction [24, 25]. Limitations of this tool include the fact that it does not address sexual dysfunction in lesbian or gay women and does not account for sexual inactivity [26]. Measurements of LH, FSH, estrogen, progesterone, and prolactin can aid in diagnosing abnormalities of the hypothalamic-pituitary-gonadal axis.

- **Treatment in Women**

  Treatment is limited as the efficacy of sexual dysfunction treatment in women with kidney disease is poorly studied and understood. Approach to treatment must include management of comorbid conditions that contribute to dysfunction, minimizing medication interactions, and addressing the symptom(s) of concern.

  1. **Comorbid Conditions**

     It is important to manage depressive disorders, diabetes mellitus, anemia, and hyperparathyroidism, as they can contribute to sexual dysfunction [1, 4, 5]. Dialysis adequacy has shown to play a role in dysfunction as well; consider adjustment of dialysis prescription if necessary.

  2. **Medication Interactions**

     Antihypertensives (aldosterone antagonists), antidepressants (selective serotonin reuptake inhibitors (SSRIs), tricyclic antidepressants (TCAs), monoamine oxidase inhibitors (MAOIs)), antipsychotics, lithium carbonate, benzodiazepines, opioids, immunosuppressants, glucocorticoids/anabolic steroids, antifungal (ketoconazole), histamine receptor antagonists (cimetidine), antiemetic (metoclopramide), and anti-estrogen/aromatase inhibitors can all be implicated in cases of sexual dysfunction [27–29].

  3. **Symptom(s) of Concern**

     (a) **General/Systemic Symptoms**

     Hyperprolactinemia: Bromocriptine has shown to improve sexual desire and function in men with ESKD; however, this is not well demonstrated or well studied in women [3, 30]. Calcitriol used in the treatment of secondary hyperparathyroidism may lower prolactin levels [31]. Recombinant human erythropoietin used in the treatment of anemia may reduce LH and FSH, increase testosterone, as well as decrease prolactin levels and has shown to improve sexual function in patients with ESKD [5, 13, 32].

     (b) **Sexual Desire/Libido and Satisfaction**

     In healthy postmenopausal women with hypoactive sexual desire disorder, characterized by interpersonal distress due to lack of desire for sexual activity, testosterone therapy can be used as a treatment option. However, there is limited data on the use of testosterone in patients with kidney disease, and majority of studies are in men [33–36].

     (c) **Vaginal Complications**

     Atrophic vaginitis may be treated with topical estrogen and lubricants [33–36].

     (d) **Menstruation**

     While progesterone can restore menstruation and potentially mitigate the unopposed effect of estrogen on the endometrium leading to endometrial hyperplasia or carcinoma, menses could worsen anemia attributed to chronic disease. Given this, progesterone may be beneficial several times a year in certain cases [37, 38]. Hormone replacement therapy should be administered on a case-by-case basis, as it is associated with several adverse side effects, including thromboembolic risks, increased circulating estrogen with risk for endometrial hyperplasia or carcinoma, and increased risk for cardiovascular events. For premenopausal women with estrogen deficiency who are on dialysis, estrogen replacement therapy is associated with menstrual restoration, improved sexual function, and increased bone density. For postmenopausal women on dialysis, estrogen replacement therapy has shown improvement in sexual desire and increased bone density [39].

Combined estrogen-progesterone therapy for healthy women has shown increased risk for cardiovascular events. Furthermore, it is not well studied in women with kidney disease and therefore could potentially increase an already elevated risk for cardiovascular complications in these patients [40, 41].

(e) **Fertility Considerations**

Women of child-bearing age with menstrual periods should be counseled on risks associated with pregnancy and offered birth control. Kidney transplantation has shown to restore fertility and should be encouraged for women who are otherwise candidates for transplantation [42–44].

13.5 Sexual Dysfunction in Men

- **Pathophysiology in Men**

  As in women, the pathophysiology of sexual dysfunction in men with kidney disease is due to hormonal disturbances that occur among all levels of the hypothalamic-pituitary-gonadal axis. To understand these derangements, it is imperative to review normal reproductive physiology.

  Reproductive Physiology: The hypothalamus secretes GnRH which stimulates the pulsatile release of LH and FSH from the anterior pituitary. LH binds to receptors on the Leydig cell stimulating testosterone production and FSH binds to Sertoli cells, when partnered with testosterone, causes release of androgen-binding protein which is needed for spermatogenesis. Negative feedback is achieved by testosterone inhibiting LH and via conversion to estradiol it inhibits GnRH, whereas FSH production of inhibition in the Sertoli cell which inhibits FSH.

  Reproductive Pathophysiology in Men with Kidney Disease: The precise processes of hormone disruption in men with kidney disease are poorly understood. Men with kidney disease have demonstrated a lack of pulsatile release of GnRH, LH, and FSH that leads to the loss of cyclic LH surge resulting in low levels of testosterone. Testicular damage due to kidney disease is another cause of low testosterone that, due to loss of negative feedback, produces elevated baseline LH levels but is not enough to surge [45–47]. Testicular failure and reduced sperm production ensue due to low testosterone synthesis. The etiology of GnRH inhibition remains ill-defined but is likely multifactorial from reduced clearance of leptin, prolactin, endorphins, and gonadotropins [12–14, 45].

- **Clinical Features in Men**
  1. **General/Systemic Symptoms**

     Hypogonadism/Low Testosterone

     General: Fatigue, decreased energy, sleep disturbances, depressive disorders, lack of secondary sexual characteristics, such as facial, axillary, and pubic hair, decreased muscle strength, and diminished bone mass [46, 48].

     Specific to sexual function: loss of libido, impotence, the presence of small soft testicles, reduced spermatogenesis causing decreased sperm count and poor semen quality, and decreased fertility [46, 48]. (See Table 13.1 for general and specific sexual symptoms in men with kidney disease.)

     Hyperprolactinemia: In men with normal kidney function, elevated prolactin levels are associated with infertility, loss of libido and low circulating testosterone levels. In men on dialysis, hyperprolactinemia causes gynecomastia which typically develops during the first few months of dialysis and subsequently improves as treatment continues [12, 49]. Successful kidney transplantation and early initiation of dialysis are associated with decreased occurrence of gynecomastia [50].
  2. **Penile Complications**

     Erectile dysfunction (ED)/impotence is defined as inability to achieve or maintain erection sufficient for satisfactory intercourse. There are multiple causes for ED [51, 52], as outlined below:
     1. Neurologic cause, manifesting with signs of neuropathy or neurogenic bladder.
     2. Vascular cause, manifesting with signs of impaired lower extremity blood flow including cramping in thighs/calves when walking, poor wound healing, coldness, numbness, and loss of hair on legs.
     3. Neurologic and vascular causes are likely to be associated with normal sized testicles.
  3. **Testicular/Fertility Considerations**
     1. Semen irregularities: Kidney disease leads to impaired spermatogenesis with semen analysis revealing decreased ejaculate volume, azoospermia, and poor sperm motility. Interestingly, upon initiation of dialysis, these abnormalities tend to improve [53].
     2. Testicular damage: Damage to seminiferous tubules, atrophy of Sertoli cells, interstitial fibrosis, and calcification [53].
     3. Infertility is an unfortunate consequence seen in men with kidney disease and is thought to be multifactorial from decreased libido, erectile dysfunction, and abnormalities in sperm production [53].
- **Evaluation of Sexual Dysfunction in Men** [52]

  The International Index of Erectile Function (IIEF-5) is a validated tool used for addressing various domains of male sexual function including erectile function, orgasmic function, sexual desire, intercourse satisfaction, and overall satisfaction [51]. Measurements of LH, FSH, testosterone, and prolactin can aid in diagnosing abnormalities of the hypothalamic-pituitary-gonadal axis [12].

In addition to hormone irregularities, men can develop sexual dysfunction due to other contributing conditions, including depressive disorders, peripheral neuropathy, and peripheral vascular disease [1, 4, 5].

1. Testing for the presence of nocturnal penile tumescence can discriminate between a psychologic and a structural cause of impotence. Patients with purely psychological causes of impotence would still experience erections while asleep, whereas the absence of an adequate erection would make a structural cause more likely.
2. Testing for neurogenic impotence is detected by a prolonged latency time of the bulbocavernosus reflex or by confirming the presence of a neurogenic bladder.
3. Testing for vascular causes of impotence includes Doppler study of penile blood flow, measurement of penile blood pressure, and penile pulse palpation.

- **Treatment in Men**

The treatment of sexual dysfunction in men is better evaluated than in women with kidney disease. As in women, approach to treatment involves management of comorbid conditions that contribute to dysfunction, minimizing medication interactions, and addressing the symptoms of concern.

1. **Comorbid conditions**

It is important to manage obesity, hypertension, depressive disorders, diabetes mellitus, anemia, and hyperparathyroidism as they can contribute to dysfunction [1, 4, 5]. Dialysis adequacy has shown to play a role in dysfunction as well; therefore, consider adjustment of prescription if necessary.

2. **Medication Interactions**

Antihypertensives (beta-blockers, aldosterone antagonists, guanethidine, reserpine, methyldopa, clonidine, propranolol, prazosin), antidepressants (selective serotonin reuptake inhibitors (SSRIs), tricyclic antidepressants (TCAs), monoamine oxidase inhibitors (MAOIs)), antipsychotics, lithium carbonate, benzodiazepines, opioids, immunosuppressants, glucocorticoids/anabolic steroids, antifungal (ketoconazole), histamine receptor antagonists (cimetidine), and antiemetics (metoclopramide, phenothiazines) can all contribute to sexual dysfunction in men [27–29]. Alternative antihypertensives such as angiotensin-converting enzyme inhibitors or angiotensin receptor blockers can be used as they are associated with a lower incidence of impotence [54].

3. **Symptom(s) of Concern**

(a) **General/Systemic Symptoms**

Hypogonadism/Low Testosterone: Treatment should be considered for men who exhibit low testosterone levels and symptoms consistent with hypogonadism. Variable improvement in sexual function and anemia have been demonstrated in the few studies on testosterone therapy in men with kidney disease [39, 55]. Risks of testosterone including stimulating prostate cancer and other anabolic effects must be taken in consideration prior to initiating therapy. Zinc deficiency due to reduced dietary intake, malabsorption, or potential removal via dialysis has been implicated as a cause of sexual dysfunction. Supplementation of zinc resulted in increased plasma testosterone levels and elevated sperm counts [56].

Hyperprolactinemia: The use of bromocriptine in the treatment of hyperprolactinemia in men with kidney disease has shown to reduce prolactin levels but has inconsistent effects on sexual desire and potency [30, 49]. Newer dopamine agonists such as cabergoline have a lower side effect profile in comparison to bromocriptine but are not studied in this population. Calcitriol used in the treatment of secondary hyperparathyroidism may lower prolactin levels [31]. Recombinant human erythropoietin (rHuEPO) used in the treatment of anemia may reduce LH and FSH, increase testosterone, as well as decrease prolactin levels [5, 13, 32]. It has shown to improve sexual function in patients with ESKD and has been recommended to prevent or treat erectile dysfunction in men with chronic kidney disease.

(b) **Penile Complications**

ED/impotence: The use of phosphodiesterase inhibitors, such as sildenafil and vardenafil, in men with kidney disease has shown promise for treatment of impotence and is associated with improvements in quality of life and depressive symptoms [57–60].

In patients with neurogenic or vascular causes, treatment options include the use of vacuum/constriction devices as well as intracavernous injection or urethral suppositories of alprostadil. In patients who fail treatment, referral and evaluation for surgical placement of a penile prosthesis can be considered.

(c) **Testicular/Fertility Considerations**

If candidates, men with kidney disease should be considered for transplantation as this has shown restoration of spermatogenesis in addition to improvement in gynecomastia, libido, impotence, and fertility [42–44, 50, 61]. It is important to recognize that many times, erectile dysfunction can worsen after kidney transplantation as well, especially if the allograft function worsens over time.

13.6 Case Vignette Analysis

This patient is likely experiencing symptoms of early ovarian failure or menopause due to ESKD. Due to lack of large clinical trials, hormone replacement therapy for menopausal women with chronic kidney disease must be evaluated on a case-by-case basis. The use of combination estrogen-progesterone therapy may be associated with increased cardiovascular events in healthy women and should be used with extreme caution as this can worsen an already elevated likelihood of adverse cardiovascular outcomes. Similar to combination therapy, estrogen as a sole hormonal therapy is associated with numerous side effects, including risk of unopposed estrogen on endometrium leading to hyperplasia or carcinoma and increased risk of thromboembolism. In this case, our patient can be considered for treatment with solo estrogen replacement as she has a history of a hysterectomy. However, given her history of lupus nephritis, it is imperative to evaluate her history/risk of thromboembolism and consider additional testing for lupus anticoagulant or antiphospholipid antibody syndrome, if indicated. In the absence of increased thromboembolic risk, say, the etiology of ESKD in this patient was due to diabetic nephropathy instead of lupus nephritis, treatment with estrogen replacement can be attempted so long as the patient understands risk-to-benefit ratio and other potential side effects and receives routine gynecological care.

Clinical Pearl

– A thorough medical evaluation must be inclusive of the patient's sexuality (including gender identity and sexual orientation), taking into consideration:
  - The context of sexual dysfunction
  - The degree of dysfunction via screening tools (FSFI or IIEF-5)
  - Performing a careful physical examination
  - Additional laboratory testing or other studies in some cases.

Recommendation

– Treatment of sexual dysfunction in chronic kidney disease should be:
  - Individualized
  - Focused on correcting coexisting medical conditions
  - Focused on recognition and reducing medication interactions
  - Focused on treatment of predominant underlying hormone imbalance(s), with close monitoring as well as collaboration with other providers.

Recommendation

– Kidney transplantation may lead to restoration of the hypothalamic-pituitary-gonadal axis and potential reversal of sexual dysfunction in patients with chronic kidney disease.

13.7 Key Takeaways

- Sexual dysfunction in chronic kidney disease is prevalent and yet is both underrecognized and underreported. It is associated with many adverse outcomes including poor self-image, impaired quality of life, psychosocial distress, and adverse cardiovascular events.
- The pathophysiology of sexual dysfunction in men and women with chronic kidney disease is due to hormonal disturbances that occur along the hypothalamic-pituitary-gonadal axis. The loss of pulsatile release of GnRH, LH, and FSH causes low concentrations of estradiol and testosterone in women and men, which accordingly have been associated with a myriad of manifestations.
- Hyperprolactinemia, hyperendorphinism, and increased leptin levels may contribute to the loss of pulsatile function and potentially play a role in the pathophysiology of sexual dysfunction in chronic kidney disease.
- A thorough medical evaluation must include the patient's sexuality (including gender identity and sexual orientation), using screening tools (FSFI or IIEF-5) as necessary, along with a careful examination, and additional laboratory testing or other studies.
- Treatment of sexual dysfunction in kidney disease should be individualized and focus on correcting coexisting medical conditions, reducing medication interactions and recognition, as well as treatment of predominant underlying hormone imbalance(s). Due to lack of large clinical trials in this population, treatment, in some cases, can be considered experimental and may require close monitoring as well as collaboration with other providers.
- Restoration of the hypothalamic-pituitary-gonadal axis and reversal of sexual dysfunction in chronic kidney disease may be seen with kidney transplantation and should be considered in patients if they are candidates.

References

1. Finkelstein F, Shirani S, Wuerth D, Finkelstein SH. Therapy insight: sexual dysfunction in patients with chronic kidney disease. Nat Clin Pract Nephrol. 2007;3:200–7.
2. Rosas S, Joffe M, Franklin E, et al. Prevalence and determinants of erectile dysfunction in hemodialysis patients. Kidney Int. 2001;59:2259–66.
3. Lim VS, Henriquez C, Sievertsen G, Frohman LA. Ovarian function in chronic renal failure: evidence suggesting hypothalamic anovulation. Ann Intern Med. 1980;93(1):21–7.
4. Anantharaman P, Schmidt RJ. Sexual function in chronic kidney disease. Adv Chronic Kid Dis. 2007;14:119–25.
5. Lawrence IG, Price DE, Howlett TA, Harris KP, Feehally J, Walls J. Erythropoietin and sexual dysfunction. Nephrol Dial Transplant. 1997;12(4):741–7.
6. Mohottige D, Lunn MR. Advancing equity in nephrology: enhancing care for LGBTQ1 patients and our workforce. Clin J Am Soc Nephrol. 2019;14(7):1094–6.
7. Ahmed SB, Saad N, Dumanski SM. Gender and CKD: beyond the binary. Clin J Am Soc Nephrol. 2020;16(1):141–3.
8. Sequeira GM, Ray KN, Miller E. CoulterRWS. Transgender youth's disclosure of gender identity to providers outside of specialized gender centers. J Adolesc Health. 2020;66(6):691–8.
9. Navaneethan SD, Vecchio M, Johnson DW, et al. Prevalence and correlates of self-reported sexual dysfunction in CKD: a meta-analysis of observational studies. Am J Kidney Dis. 2010;56(4):670–85.

10. Lim VS. Reproductive function in patients with renal insufficiency. Am J Kidney Dis. 1987;9(4):363–7.
11. Adams JM, Taylor AE, Schoenfeld DA, Crowley WF Jr, Hall JE. The midcycle gonadotropin surge in normal women occurs in the face of an unchanging gonadotropin-releasing hormone pulse frequency. J Clin Endocrinol Metab. 1994;79(3):858–64.
12. Gomez F, de la Cueva R, Wauters JP, Lemarchand-Beraud T. Endocrine abnormalities in patients undergoing long-term hemodialysis. The role of prolactin. Am J Med. 1980;68(4): 522–30.
13. Palmer BF. Sexual dysfunction in men and women with chronic kidney disease and end-stage kidney disease. Adv Ren Replace Ther. 2003;10(1):48–60.
14. Sharma K, Considine RV, Michael B, et al. Plasma leptin is partly cleared by the kidney and is elevated in hemodialysis patients. Kidney Int. 1997;51(6):1980–5.
15. Weisinger JR, Bellorin-Font E. Outcomes associated with hypogonadism in women with chronic kidney disease. Adv Chronic Kidney Dis. 2004;11(4):361–70.
16. Pastan S, Bailey J. Dialysis therapy. N Engl J Med. 1998;338(20):1428–37.
17. Alvarez-Villarreal M, Velarde-Garcia JF, Chocarro-Gonzalez L, Perez-Corrales J, Gueita-Rodriguez J, Palacios-Cena D. Body changes and decreased sexual drive after dialysis: a qualitative study on the experiences of women at an ambulatory dialysis unit in Spain. Int J Environ Res Public Health. 2019;16(17):3086.
18. Raymond JP, Isaac R, Merceron RE, Wahbe F. Comparison between the plasma concentrations of prolactin and parathyroid hormone in normal subjects and in patients with hyperparathyroidism or hyperprolactinemia. J Clin Endocrinol Metab. 1982;55(6):1222–5.
19. Semmens JP, Wagner G. Estrogen deprivation and vaginal function in postmenopausal women. JAMA. 1982;248(4):445–8.
20. Holley JL, Schmidt RJ, Bender FH, Dumler F, Schiff M. Gynecologic and reproductive issues in women on dialysis. Am J Kidney Dis. 1997;29(5):685–90.
21. Ginsburg ES, Owen WF Jr. Reproductive endocrinology and pregnancy in women on hemodialysis. Semin Dial. 1993;6:105–16.
22. Gill JS, Zalunardo N, Rose C, Tonelli M. The pregnancy rate and live birth rate in kidney transplant recipients. Am J Transplant. 2009;9(7):1541–9.
23. Hladunewich MA. Chronic kidney disease and pregnancy. Semin Nephrol. 2017;37(4): 337–46.
24. Rosen R, Brown C, Heiman J, et al. The Female Sexual Function Index (FSFI): a multidimensional self-report instrument for the assessment of female sexual function. J Sex Marital Ther. 2000;26(2):191–208.
25. Basok EK, Atsu N, Rifaioglu MM, Kantarci G, Yildirim A, Tokuc R. Assessment of female sexual function and quality of life in predialysis, peritoneal dialysis, hemodialysis, and renal transplant patients. Int Urol Nephrol. 2009;41(3):473–81.
26. Mor MK, Sevick MA, Shields AM, et al. Sexual function, activity, and satisfaction among women receiving maintenance hemodialysis. Clin J Am Soc Nephrol. 2014;9(1):128–34.
27. Bailie GR, Elder SJ, Mason NA, et al. Sexual dysfunction in dialysis patients treated with antihypertensive or antidepressive medications: results from the DOPPS. Nephrol Dial Transplant. 2007;22(4):1163–70.
28. Turner HE, Wass JA. Gonadal function in men with chronic illness. Clin Endocrinol. 1997;47(4):379–403.
29. Schmidt A, Luger A, Horl WH. Sexual hormone abnormalities in male patients with renal failure. Nephrol Dial Transplant. 2002;17(3):368–71.
30. Muir JW, Besser GM, Edwards CR, et al. Bromocriptine improves reduced libido and potency in men receiving maintenance hemodialysis. Clin Nephrol. 1983;20(6):308–14.
31. Leavey SF, Weitzel WF. Endocrine abnormalities in chronic renal failure. Endocrinol Metab Clin N Am. 2002;31(1):107–19.
32. Kokot F, Wiecek A, Schmidt-Gayk H, et al. Function of endocrine organs in hemodialyzed patients of long-term erythropoietin therapy. Artif Organs. 1995;19(5):428–35.
33. Shifren JL, Davis SR, Moreau M, et al. Testosterone patch for the treatment of hypoactive sexual desire disorder in naturally menopausal women: results from the INTIMATE NM1 study. Menopause. 2006;13(5):770–9.

34. Simon J, Braunstein G, Nachtigall L, et al. Testosterone patch increases sexual activity and desire in surgically menopausal women with hypoactive sexual desire disorder. J Clin Endocrinol Metab. 2005;90(9):5226–33.
35. Somboonporn W, Davis S, Seif MW, Bell R. Testosterone for peri- and postmenopausal women. Cochrane Database Syst Rev. 2005;4:CD004509.
36. Shifren JL, Davis SR. Androgens in postmenopausal women: a review. Menopause. 2017;24(8):970–9.
37. Anantharaman P, Schmidt RJ. Sexual function in chronic kidney disease. Adv Chronic Kidney Dis. 2007;14(2):119–25.
38. Palmer BF, Clegg DJ. Gonadal dysfunction in chronic kidney disease. Rev Endocr Metab Disord. 2017;18(1):117–30.
39. Holley JL, Schmidt RJ. Changes in fertility and hormone replacement therapy in kidney disease. Adv Chronic Kidney Dis. 2013;20(3):240–5.
40. Rossouw JE, Anderson GL, Prentice RL, et al; Writing Group for the Women's Health Initiative Investigators. Risks and benefits of estrogen plus progestin in healthy postmenopausal women: principal results from the Women's Health Initiative randomized controlled trial. JAMA. 2002;288(3):321–33.
41. Hulley S, Grady D, Bush T, et al. Randomized trial of estrogen plus progestin for secondary prevention of coronary heart disease in postmenopausal women. JAMA. 1998;280:605–13.
42. Tsujimura A, Matsumiya K, Tsuboniwa N, et al. Effect of renal transplantation on sexual function. Arch Androl. 2002;48(6):467–74.
43. Saha MT, Saha HH, Niskanen LK, Salmela KT, Pasternack AI. Time course of serum prolactin and sex hormones following successful renal transplantation. Nephron. 2002;92(3):735–7.
44. Wang GC, Zheng JH, Xu LG, et al. Measurements of serum pituitary-gonadal hormones and investigation of sexual and reproductive functions in kidney transplant recipients. Int J Nephrol. 2010;2010:612126.
45. Lim VA. Reproductive function in patients with renal insufficiency. Am J Kidney Dis. 1987;9(4):363–7.
46. Schmidt A, Luger A, Hörl WH. Sexual hormone abnormalities in male patients with renal failure. Nephrol Dial Transplant. 2002;17(3):368–71.
47. Holdsworth S, Atkins RC, de Kretser DM. The pituitary-testicular axis in men with chronic renal failure. N Engl J Med. 1977;296(22):1245–9.
48. Zitzmann M, Faber S, Nieschlag E. Association of specific symptoms and metabolic risks with serum testosterone in older men. J Clin Endocrinol Metab. 2006;91:4335–43.
49. Degli Esposti E, Sturani A, Santoro A, Zuccalà A, Chiarini C, Zucchelli P. Effect of bromocriptine treatment on prolactin, noradrenaline and blood pressure in hypertensive haemodialysis patients. Clin Sci (Lond). 1985;69(1):51–6.
50. Akbari F, Alavi M, Esteghamati A, et al. Effect of renal transplantation on sperm quality and sex hormone levels. BJU Int. 2003;92(3):281–3.
51. Rosen RC, Cappelleri JC, Smith MD, Lipsky J, Peña BM. Development and evaluation of an abridged, 5-item version of the International Index of Erectile Function (IIEF-5) as a diagnostic tool for erectile dysfunction. Int J Impot Res. 1999;11(6):319–26.
52. Yafi FA, Jenkins L, Albersen M, et al. Erectile dysfunction. Nat Rev Dis Primers. 2016;2:16003.
53. Levitan D, Moser SA, Goldstein DA, Kletzky OA, Lobo RA, Massry SG: Disturbances in the hypothalamic-pituitary-gonadal axis in male patients with acute renal failure. Am J Nephrol. 1984;4:99–106.
54. Nunes KP, Labazi H, Webb RC. New insights into hypertension-associated erectile dysfunction. Curr Opin Nephrol Hypertens. 2012;21(2):163–70.
55. Snyder G, Shoskes DA. Hypogonadism and testosterone replacement therapy in end-stage renal disease (ESRD) and transplant patients. Transl Androl Urol. 2016;5(6):885–9.
56. Mahajan SK, Abbasi AA, Prasad AS, Rabbani P, Briggs WA, McDonald FD. Effect of oral zinc therapy on gonadal function in hemodialysis patients. A double-blind study. Ann Intern Med. 1982;97(3):357–61.

57. Sharma RK, Prasad N, Gupta A, Kapoor R. Treatment of erectile dysfunction with sildenafil citrate in renal allograft recipients: a randomized double-blind, placebo-controlled, cross-over trial. Am J Kidney Dis. 2006;48:128–33.
58. Procci WR, Goldstein DA, Adelstein J, Massry SG. Sexual dysfunction in the male patients with uremia: a reappraisal. Kidney Int. 1981;19:317–23.
59. Papadopoulou E, Varouktsi A, Lazaridis A, Boutari C, Doumas M. Erectile dysfunction in chronic kidney disease: from pathophysiology to management. World J Nephrol. 2015;4(3):379–87.
60. Lasaponara F, Sedigh O, Pasquale G, et al. Phosphodiesterase type 5 inhibitor treatment for erectile dysfunction in patients with end-stage renal disease receiving dialysis or after renal transplantation. J Sex Med. 2013;10(11):2798–814.
61. Perri A, Izzo G, Lofaro D, et al. Erectile dysfunction after kidney transplantation. J Clin Med. 2020;9(6):1991.

Psychotoxicity of Immunomodulators: Corticosteroids, Mycophenolate, Tacrolimus, Cyclophosphamide, and Hydroxychloroquine

14

Stanislav Pasyk, Shyam Maharaj, and James A. Bourgeois

14.1 Corticosteroids

14.1.1 Overview

Corticosteroids are potent anti-inflammatory drugs that are often a key element of treatment in a variety of renal pathologies, including nephritis associated with systemic lupus erythematosus, systemic vasculitis, and other forms of glomerulonephritis. While corticosteroids are highly therapeutic, they may also come with a vast array of possible systemic side effects. Unfortunately, psychiatric complications related to corticosteroid use are common and often overlooked. Prevalence of clinically significant psychiatric symptoms is typically reported to be between 5 and 10% of patients using corticosteroids [1]. Possible side effects include a substantial range of psychiatric disturbances, including anxiety, delirium, insomnia, cognitive impairment, depressive disorders, and psychotic

S. Pasyk (✉)
Department of Psychiatry and Behavioural Neurosciences, Michael G. DeGroote School of Medicine, McMaster University, Hamilton, ON, Canada
e-mail: stanislav.pasyk@medportal.ca

S. Maharaj
Department of Medicine, McMaster University, Hamilton, ON, Canada
e-mail: maharass@mcmaster.ca

J. A. Bourgeois
Department of Psychiatry, Baylor Scott & White Health, Central Texas Division, Department of Medical Education, College of Medicine, Texas A&M University Health Science Center, Temple, TX, USA
e-mail: james.bourgeois@BSWHealth.org

A. Hategan et al. (eds.), *Psychonephrology*,
https://doi.org/10.1007/978-3-030-84740-1_14

disorders. In some instances, the burden of a corticosteroid-induced mood or psychotic disorder can be severe and warrant psychiatric admission for definitive management.

Clinical Pearl

- The overall risk of developing psychiatric side effects related to corticosteroid use is estimated to be between 5 and 10%.

14.1.2 Range of Psychiatric Side Effects of Corticosteroids

For decades, corticosteroid-related psychiatric side effects have been reported [1]. Efforts to precisely characterize the psychiatric risk associated with corticosteroids have been challenging, in part due to the heterogeneity and often poorly demarcated nature of acute psychiatric reactions. Many factors likely influence the nature and severity of a psychiatric reaction, including corticosteroid dosage, chronicity of corticosteroid use, nature of chronic inflammatory illness, comorbid psychiatric illnesses, and psychosocial/environmental factors. Despite multiple confounding variables, there is a general understanding of the psychiatric risks associated with corticosteroids.

The most common psychiatric sequelae of corticosteroid use are mood disturbances, accounting for up to 70% of all psychiatric reactions [1]. Corticosteroid use can precipitate de novo symptoms of depression, mania, or both (mixed states). In various studies focusing on patients who experienced a psychiatric complication of corticosteroids, depression has been reported in 28–40% of cases, mania in 28–35%, and mixed mood states in 7.5–12% [1]. Beyond mood disorders,11% of patients with a psychiatric complication experienced psychosis *without* a concurrent mood disturbance. The remaining cases were those with delirium (reported in 10–13% of cases) [1, 2].

A three-tier grading system has been proposed to characterize the severity of the most common reactions. *Grade 1* represents a subclinical mild euphoria, *grade 2* a reversible acute or subacute mania and/or depression only in the context of corticosteroids, and *grade 3* representing an unmasking of a bona fide bipolar disorder with relapses possible even without corticosteroid induction [2].

Clinical Pearl

- Psychiatric side effects of corticosteroids are most often depression and/or mania.
- Less common side effects include delirium and psychosis.

14.1.3 Timing of Symptom Onset

Adverse psychiatric events attributable to corticosteroid use generally have a rapid onset. The majority of psychiatric side effects become evident within the first 2 weeks of treatment. Symptom onset has been reported as early as day 1 of treatment, though it can occur as late as 2 months. In cases of treatment with corticosteroids with long half-lives (e.g., dexamethasone, betamethasone), psychiatric symptom onset has been reported even *after* discontinuation of the drug.

While depression and mania are the most common psychiatric side effects associated with corticosteroids, there appears to be a difference in the timing of onset of these symptoms. Studies suggest that corticosteroid-induced mania and psychosis have onset *early* in the course of treatment, whereas the risk of developing depression is associated with more *prolonged or chronic* exposure [1].

14.1.4 Dose Dependence

Psychiatric complications associated with corticosteroids have been demonstrated to be dose dependent. While psychiatric symptoms may develop at *any* dose of corticosteroid, a commonly cited dose threshold is 40 mg per 24 hours of prednisone, above which psychiatric symptoms become far more likely [2]. Based on the Boston Collaborative Drug Surveillance Project, the incidence of psychiatric events is 1.3% at doses under 40 mg per 24 hours, 4.6% between 41 and 80 mg per 24 hours, and 18.4% for doses of 80 mg per 24 hours and above [3]. This highlights the rapidly escalating risk associated with increased dosage. With this dose dependence in mind, it can often be a challenging risk-benefit balance to achieve the desired therapeutic effect of corticosteroids while minimizing the psychiatric and other risks.

Clinical Pearl
- Clinical tools are available for estimating probability of adverse drug reactions, including the Naranjo Adverse Drug Reaction Probability Scale [4].

Recommendation
- The risk of psychiatric reactions associated with corticosteroids is dose dependent.
- To minimize this risk, the corticosteroid dose should be kept below the prednisone equivalent of 40 mg per 24 hours.

14.1.5 Risk Factors

Given how common psychiatric side effects are in the context of corticosteroid use, it is useful to have a strategy to predict who is at risk. Unfortunately, aside from corticosteroid dose, no clear risk factors have been identified.

Paradoxically, current evidence suggests that a history of previous psychiatric disorders does *not* appear to increase the risk of an adverse psychiatric event from corticosteroids. Previous psychiatric history is *not* an absolute contraindication to corticosteroid therapy [1]. Additionally, patients who have had a *previous* adverse psychiatric reaction to corticosteroids do *not* appear to be at an increased risk for a second such reaction, though this has not been comprehensively addressed in literature, and some have challenged this assertion [5]. The risk of a recurrence of a psychiatric side effect during subsequent courses of corticosteroids has not been well defined in the literature.

Age is another risk factor that has been reported. Unsurprisingly, older adults taking corticosteroids are at an increased risk of developing delirium. With the current evidence, there does *not* appear to be a clear association between age and the risk of developing depressive, manic, or psychotic symptoms. There is limited evidence suggesting that females are at a slightly greater risk of developing a corticosteroid-induced psychosis though this has not been consistently demonstrated [2].

Clinical Pearl

- Past psychiatric history does not appear to increase the risk of a corticosteroid-induced psychiatric reaction.

14.1.6 Pathophysiology

The pathophysiology underpinning the psychiatric complications of corticosteroid use remains unclear. Multiple hypotheses have been postulated, though there is no current working hypothesis to explain the various psychiatric events related to treatment with corticosteroids.

On a conceptual level, there is a clear common factor between corticosteroids and psychiatric symptoms: stress. Broadly speaking, stress is a disturbance in homeostasis. Endogenous glucocorticoids are important mediators in the stress response pathway, and stress is a potent risk factor for developing certain psychiatric illnesses. Regulation of the hypothalamic-pituitary-adrenal (HPA) axis can be disrupted by chronic stress, which in turn can impair the feedback sensitivity for endogenous glucocorticoids. Dysregulation of the HPA axis is a common feature of many stress-related psychiatric disorders.

Corticosteroids have also been demonstrated to have a broad range of effects on neuronal transmission, which likely plays into the pathophysiology of adverse psychiatric symptoms. These effects include a decrease in serotonin release, impacts on dopaminergic and cholinergic systems, and toxic effects on hippocampal neurons [2]. Any combination of these observed steroid effects may contribute to the complex, heterogeneous psychiatric events, which can occur during treatment with corticosteroids.

14.1.7 Treatment of Corticosteroid-Induced Psychiatric Reactions

The preferred treatment for a corticosteroid-induced psychiatric reaction is tapering and/or discontinuation of the offending corticosteroid. Tapering the dose of a corticosteroid to a prednisone equivalent of 40 mg per 24 hours or lower is thought to minimize the impact of a corticosteroid-induced psychiatric reaction, though a taper

Table 14.1 Pharmacological treatment of persistent corticosteroid-induced psychiatric symptoms [1, 2]

Symptoms	Primary strategy	Secondary strategy (persistent symptoms, taper not feasible)
Depression	Taper or discontinue corticosteroid	SSRI or mood stabilizer
Mania/ hypomania	Taper or discontinue corticosteroid	Mood stabilizer and/or second- or third-generation antipsychotic
Psychosis	Taper or discontinue corticosteroid	Second- or third-generation antipsychotic

Note: *SSRI* selective serotonin reuptake inhibitor

to full discontinuation is typically a more effective means to treat these symptoms. Careful clinical judgment is necessary to balance the risks and benefits of ongoing steroid exposure.

Discontinuation of steroid therapy can be an effective strategy in treating an acute adverse psychiatric reaction; however, full resolution of symptoms often takes several weeks. In the case of corticosteroid-induced psychosis, about 50% of cases resolve within 4 days of corticosteroid discontinuation, with the most persistent cases resolving by 14 days. Corticosteroid-induced mania is reported to persist for up to 3 weeks, whereas depressive symptoms attributable to steroids are thought to resolve by 4 weeks in the absence of psychopharmacological interventions [1]. Resolution of corticosteroid-associated delirium typically occurs within days of withdrawal of corticosteroids.

Psychopharmacological treatment of corticosteroid-induced psychiatric symptoms is generally reserved for more severe cases, persistent symptomatology, or in patients for whom a taper from corticosteroids is not medically appropriate. Treatment of corticosteroid-induced psychiatric symptoms with psychopharmacological agents is considered an off-label use; however, the rationale for utilizing psychotropic medications to alleviate burdensome psychiatric symptoms is intuitive and well precedented [2]. The use of second- or third-generation antipsychotics, antidepressants, and mood stabilizers has been recommended in the literature [1, 2]; the choice of medication should be guided by the specific manifest psychiatric symptoms. Lithium has received attention in the literature for use in the prevention and treatment of psychiatric adverse events related to corticosteroids [2]; however, evidence for this is limited, and treatment with lithium should be avoided in patients with renal disease.

A brief summary of the pharmacological strategies of corticosteroid-induced psychiatric symptoms is listed in Table 14.1.

14.1.8 Case Vignette: Corticosteroid-Induced Psychiatric Symptoms

A 38-year-old female patient with lupus nephritis was treated with a prednisone dose of 60 mg per 24 hours. Within 2 days of initiating treatment, she started to exhibit manic-type symptoms including pressured speech, decreased sleep, irritability, increased energy, impulsive disinhibition, and cognitive impairment. Her symptoms were treated empirically with olanzapine 5 mg at bedtime which resulted in a rapid recovery of her baseline mental status. Her prednisone was tapered to 20 mg daily. After 1 week of treatment with olanzapine, it was discontinued. Her symptoms did not recur, and she did not require any maintenance treatment with olanzapine once her prednisone dose was lowered.

Clinical Pearl

- Preferential treatment of corticosteroid-induced psychiatric reactions is withdrawal of the offending agent, though empiric psychopharmacological approaches may be warranted depending on clinical context.

14.2 Mycophenolate

Mycophenolate is an immunosuppressive agent used for the prevention of allogeneic organ transplant rejection and continues to be evaluated for treatment of various autoimmune disease states. Mycophenolate is used as a steroid-sparing agent to avoid the adverse effects of steroids, including the psychiatric side effects. Mycophenolate can cross the blood-brain barrier and may conferred neuropsychiatric complications. Depressive and anxiety symptoms are listed as possible side effects in the product monograph, though it seems to be an uncommon phenomenon (less than 10% occurrence) [6].

Few case reports document depressive symptoms secondary to mycophenolate use. In a case series of 38 adults treated with mycophenolate, there was one patient who developed depressive symptoms which were thought to be attributable to the drug [7]. In one case report, a 64-year-old woman was treated for myasthenia gravis with mycophenolate and developed severe depression 4 days after initiating the drug. The severity of her symptoms led to a psychiatric inpatient admission. Her symptoms resolved within 2 days of discontinuation of mycophenolate but recurred within 2 days of a rechallenge [8].

Two case reports of psychiatric side effects attributed to mycophenolate are available to date in the pediatric population. In the first, an adolescent male reported severe anxiety, panic attacks, and inconsolable crying upon initiation of mycophenolate 500 mg twice daily, which resolved upon days of discontinuation. In the second, a female patient taking mycophenolate 500 mg twice daily developed significant irritability and anhedonia after 8 weeks of mycophenolate initiation. Her symptoms fully resolved within 6 weeks of mycophenolate discontinuation, and there was no recurrence of symptoms within 4 years of subsequent follow-up [9].

Psychiatric side effects reported in the context of mycophenolate use appear to be isolated to symptoms of depression and anxiety. There is no readily available literature describing case reports of mania or psychosis attributable to therapy with mycophenolate. Based on the available evidence, mycophenolate is considered safe with respect to psychiatric side effects, though patients should be made aware of the remote possibility of reversible mood and anxiety side effects.

14.3 Tacrolimus

14.3.1 Overview

Tacrolimus is an immunosuppressive agent most commonly used to prevent rejection after allogeneic organ transplant, though its immunosuppressive properties have been studied in a variety of other medical applications. In nephrology, a recent randomized controlled trial demonstrated the efficacy of tacrolimus monotherapy as an alternative to corticosteroid therapy in the treatment of minimal change disease (which is a renal disorder with intense proteinuria that can lead to nephrotic syndrome) [10].

Like other common immunosuppressive agents, tacrolimus does have some potential to cause neuropsychiatric side effects. It has been reported that about 40–60% of patients on tacrolimus may develop mild to moderate neurotoxic effects including headaches, paresthesias, tremors, and sleep disturbance [11]. More severe neurotoxic effects are found in 5–9% of patients, including confusion, lethargy, dysarthria, seizures, coma, and posterior reversible encephalopathy syndrome. Tacrolimus-induced encephalitis can have a clinically variable presentation. Catatonia and psychosis have been described as rare sequelae of tacrolimus therapy, even when blood levels are apparently therapeutic. Tacrolimus can also contribute to delirium risk, with older adults being particularly vulnerable [11].

14.3.2 Tacrolimus-Induced Catatonia

There are multiple case reports describing tacrolimus-induced neuropsychiatric syndromes satisfying DSM-5 criteria for catatonia [11, 12]. Catatonia, as defined by DSM-5, is characterized by three or more of the following symptoms: (i) catalepsy, (ii) waxy flexibility, (iii) stupor, (iv) agitation, (v) mutism, (vi) negativism, (vii) posturing, (viii) mannerism, (ix) stereotypies, (x) grimacing, (xi) echolalia, and (xii) echopraxia. These mental status changes have been reported even in the context of apparently "therapeutic" serum tacrolimus levels. Long-standing use of tacrolimus without catatonic symptoms does *not* preclude the possibility of developing new onset neuropsychiatric side effects. Sikavi et al. describe an acute onset catatonia after 16 years of exposure to tacrolimus, which resolved within 1 week of switching to an alternative immunosuppressant [12].

Treatment of tacrolimus-induced catatonia includes reducing the dose of tacrolimus, or substitution with a different immunosuppressive agent. Acute management of catatonia should also include regular scheduled doses of benzodiazepines (e.g., lorazepam 1 mg IV q6h, titrated to 3–4 mg IV q6h as needed based on the clinical presentation, to an upper limit of 16–24 mg per 24 hours) to provide relief from catatonic symptoms. High doses of benzodiazepines are often required to confer maximum therapeutic benefit. If symptoms of catatonia are not relieved within 48–72 hours of optimized medical management, electroconvulsive therapy (ECT) should be considered as it is regarded to be the most effective treatment for catatonic syndromes.

14.3.3 Tacrolimus-Induced Psychosis

While psychosis is described in the product monograph as a possible adverse effect [13], there are limited publications describing this [14–16]. Krishna et al. describes a 43-year-old male with no past psychiatric history who developed psychosis after starting tacrolimus [14]. Obayi described a 21-year-old female with no past psychiatric history who developed psychosis, which resolved completely after withdrawal of the medication [15]. Bersani et al. described mania with psychotic symptoms in a 46-year-old male 17 years post-transplant [16]. In this case, the patient's serum tacrolimus level was supratherapeutic. Symptoms resolved gradually with a reduction of dose [16].

The heterogeneous case reports highlight the imprecision regarding risk factors for developing tacrolimus-induced psychosis. These cases underscore the importance of routine monitoring of mental status during treatment with tacrolimus. Psychosis is a rare side effect but one that develops at any time during treatment with tacrolimus, regardless of whether tacrolimus blood levels are therapeutic or toxic.

Treatment recommendations include reduction of dose or substitution for an alternative immunosuppressive agent. Second- or third-generation antipsychotics have also been used successfully in the treatment of tacrolimus-induced psychosis [15, 16].

14.3.4 Psychotoxic Effects of Tacrolimus in Pediatrics

In a case series of 20 pediatric renal transplantation patients, 75% tolerated tacrolimus well, while others developed a range of clinically significant behavioral and psychiatric symptoms including depression, anorexia nervosa-like symptoms, and severe insomnia. One patient (the only one with a toxic blood level of tacrolimus) developed significant anxiety and aggressive behavior. These effects were all fully reversible after discontinuation of tacrolimus. This study may suggest slightly different psychiatric vulnerabilities in pediatric patients while receiving tacrolimus treatment as compared to the adult population [17].

14.3.5 Pathophysiology

Details regarding the neurobiological basis of the psychiatric effects of tacrolimus are largely unknown. Tacrolimus inhibits the glutamate/N-methyl-D-aspartate receptor (NMDA) excitatory system, which has been postulated to result in compromise of complex cognition [18].

14.3.6 Case Vignette 1: Tacrolimus-Induced Psychosis

A 44-year-old male patient post-renal transplant treated with tacrolimus 6.5 mg daily developed religious delusions of being the "Messiah" on a special mission, euphoric affect, decreased sleep, and intermittent agitation. His tacrolimus levels were in the therapeutic range. He was treated empirically with olanzapine 7.5 mg at bedtime. Over the course of 2 weeks, the patient's agitation and insomnia improved; however, he continued to experience delusions. His tacrolimus was discontinued completely in favor of treatment with mycophenolate, after which his delusional ideas gradually disappeared. Olanzapine was discontinued after symptom resolution, and he did not experience any recurrence of his symptoms.

14.3.7 Case Vignette 2: Tacrolimus-Induced Catatonia

A 59-year-old male treated with tacrolimus 2.5 mg daily and prednisone 5 mg daily developed neuropsychiatric symptoms including mutism, negativism, and waxy flexibility diagnosed as catatonia (Bush-Francis Catatonia Rating Scale score of 13). At the time of symptom onset, he had therapeutic levels of tacrolimus. His tacrolimus was discontinued and mycophenolate was started. Intravenous lorazepam was administered and titrated up to 16 mg per day over 4 days with only partial resolution of his catatonic symptoms, at which time ECT was initiated leading to complete symptom resolution after three bilateral treatments.

14.4 Cyclophosphamide

Cyclophosphamide is an alkylating agent used commonly in cancer chemotherapy and for immunosuppression. Cyclophosphamide has some significant systemic side effects, but no significant psychiatric side effects are cited in the literature and product monographs [19]. No case studies have been published that describe psychiatric reactions directly attributable to treatment with cyclophosphamide. A scarcity of documented reports describing psychiatric side effects does not necessarily imply that cyclophosphamide is devoid of any potential for catalyzing a psychiatric reaction; however, its widespread use since it was first approved in the USA in 1959 without reports of psychiatric reactions is reassuring.

14.5 Hydroxychloroquine

14.5.1 Overview

Hydroxychloroquine, originally developed as an antimalarial, is used to suppress inflammatory responses and slow the progression of autoimmune diseases. The most common psychiatric side effects associated with hydroxychloroquine are affective lability (reported in 1–10%) and rare reports of nightmares, suicidal behavior, and psychosis. Since first approved for medical use in 1955, there have been multiple case reports describing a variety of psychiatric events related to treatment with hydroxychloroquine including reports of psychosis, depression, mania, and delirium [20, 21]. With the limited case reports available and with heterogeneous presentations, it is difficult to define specific risk factors for the development of psychiatric side effects related to hydroxychloroquine. Numerous case reports describe new onset psychiatric symptoms in individuals with no past psychiatric history [20]. Treatment generally involves withdrawal of hydroxychloroquine and/or treatment with a symptom-appropriate psychopharmacological agent.

Despite these multiple case reports of psychosis and mood symptoms associated with hydroxychloroquine, recent larger-scale studies have not consistently reported any significant risk for these side effects [21]. Pharmacovigilance related to adverse outcomes associated with hydroxychloroquine intensified in the year 2020 after it garnered much interest as a potential therapeutic agent to treat severe COVID-19 infections. One major study accessed the US Food and Drug Administration (FDA) reporting system to investigate over 2.3 million adverse event cases associated with chloroquine and hydroxychloroquine, only 520 of which involved psychiatric symptoms. Sato et al. concluded that there was no significant association between chloroquine and hydroxychloroquine treatment and suicide, psychosis, confusion, or agitation [21]. The authors did identify a significant but very weak association between these chloroquine agents and delirium and depression [16]. A multinational network cohort study including over 900,000 hydroxychloroquine users compared the risk of patients being treated from rheumatoid arthritis with hydroxychloroquine to those treated with sulfasalazine [22]. The study found no significant differences in rates of depression, suicidal behavior, or psychosis between the two drugs, suggesting that hydroxychloroquine confers no greater psychiatric risk than that of sulfasalazine [22].

Overall, emotional lability is the only common psychiatric side effect associated with hydroxychloroquine use. Other psychiatric conditions including psychosis, suicidal behavior, and depression should be considered possibly related; however, despite scant case reports [23, 24], the most recent body of evidence suggests that these conditions are exceedingly very rare complications of hydroxychloroquine.

14.5.2 Case Vignette: Hydroxychloroquine-Induced Psychiatric Symptoms

A 54-year-old woman with lupus nephritis began treatment with hydroxychloroquine 100 mg daily and developed new onset mood lability, irritability, and anxiety. Her symptoms were empirically treated with sertraline 50 mg daily and discontinuation of hydroxychloroquine. There was a rapid resolution of symptoms attributed primarily to the discontinuation of hydroxychloroquine, as the response was too prompt to be fully accounted for by the usual onset of therapeutic effects of serotonergic antidepressants. Upon recovery, sertraline was discontinued with further monitoring of her mood state.

14.6 Key Takeaways

Corticosteroids

- Psychiatric side effects related to corticosteroid treatment are common.
- The most common psychiatric side effects are depression and mania, followed by mixed mood disorders, psychosis, and delirium.
- Corticosteroid dosage is the only known risk factor for psychiatric events related to corticosteroids.
- Withdrawal of corticosteroid medication and empiric psychopharmacological intervention are the most effective treatment options.

Mycophenolate

- Psychiatric adverse drug events with mycophenolate are rare; however, case reports of depressive symptoms and anxiety symptoms associated with mycophenolate have been documented.
- Patients should be made aware of the possibility of rare and reversible mood and anxiety side effects with mycophenolate.

Cyclophosphamide

- No common or serious psychiatric adverse reactions are associated with cyclophosphamide.

Hydroxychloroquine

- The only relatively common psychiatric side effect of hydroxychloroquine is emotional lability.
- Other psychiatric side effects are very rare but may include psychosis, suicidal behavior, and depression.

References

1. Kenna HA, Poon AW, de los Angeles CP, Koran LM. Psychiatric complications of treatment with corticosteroids: review with case report. Psychiatry Clin Neurosci. 2011;65(6):549–60.
2. Parasher A, Bez J. Steroid induced psychiatric adverse effects: An overview of risk factors, clinical features and management. Int J Res Med Sci. 2020;8(6):2365.
3. Boston Collaborative Drug Surveillance Program. Acute adverse reactions to prednisone in relation to dosage. Clin Pharmacol Ther. 1972;13(5 part 1):694–8.
4. Naranjo CA, Busto U, Sellers EM, Sandor P, Ruiz I, Roberts EA, Janecek E, Domecq C, Greenblatt DJ. A method for estimating the probability of adverse drug reactions. Clin Pharmacol Ther. 1981;30(2):239–45.
5. Judd LL, Schettler PJ, Brown ES, et al. Adverse consequences of glucocorticoid medication: psychological, cognitive, and behavioral effects. Am J Psychiatry. 2014;171(10):1045–51.

6. Myfortic. Dorval (QC). [Updated 2016 Oct 06; Cited 2021 Feb 7]. Available from: www.sandoz.ca.
7. Chaudhry V, Cornblath DR, Griffin JW, O'Brien R, Drachman DB. Mycophenolate mofetil: a safe and promising immunosuppressant in neuromuscular diseases. Neurology. 2001;56(1):94–6.
8. Draper HM. Depressive disorder associated with mycophenolate Mofetil. Pharmacotherapy. 2008;28(1):136–9.
9. Arkin L, Talasila S, Paller AS. Mycophenolate Mofetil and mood changes in children with skin disorders. Pediatr Dermatol. 2016;33(3):e216–7.
10. Medjeral-Thomas NR, Lawrence C, Condon M, et al. Randomized, controlled trial of tacrolimus and prednisolone monotherapy for adults with de novo minimal change disease: a multicenter, randomized, controlled trial. Clin J Am Soc Nephrol. 2020;15(2):209–18.
11. Chopra A, Das P, Rai A, Kuppuswamy PS, Li X, Huston J, Philbrick K, Sola C. Catatonia as a manifestation of tacrolimus-induced neurotoxicity in organ transplant patients: a case series. Gen Hosp Psychiatry. 2012;34(2):209–e209.
12. Sikavi D, McMahon J, Fromson JA. Catatonia due to tacrolimus toxicity 16 years after renal transplantation: case report and literature review. J Psychiatr Pract. 2019;25(6):481–4.
13. Sandoz Tacrolimus, Boucharville (QC) [Updated 2018 July 31; cited 2021 Feb 7]. Available from: www.sandoz.ca.
14. Krishna N, Chiappelli J, Fischer BA, Knight S. Tacrolimus-induced paranoid delusions and fugue-like state. Gen Hosp Psychiatry. 2013;35(3):327.e5–6.
15. Obayi ON. Acute schizophrenia-like psychotic disorder associated with immunosuppressive agent use three years after renal transplantation: a case report. Int J Sci Rep. 2018;4(7):192.
16. Bersani G, Marino P, Valeriani G, Cuoco V, Zitelli C, Melcore C, Bersani FS. Manic-like psychosis associated with elevated trough tacrolimus blood concentrations 17 years after kidney transplant. Case Rep Psychiatry. 2013;2013:926395.
17. Kemper MJ, Spartà G, Laube GF, Miozzari M, Neuhaus TJ. Neuropsychologic side-effects of tacrolimus in pediatric renal transplantation. Clin Transplant. 2003;17(2):130–4.
18. Beresford TP. Neuropsychiatric complications of liver and other solid organ transplantation. Liver Transpl. 2001;7(11):S36–45.
19. Procytox, Mississauga (ON) [Updated 2012 Sept 7; cited 2021 Feb 07]. Available from: www.baxter.ca.
20. Mascolo A, Berrino PM, Gareri P, Castagna A, Capuano A, Manzo C, Berrino L. Neuropsychiatric clinical manifestations in elderly patients treated with hydroxychloroquine: a review article. Inflammopharmacology. 2018;26(5):1141–9.
21. Sato K, Mano T, Iwata A, Toda T. Neuropsychiatric adverse events of chloroquine: a real-world pharmacovigilance study using the FDA Adverse Event Reporting System (FAERS) database. Biosci Trends. 2020;14(2):139–43.
22. Lane JC, Weaver J, Kostka K, et al. Risk of depression, suicide and psychosis with hydroxychloroquine treatment for rheumatoid arthritis: a multinational network cohort study. Rheumatology (Oxford). 2020;keaa771. Online ahead of print.
23. Hsu W, Chiu N, Huang S. Hydroxychloroquine-induced acute psychosis in a systemic lupus erythematosus female. Acta Neuropsychiatr. 2011;23(6):318–9.
24. Kwak YT, Yang Y, Park SY. Chloroquine-associated psychosis mimicking very late-onset schizophrenia: case report. Geriatr Gerontol Int. 2015;8(15):1096–7.

15 Psychological Aspects of Adaptation to Critical Care Nephrology, Dialysis, and Transplantation for the Patient and the Caregiver

Joseph R. Pellizzari

15.1 Introduction

Understanding the psychological aspects of adaptation to various important medical events during the course of chronic, progressive renal disease provides the clinician with rich information to enhance case formulation. This massive content area could conceivably traverse conceptual models such as Engel's biopsychosocial model of health [1], Lazarus and Folkman's model of stress and coping [2], and Leventhal's common-sense model of self-regulation [3], to name a few. A comprehensive review of all these areas is beyond the scope of this chapter. The intention is to pull from some of those models a concise and practical resource to introduce the clinician to this important topic of psychological adaptation to renal disease. This is a topic that can highlight important psychological influences on the course of renal disease morbidity and mortality.

We begin by providing a brief review of concepts and constructs that have emerged in the study of models of adjustment and adaptation to health conditions. Application to people living with renal disease will be highlighted, with special consideration within major disease course encounters – critical care, dialysis, and transplantation. Lastly, the important role of the caregiver (e.g., spouse, partner) is featured as considerations around dyadic coping (coping within patient-caregiver pairs) are presented.

J. R. Pellizzari (✉)
St. Joseph's Healthcare Hamilton, McMaster University, Hamilton, ON, Canada
e-mail: jpellizz@stjosham.on.ca

A. Hategan et al. (eds.), *Psychonephrology*,
https://doi.org/10.1007/978-3-030-84740-1_15

15.2 Case Vignette – "Brenda in Renal Crisis: Critical Care Nightmare"

Brenda, a 59-year-old woman with end-stage renal disease (ESRD) on hemodialysis, was recovering from an acute respiratory illness. Her hospital course included a 10-day stay in the intensive care unit (ICU) with a brief period of intubation. As she recovered on the general nephrology ward, John, her partner of 25 years, commented "she's still not right." Pronounced fears and anxieties were noticed around various aspects of her recovery, particularly eating, mobilization, and cognition. John had witnessed her episode of delirium in the ICU and had thought that she was dying. He was also feeling very worn down. Now recovered from her critical illness, Brenda and John began a new adjustment phase with hopes of leaving hospital and returning to the usual "grind" of outpatient dialysis. Transplant was on hold temporarily but continued to be "the light at the end of the tunnel." John was cleared to be Brenda's donor, and they both imagined a life that could return to some stability – enjoying travel and visits with their two adult children who lived in different cities several hundred kilometers away. This case vignette is later developed to highlight various aspects of Brenda and John's psychological adaptation to these various renal disease settings and encounters.

15.3 Psychological Adjustment and Adaptation in Chronic Illness

Literature reviews of psychological adjustment to chronic illness point to a complex array of pertinent constructs and factors [4, 5]. Some general conclusions from these reviews are listed below:

- *Impact on quality of life*: Multiple domains of life functioning are impacted, such as employment roles, relational dynamics, and the development of leisure pursuits.
- *Lifelong processes*: Across the lifespan, there are demands for adjustment and adaptation that have important impacts on psychological and social development. Consider the changes to one's sense of self from childhood to older adulthood as a result of experiencing acute medical events, depending on arduous treatments such as dialysis to stay alive, and navigating the "terrain" of transplant.
- *Variability*: There is considerable variability or heterogeneity across individuals, within patient-partner dyads in adjustment and adaptation styles, and across specific disease processes that lead to renal failure.
- *Multiple, interrelated domains*: Adjustment to chronic illness is multifaceted and involves multiple, interrelated domains of psychological functioning:
  - Interpersonal (e.g., development of relationships, dyadic coping – patient-partner).
  - Cognitive (e.g., appraisal processes such as threat or challenge, maintaining self-esteem, opportunities for personal growth).

  - Emotional (e.g., both positive and negative affective outcomes).
  - Physical (e.g., pain, fatigue, bodily changes).
  - Behavioral (e.g., medication adherence, adherence to diet and lifestyle changes).
- *Dynamic*: Adjustment to chronic illness is extremely dynamic and often unpredictable. There are many twists and turns and ups and downs during the renal disease course such as:
  - Changes in symptom acuity and severity over time.
  - Changes in prognosis.
  - Medication responses and side effects.
  - Impact of different modes of renal replacement therapies (e.g., home or hospital based).
  - Demands for lifestyle changes, such as diet and nutrition.
  - Dealing with acute events such as renal crises that may require acute hospitalization or critical care.
  - Considerations related to organ transplantation such as the relational dynamics of living-organ donation and the demands for adherence to lifelong post-transplant medication regimens and clinical surveillance.
  - Complex medical decision-making, including therapeutic modality decision-making and decisions around conservative management or discontinuing dialysis.

In reviewing more specific factors, determinants, and contributors to psychological adjustment in chronic illness, many models have been proposed and studied such as stress coping, self-regulation, and personality/social psychology theories [4, 5]. Reviews tend to cluster these determinants (many of these are presented in other chapters) according to whether they are more distal (indirectly affecting) or proximal (directly affecting) in nature as outlined below.

- Distal determinants of adjustment to chronic illness:
  - Socioeconomic status
  - Ethnicity
  - Gender
- Proximal determinants of adjustment to chronic illness:
  - Interpersonal or dyadic processes (e.g., patient-caregiver dynamics, relationships with complex networks of care providers)
  - Personality factors (e.g., levels of neuroticism, extraversion, and optimism that play out in many aspects of care management and decision-making)
  - Cognitive appraisals (e.g., interpretations of events and symptoms)
  - Coping processes (e.g., those intentional efforts to adjust and adapt)

Furthermore, efforts have been made to integrate previous theoretical and research findings in the area of adjusting and adapting to chronic illness. Moss-Morris has argued for a unified and consistent model based on empirical findings and qualitative studies across chronic illness populations [6]. Background and illness-specific factors influence the experience of both key critical events and ongoing chronic illness stressors. Fundamentally, this results in a state of a disrupted emotional equilibrium and an impact on one's quality of life, which requires adaptation and adjustment. For critical or acute events, successful adjustment implies a return to equilibrium, while for ongoing stressors of the chronic condition, successful adjustment requires the maintenance of equilibrium. The result is either good or poor adjustment across psychological, physical, and social spheres. In the sections below, each component of this unified model is presented, and applications to the patient with renal disease are offered.

- Background and illness-specific factors
  - *Personal background factors* – These factors include influences such as early life experiences, personality characteristics, values, and age. Some examples in renal populations where these factors are highlighted are in genetic disorders such as polycystic kidney disease, where there may be multi-generational influences on how one approaches the illness. Patients with those conditions will have typically learned about or witnessed a wide range of adjustment responses among important role models. These can have important influences on the individual in developing their own adjustment repertoires. Clearly, the influence of personality characteristics can be seen in renal clinics, as those with more optimistic personalities adjust differently than those with more neurotic or anxious temperaments. The age factor is also especially important as one considers developmental influences on adjustment. Observing individuals in the transitional age period (moving from child-adolescent care models to adult care models) reveals particular dynamic adjustments, including the navigation from dependency to autonomy in medical decision-making.
  - *Illness-specific factors* – These factors include aspects of symptoms (e.g., pain, fatigue) and their impact on function. Renal replacement therapies and medication treatments have many side effects that can have a wide range of influence in adjustment to renal disease (e.g., physical appearance changes). As treatments initiate and progress, aspects of illness prognosis and uncertainty become additional challenging elements.
  - *Social and environmental factors* – Social determinants of health are increasingly appreciated as major factors in how one adapts to renal disease. These include factors such as socioeconomic and the availability of healthcare resources (e.g., proximity to dialysis centers). Social support is a major factor in this category. Quite simply, those without strong networks of support (partners, family, friends, and positive relationships with healthcare providers) fare more poorly.
- Critical events and ongoing stressors
  - *Critical events* – Key time points in the journey of renal disease will require the demands of adaption from the initial onset of acute symptoms, diagnosis, acute and/or critical illness episodes requiring hospitalization, mortality concerns, and the ongoing changes in one's self-identity as the course of illness proceeds.

- *Ongoing illness stressors* – The chronicity of the disease imparts ongoing stressors that need to be managed constantly over time. These include how one navigates their social relationships for demands such as travel to and from dialysis sessions or to clinic appointments. Developing long-standing relationships with healthcare providers requires regular attention, as providers come and go and resources go through periods of changes. Living life as fully as possible is attempted as one faces an uncertain future. This includes trying to maintain a strong sense of self-identity while autonomy can be frequently challenged and stressful and ongoing treatments become part of one's lifestyle. Chronic illness management becomes important, as changes to many life domains occur (e.g., employment, leisure), along with sometimes frequent changes to levels of independence and abilities.

- Adjustment and adaptation
  - *Successful adjustment (return to equilibrium)* – Moss-Morris lists factors to be studied within disease groups that can be *helpful* for adjustment [6]. *Cognitive* factors include maintaining a sense of control and/or self-efficacy around disease and treatment management (e.g., renal replacement therapies), acceptance of illness, acquiring a sense of high perceived social support, and having coping styles that encompass aspects of meaning making or benefit finding. *Behavioral* factors include aspects of problem focused coping, purposeful planning, seeking out social or health-related supports, adherence to medical treatments and diet/lifestyle modifications, staying active (physically, socially, recreationally), and healthy expression of emotions (e.g., anger, frustrations, sadness, fears).
  - *Adjustment difficulties (ongoing disequilibrium)* – Similarly, Moss-Morris lists factors to be studied within disease groups that can be *unhelpful* for adjustment [6]. *Cognitive* factors include high levels of perceived stress, denial or having unreasonable expectations, negative illness and symptom representations, unhelpful thinking styles (e.g., all-or-none thinking, catastrophizing), adopting stances of helplessness or hopelessness, and emotional repression. *Behavioral* factors include avoidance coping, unhelpful responses to symptoms (e.g., pain, fatigue) such as activity avoidance or excessive rest, hyper-vigilance with respect to somatic symptoms or the environment, and unhelpful approaches to regulating emotions such as excessive venting/reactivity and alcohol or other substance use.
- Outcomes
  - *Good adjustment (psychological, physical, and social)* – Better adaptation or adjustment outcomes include less emotional distress, less interference with important quality of life domains such as employment status and social relationships, better chronic disease management behaviors, acceptance, self-compassion, and more positive emotionality.
  - *Poor adjustment (psychological, physical, and social)* – Poorer adaptation or adjustment outcomes include high levels of emotional distress, severe interference with functional life goals and domains such as relationships and work, poor disease management including medical non-adherence behavior, and lower positive emotionality.

Clinical Pearl

- **Ways of coping**: Aldwin and Yancura [7] in their comprehensive review of coping with stress and trauma outline five broad categories. In thinking of how your patient may be adjusting to their renal disease during encounters of critical care, dialysis, and transplantation, consider these five categories that are not mutually exclusive:
  - Problem-focused coping (e.g., adherence efforts, purposeful planning, seeking out health information)
  - Emotion-focused coping (e.g., healthy expression of emotions such as sadness, frustrations, anger, and anxiety, limiting avoidance and withdrawal, limiting substance use)
  - Social support (e.g., maintaining positive support networks within families and health-provider networks, having someone reliable to talk to in a validating way)
  - Faith-based coping (e.g., maintaining prayer and religious practices, developing a philosophy in life)
  - Meaning making (e.g., benefit finding such as finding "silver linings," "giving back," and volunteering, opportunities for personal growth)

Clinical Pearl

- **Adaptive tasks**: Moos and Holahan [8] in their conceptual model of adjusting to chronic illness and disability identify seven tasks that are encountered by patients and families (both illness specific and more general). Consider these tasks as you evaluate how well (or poorly) your patient is coping.
  - Managing symptoms (e.g., fatigue, different kinds of pain, bodily changes, sexual dysfunction)
  - Managing treatments (e.g., getting to–from dialysis; post-transplant medication adherence)
  - Managing emotions (e.g., strong emotional reactions are normal in the context of the stressors faced by renal patients and require healthy approaches to expression)
  - Maintaining a positive self-image (e.g., revising one's self-identity, managing dependency needs, dealing with body image issues resulting from fistula creations or immunosuppression facial changes, dealing with negative beliefs such as "I am broken" or "I am unlovable," dependence on machines for life support)
  - Relating to family members and friends (e.g., developing effective communication styles, dealing with thoughts of "perceived burden," managing demands for instrumental and emotional supports from loved ones)

- Preparing for an uncertain future (e.g., purposeful planning for controllable issues such as preparing wills and advance care planning, balancing hope with realistic expectations around a life-limiting disease)
- Forming relationships with healthcare providers (e.g., developing effective partnerships with the complex array of renal health providers such as nurses, pharmacists, social workers, nephrologists, technicians)

15.4 Case Vignette – "Brenda and John in Recovery: Adjustment Post-critical Illness"

Brenda and John benefitted immensely from visits from the consultation-liaison psychiatry team while she was on the nephrology ward ("critical event"). They learned that their reactions were rather normal and were intrigued about the education around "post-intensive care syndrome" [9]. They could definitely both relate to the cognitive (memory, executive functioning), psychological (depression, anxiety, and post-traumatic stress symptoms), and physical (weakness) components of the syndrome. John and Brenda looked up more information on the topic and began keeping a diary ("problem-focused coping," "emotion-focused coping"), and they started to feel better as a couple ("return to equilibrium"). They also had a productive session with the unit social worker around advance care planning ("preparing for an uncertain future"). As her mobilization and cognition improved, her emotional well-being shifted ("emotion-focused coping"). She had increased confidence about returning to some functional ability, and this enhanced her self-esteem ("cognitive"). She found that approaching her fears of falling lessened her anxiety and brightened her mood ("emotion-focused coping"). Visits with the nephrology team addressed ongoing discrepancies between them on expectations for recovery, and they seemed to be having fewer disputes around her engagement in care ("social support").

15.5 Qualitative Studies of Adjustment in Patients with End-Stage Renal Disease

While adjustment has historically been defined as the absence of psychopathology, clear limitations of this approach are apparent. There are several chapters in this volume that address diagnosable psychiatric illnesses such as depressive, anxiety, and sleep disorders that may develop comorbidly with ESRD, are highly prevalent, and have important influences on both morbidity and mortality. These conditions could be viewed as being the outcomes of poor or mal-adjustment to illness, among other mechanisms.

However, there are levels of psychological distress that are clinically important with respect to illness management but may not meet the diagnostic threshold of "disorder." Frequently, this is referred to those with "sub-threshold" clinical distress or those with mild or moderate levels of emotional distress. Considering adjustment as a dynamic process incorporating aspects of responses to both acute events and chronic disease stressors, previously identified models and constructs have been explored according to a continuum of outcomes from normal sadness, fears, vulnerabilities, and demoralization to disabling conditions involving clinical episodes of depression and anxiety.

On balance, more interventional focus is placed on those with more severe conditions, but it is becoming increasingly apparent that there can be risks in under-detecting and under-recognizing those with milder and moderate levels of distress that may also have important impacts on disease outcomes [10]. In a qualitative study of UK patients with ESRD ($n = 46$) who endorsed mild or moderate levels of distress (on distress or emotion thermometers), insights into adjustment-related phenomena were captured. The five identified themes clearly mapped onto many of the pertinent components in the conceptual models of adjustment to chronic illness presented previously. The themes were divided according to patients' experiences of distress and aspects of the kidney unit and support. They are described here briefly [10].

- *The emotional burden of distress:* Descriptions of difficult emotional states (often unanticipated) were highlighted including anger, frustration, feelings of helplessness, and loss of control. The theme of experiencing a "rollercoaster of emotions" was identified. Changes to sense of self and the ability to live a normal life were also captured here. With the dependency on renal replacement therapies and frequent impact on functional domains such as work, the statement "I don't know who I am anymore" is one that is frequently encountered in clinic.
- *Patient's relationship with treatment:* Descriptions around a difficult, conflictual, and paradoxical relationship with dialysis were captured here. Issues such as related medication regimens, side effects, fatigue, lifestyle restrictions, and dietary and fluid restrictions were identified. Perceived loss of control and elements of dissatisfaction around modality decision-making were also raised. All of these elements were expressed with full knowledge that the dialysis treatments were life sustaining.
- *Coping and adjustment:* Mention of emotion-focused and problem-focused strategies were included in this theme along with social support. Social support was cited both within the dialysis units and within the network of family and friends as a positive modality of coping. Indeed, patients frequently comment on the positive development of social supports with unit staff – sometimes occurring over many years.
- *Patient-staff interaction and kidney-unit support:* A wide range of experiences were captured here including positive and highly complementary (development of strong relationships with some staff that was conducive to disclosures around emotional well-being; elements of "being heard") to negative (environments that had staff who did not have clinical competencies nor time around the psychosocial aspects of adjustment). Even in those units that had dedicated psychosocial resources, it was expressed that those were sometimes highly restricted.

- *Impact of the treatment environment:* Issues such as the lack of privacy and attempts to make the environment lighthearted, jovial, and more casual were experienced differently (ranging from positive to negative) by participants with respect to addressing psychosocial aspects of adjustment.

15.6 Case Vignette – "Brenda and John in Dialysis: Back to the Grind"

After discharge from hospital, Brenda resumed dialysis treatments three times per week at their local center. They had the opportunity to visit with their adult children ("social support") and adjusted to their "new normal" ("ongoing illness stressors"). The dialysis center was in the process of rebuilding, and they found the frequent disruptions difficult ("return to disequilibrium"). They reminded each other that the changes were only temporary ("patient's relationship with treatment"). They were approached to see if they would be interested in joining a new online support group for dialysis patients and their partners and they accepted ("kidney-unit support"). In fact, after a couple of months, John volunteered to be a peer facilitator of the group, and he felt really good about "giving back" ("meaning making"). They both felt that the group enhanced their coping as a couple ("coping and adjustment") and also enhanced their relationships with center staff. They felt that they belonged to caring community ("patient-staff interaction," "impact of treatment environment," "social support"). As the months went on, they circled back to their modality education binder and decided to move forward with renal transplant. They wished to have more freedom for travel, and the burden of fatigue was increasing for Brenda ("managing symptoms," "managing treatments").

15.7 Post-transplant Adjustment

The quality of life and health benefits of renal transplantation are widely known, such that it is frequently described as the preferred "modality" following the determination of ESRD [11]. However, complications do arise that can lead to poor outcomes and graft loss. Patients often look forward to a state of "normalcy" following sometimes years of dialysis, while others may think that they are simply trading one set of problems with another. In considering the unique adjustments and adaptations for people following transplantation, studies with mixed methodologies have pointed to a range of complex findings. For example, patients have reported preferences that they would rather experience severe adverse treatment reactions than experience graft loss, patients have ranked experiencing graft loss worse than death, and patients have been found to overestimate quality-of-life gains post-renal transplant [12].

One recent study examined open-ended survey responses from approximately 400 US participants [13]. Questions included "How has your life changed since having a kidney transplant?" and "What concerns you most about your health care and future quality of life?" Identified themes again map nicely onto previously identified constructs and concepts from the larger coping with chronic illness literature. Life changes post-transplant were captured under the following themes, one of which was "no change":

- Improved quality of life and return to "normalcy" (e.g., improved functioning in lifestyle, family relations, employment, relief from no longer requiring the grind of dialysis)
- Better health and more energy (e.g., feeling better overall, having more energy, feeling more active, brighter outlook on life, more optimistic)
- Gratitude and enhanced sense of purpose in life or freedom (e.g., more time and freedom to travel, "second chance for life," more positive and purposeful outlook)
- Burdens of post-transplant regimens (fears of losing kidney, taking multiple medications, dietary restrictions)
- Worsened and less energy (more stressful with post-transplant regimens, ongoing disability)

Concerns about health care and future quality of life were represented under six themes, one including "no concerns":

- Kidney-related health issues (e.g., concerns and uncertainties around graft failure – if or when, concerns around a return to dialysis in the event of graft failure, concerns around eligibility for future transplants)
- Comorbidities and quality of life (concern for ongoing comorbidity management such as with diabetes mellitus, concerns around maintaining quality of life, fears of acute hospitalizations)
- Quality and cost of healthcare (insurance and financial concerns)
- Family and support systems (concern around graft failure and the impact/burden on family)
- Lifestyle changes (desire to increase mobility and energy, concerns around returning to functional roles such as employment)

Overall, the wide variety of adjustments and adaptations to post-transplant life speak to the complex and extremely dynamic nature of adjustment processes that are influenced by so many background and contextual factors. Many patients feel a profound responsibility and duty to care for their donated organs (i.e., "the gift of life"), especially those that involve family members. This can add to increased emotional burdens for post-transplant patients who fear the guilt and shame that may occur when donated organs fail. On the other hand, the same complex mix of adjustment factors may lead to non-adherence behavior that results in graft failure, particularly in the transition-aged groups [14].

15.8 Caregiver Roles and Adjustments

The demands for adjustment and adaptation are equally as challenging for the caregiver (spouse, partner, family member, friend) of the renal patient. Caregivers are essential in providing social support for patients in the form of instrumental, emotional, and various other aspects of psychosocial adaptation. The demands for these supports vary across the disease course and lifespan including acute events requiring hospitalization, dialysis, and transplantation. Some examples include:

- Managing complex treatment regimens of immunosuppression post-transplant
- Administration of medications
- Assistance with symptom monitoring such as blood pressure
- Managing the scheduling arrangements for dialysis, testing, and clinic appointments
- Assisting in transportation and attending medical appointments
- Managing the arrangements and the complexities of home-based dialysis
- Supporting the patient with medical decision-making
- Managing changes to diet and lifestyle that affect the entire family
- Managing household finances which can become very challenging in the context of disability
- Coping with changes in relationship dynamics including intimacy and communication
- Advocacy
- Donating a kidney and all that it entails from physical, psychological, and social perspectives

All of the processes and concepts presented in models of adjustment (cognitive, emotional, behavioral) are equally applied to the caregiver of the patient with ESRD. There are coping strategies enacted by both members of the dyad, and they can influence each other, vary over the course of the illness, and also vary according to the development of the relationship over time. The demands for caregivers are very heavy, and outcomes can be poor with respect to depression, anxiety, fatigue, physical health, quality of life, social isolation, and post-traumatic stress symptoms for those whose partners experience critical illness. On the other hand, caregiver support has known benefits to both patients and the renal care teams with respect to important outcomes such as improved self-management and enhanced adherence. Some caregivers may also have opportunities for enhancements in self-worth and personal growth. Nonetheless, it is becoming increasingly documented that the support needs for caregivers are largely unmet in the context of renal disease [15–17].

DePasquale and colleagues offer excellent recommendations following their qualitative study of family members caring for patients on dialysis or who have had a renal transplant [16]. We have adapted and summarized below:

- Disseminate *family-centered* information on treatment – there can often be a mismatch in priorities between healthcare providers and family members on information to be shared.
- Facilitate discussions with family members about responsibilities or care activities that are required. Prepare family members to be care partners by including discussions of events or circumstances that may arise such as:
  - Sleep disruptions (e.g., in the case of home-based modalities)
  - Psychological reactions to treatments (e.g., mood changes)
  - Information around treatments in various settings from the dialysis unit, to acute hospitalization, to critical care
  - Information around medication management of complex regimens
  - Inconveniences that will arise such as the management of supplies for home-based modalities
  - Information around comorbidities and related health problems that can arise from dialysis and transplantation
  - Understanding and managing fatigue in their partner.
- Enhance education to family members and partners to explicitly include the impact on caregivers of various treatment decisions.
- Prepare family members to manage their own psychological reactions such as managing uncertainty, anxiety, and demoralization.
- Consider introducing family-based interventions to enhance coping skills such as problem-focused and emotion-focused strategies.
- Consider aspects of communication between dyads to address potential discrepancies.
- Prepare families in managing expectations, validate difficult aspects of adjustment and adaptation, and promote disclosures around emotional and psychological aspects of adjustment.

15.9 Case Vignette – "Brenda and John in Transplant: Walking into the Sunset – Not!"

Brenda and John had this image of walking out of the hospital after her transplant, clicking their heels, feeling "on top of the world," and walking into the sunset of the next phase of their marriage. John found the presurgical workup very stressful as he struggled to juggle work demands and the multiple tests and visits with the transplant team, the social worker, the psychologist, and the surgeon ("problem-focused coping"). There was a new cast of providers to work with ("patient-staff interaction"). There were potentially some concerns around his candidacy, and the uncertainty started generating some anxiety and conflict between them ("ongoing disequilibrium"). Brenda's fatigue seemed to be worsening, and she was becoming more hopeless about a positive outcome ("coping and adjustment").

Fortunately, John was cleared to proceed with donation, and a few weeks later, Brenda received a living donor kidney from John. John's acute pain subsided quickly, and he was able to pay Brenda a visit on the ward. Unfortunately, she developed an infection, and concerns about surgical complications were being raised. John was devastated and wondered if he had "done this for nothing" ("cognitive factors"). They were able to engage again with the consultation-liaison psychiatry service that remembered them well ("patient-staff interaction").

Supportive visits to monitor both their mood and anxiety levels were helpful. Brenda's appetite returned, her infection was successfully treated, and her renal function improved with her new organ. They were able to be discharged with close monitoring. Their walk out of the hospital was not as pleasant as they expected. Brenda continued to be very nauseated, and the immunosuppressive medications were making her feel very edgy and irritable. They had heard about this and knew that it would get better over time as steroids were tapered ("coping and adjustment").

In the period post-transplant, there were many visits for testing and monitoring, and the medication regimen became overwhelming to manage. John consulted with the pharmacist who was able to prepare blister packs to enhance medication adherence ("problem-focused coping"). Over time, their adjustment improved ("return to equilibrium").

Detecting a gap in support for couples post-transplant, John and Brenda initiated a meeting with the clinic leadership and were able to organize a peer-facilitated service to assist couples in managing expectations during the transplant process ("kidney unit-support," "social support"). In meeting with other donors, John felt especially proud that he had been able to donate ("meaning making"). They did miss their dialysis community but were able to develop new networks of support and resume more regular visits with their adult children ("social support"). Brenda's condition post-transplantation continued to improve, and there was a return to some renewed energy. Brenda and John's relationship continued to grow, and their new treatment team continued to be attuned to how both of them were coping together with yet another "new normal" ("impact of the treatment environment"). Together, there was a renewed sense of purpose in life.

15.10 Key Takeaways

- *Adjustment is complex and dynamic* – Appreciate the extremely complex and dynamic concepts and processes involved in adjusting to renal disease across acute and critical episodes, periods of dialysis, and the transplantation.
- *Develop knowledge* – Building knowledge around factors leading to good adjustment (e.g., cognitive factors such as improving sense of control, enhancing acceptance of one's illness, developing higher levels of social support and behavioral factors such as enhancing adherence, positive health behaviors around activity, diet, problem-focused coping) can enhance case formulation across the distress continuum and across the lifespan.
- *Education* – Enhancing pre-dialysis education to include both the physical, psychological/emotional, and social adjustments to treatment may assist in managing patients' expectations and prepare patients more fully so they do not feel like those reactions occur "unexpectedly."

- *Validate and normalize* – Development of supportive care environments can promote the discussion of adjustments (both difficult and positive aspects) to reduce stigma around disclosures of emotional challenges and seeking of support.
- *Focus on caregivers* – The demands for adjustment and adaptation are equally as challenging for the caregiver (spouse, partner, family member, friend) of the renal patient. Caregivers are essential in contributing to important adjustment and health outcomes for the patient. Include them as much as possible in all aspects of care and attend to their unique adjustment needs.
- *Intervention* – Consider the development of educational or psychosocial treatment packages to help build healthy coping and adjustment mechanisms for both patients and their caregivers.
- *Encourage peer supports* – Peer support networks or groups enhance important elements of all types of coping, especially social support.
- *Staff training* – Consider in-services and other teaching modalities around understanding, identifying, and responding to emotional distress and adjustment reactions across the continuum from mild to moderate to severe.
- *Treatment environment* – Enhance treatment environments that are conducive to patients discussing psychological and emotional concerns that may range from offering informal, casual, supportive conversations with staff to more formal treatment consultations with specialists (e.g., renal psychologists or social workers, consultation-liaison psychiatrists).

References

1. Engel GL. The clinical application of the biopsychosocial model. Am J Psychiatry. 1980;137:535–44.
2. Lazarus RS, Folkman S. Stress, appraisal and coping. New York: Springer; 1987.
3. Leventhal H, Phillips LA, Burns E. The Common-Sense model of self-regulation (CSM): a dynamic framework for understanding illness self-management. J Behav Med. 2016;39:935–46.
4. Stanton AL, Revenson TA, Tennen H. Health psychology: psychological adjustment to chronic disease. Annu Rev Psychol. 2007;58:565–92.
5. Stanton AL, Hoyt MA. Psychological adjustment to chronic disease. In: Guillemin F, Briancon S, Spitz E, Coste J, editors. Perceived health and adaptation in chronic disease. Routledge; 2018. p. 46–59.
6. Moss-Morris R. Adjusting to chronic illness: time for a unified theory. Br J Health Psychol. 2013;18:681–6.
7. Aldwin CM, Yancura LA. Coping and health: a comparison of the stress and trauma literatures. In: Schnurr PP, Green BL, editors. Trauma and health: physical health consequences of exposure to extreme stress. American Psychological Association; 2004. p. 99–125.
8. Moos RH, Holahan CJ. Adaptive tasks and methods of coping with illness and disability. In: Martz E, Livneh H, editors. Coping with chronic illness and disability: theoretical, empirical, and clinical aspects. Springer; 2007. p. 107–26.
9. Harvey MA, Davidson JE. Postintensive care syndrome. Crit Care Med. 2016;44(2):381–5.

10. Sein K, Damery S, Baharani J, Nicholas J, Combes G. Emotional distress and adjustment in patients with end-stage kidney disease: a qualitative exploration of patient experience in four hospital trusts in the West Midlands, UK. PLoS One. 2020;15(11):e0241629.
11. Kostro JZ, Hellmann A, Kobiela J, Skóra I, Lichodziejewska-Niemierko M, Dębska-Ślizień A, et al. Quality of life after kidney transplantation: a prospective study. Transplant Proc. 2016;48:50–4.
12. Howell M, Tong A, Wong G, Craig JC, Howard K. Important outcomes for kidney transplant recipients: a nominal group and qualitative study. Am J Kidney Dis. 2012;60:186–96.
13. Tucker EL, Smith AR, Daskin MS, et al. Life and expectations post-kidney transplant: a qualitative analysis of patient responses. BMC Nephrol. 2019;20:175.
14. Dallimore DJ, Neukirchinger B, Noyes J. Why is transition between child and adult services a dangerous time for young people with chronic kidney disease? A mixed-method systematic review. PLoS One. 2018;13(8):e0201098.
15. Hoang VL, Green T, Bonner A. Informal caregivers' experiences of caring for people receiving dialysis: a mixed-methods systematic review. J Ren Care. 2018;44(2):82–95.
16. DePasquale N, Cabacungan A, Ephraim PL, Lewis-Boyér L, Powe NR, Boulware LE. Family members' experiences with dialysis and kidney transplantation. Kidney Med. 2019;1(4):171–9.
17. Berg CA, Upchurch R. A developmental-contextual model of couples coping with chronic illness across the adult life span. Psychol Bull. 2007;133(6):920–54.

16 Palliative, End-of-Life, and Psychiatric Care of Patients with Advanced Renal Disease

Margaret Leung and April Zehm

16.1 Introduction

Patients with serious or life-limiting illness, such as advanced kidney disease, experience multiple changes physically, emotionally, socially, and spiritually. As they live through functional loss related to increasing symptom burden, they may struggle with finding meaning and purpose while worrying about the impact of their illness on their loved ones. Common psychiatric diagnoses such as depressive disorder, anxiety disorder, and delirium may be difficult to distinguish in the setting of serious illness. Vascular risk factors seen in patients with chronic kidney disease (CKD) pose further risk for the development of cognitive impairment including major neurocognitive disorder. A palliative care approach to caring for patients and their families facing chronic disease can help patients live as well as possible in the setting of an ever-evolving disease course. This chapter has three objectives: (a) to provide non-palliative care providers with a palliative care framework to support CKD patients, with an emphasis on excellent communication skills; (b) to identify common psychiatric needs in the palliative care setting; and (c) to offer guidance on managing common symptoms for patients at end of life.

M. Leung (✉)
Department of Palliative Care Services, Kaiser Permanente, Roseville, CA, USA
e-mail: margaret.w.leung@kp.org

A. Zehm
Department of Medicine, Division of Geriatric and Palliative Medicine, Medical College of Wisconsin, Milwaukee, WI, USA
e-mail: azehm@mcw.edu

A. Hategan et al. (eds.), *Psychonephrology*,
https://doi.org/10.1007/978-3-030-84740-1_16

16.2 Case Vignette[1]

Ms. X, a 72-year-old female with long-standing type 2 diabetes mellitus complicated by proteinuric diabetic kidney disease, was referred to nephrology for stage 5 CKD. She worried how her CKD would impact her life moving forward. She was increasingly despondent over her shortened life expectancy and became increasingly depressed and anxious. Over the next few clinic visits, her nephrologist explored Ms. X's goals and priorities to further guide decision-making. She was willing to accept potentially burdensome treatments if it could help her live longer to maximize time with her family. Given her goals, her nephrologist recommended hemodialysis. Her uremic symptoms and mood improved after seeing the benefits of hemodialysis, and she enjoyed time at home with her son and young grandchildren.

Two years later, Ms. X developed ischemic cardiomyopathy and end-stage heart failure. Due to recurring hemodynamic instability during hemodialysis, she was hospitalized four times in 3 months. Her depression returned and was more pronounced. She skipped several hemodialysis sessions because she did not feel it would make a difference: "I'm just going to die anyway." Her functional status declined precipitously, now spending most of her time in bed or in her reclining chair. She also experienced increasing symptom burden, including anorexia, fatigue, and dyspnea with minimal exertion, which she refused medications for.

On her fourth hospital admission, she vacillated about whether to stop hemodialysis and became more withdrawn. Her son expressed concern that her depression impaired her capacity to make medical decisions. A psychiatrist met with Ms. X who determined that her depressive disorder was not impairing her medical decision-making capacity based on patient autonomy and desire to reduce physical suffering, though she recommended starting sertraline 50 mg per day. The medical team consulted the palliative care team and coordinated an interdisciplinary family meeting involving the patient, her son, cardiologist, nephrologist, palliative medicine specialist, psychiatrist, case manager, and nurse. During this discussion, Ms. X and her son were surprised to hear her prognosis measured in "weeks to months" rather than "years." The ongoing difficulties with hemodialysis tolerance and her declining heart function were reviewed in detail. She expressed frustration with repeated hospitalizations and a desire to be home, although she remained determined to continue hemodialysis for "as long as possible." A time-limited trial of continued outpatient hemodialysis was suggested, with her clinicians outlining that if this became unsafe or no longer medically indicated, it would no longer be offered.

Over the coming days, Ms. X was unable to complete hemodialysis due to hemodynamic compromise. Her nephrologist now recommended discontinuing hemodialysis because the harms outweighed the benefits. During this time, Ms. X and her son discussed the situation further with the palliative care team. She shared her grief around losing her independence, feeling abandoned by God, and terrified of "suffocating" at the end of life, as her dyspnea had progressively worsened over months.

[1] The authors wish to acknowledge Aaron Dall, MD, for his review of the case.

Based on her worsening quality of life and functional decline, Ms. X agreed to stop hemodialysis. The palliative care team recommended a bedside fan and initiating low-dose hydromorphone as needed for pain and dyspnea. She was discharged to a hospice facility and died peacefully 5 days later.

16.3 Palliative Care Principles

Palliative care is specialized medical care for people living with serious illness, focused on providing relief from the symptoms and stress of the illness or its treatments and improving quality of life for patients and their families [1]. While often confused with strictly "end-of-life" care, palliative care is appropriate at any age and any stage of a serious illness; it can and should be delivered alongside curative or life-prolonging treatments (Fig. 16.1).

Palliative care specialists offer expertise in several clinical domains including (a) complex physical and psychological symptom management; (b) skilled communication about patients' goals and values, complex medical decision-making throughout the illness trajectory, contingency planning, or navigating conflict or ethical dilemmas; and (c) coordination and communication of care plans among patients and clinicians [1].

Growing numbers of patients with advanced kidney disease are living longer with serious illness, resulting in an increased demand for palliative care that exceeds

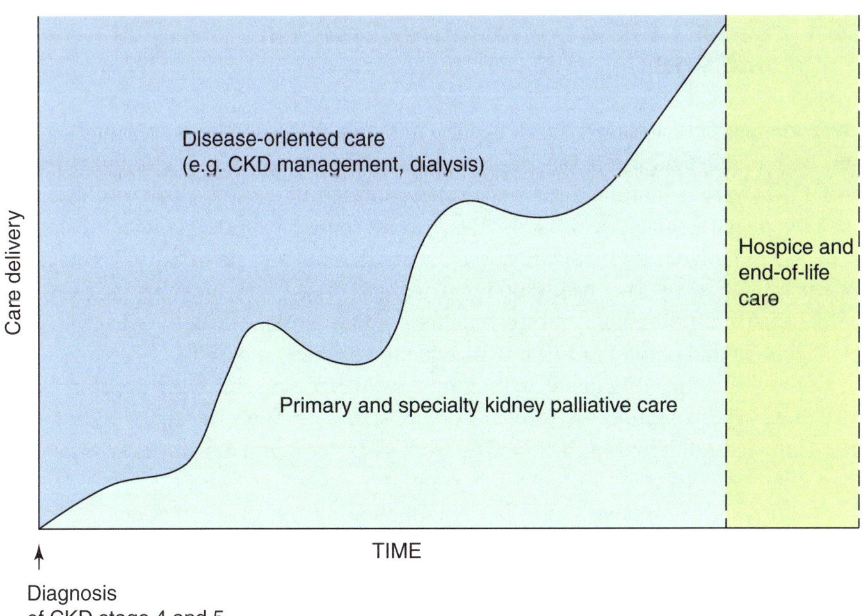

Fig. 16.1 Early, integrated model of palliative care in chronic kidney disease (CKD)

Table 16.1 Areas of domain in primary and specialty palliative care in nephrology

Palliative care domain	Primary palliative care addressed by nephrology team	Specialty-level palliative care consultation
Symptom management	Routine symptom assessment and treatment	Refractory symptom management
Serious illness communication and decision-making	Basic discussions about prognosis, goals of treatment, dialysis modalities/risks/benefits, advance care planning, and code status	Navigating complex goals of care or interpersonal dynamics, patient/family/team conflict, challenging ethical issues
Interdisciplinary team support	Screening for psychosocial or spiritual distress	Management of existential distress, including access to trained social workers, chaplains, and other clinicians to address nonphysical aspects of suffering
Conservative care	Medical management of CKD or ESRD with a focus on quality of life, referral to hospice when appropriate	Assistance with advance care planning, end-of-life care, bereavement

what the limited specialist-level workforce can supply. For patients living with CKD or end-stage renal disease (ESRD), kidney or renal palliative care is provided via collaboration among nephrologists (who use primary palliative care skills) and palliative care specialists [2, 3] (Table 16.1).

16.4 Serious Illness Conversations Establish Patient Values and Goals

Over the last two decades, the dialysis population has become increasingly older and with a substantial number of serious comorbid conditions [4]. Patients living with CKD have a shortened life expectancy, and the illness trajectory is characterized by psychological distress, high symptom burden similar to that of cancer patients, and increasing medicalization that escalates at the end of life [5]. Given the extensive palliative care needs of renal patients that often manifest many years before death, all clinicians caring for this population need expertise in symptom management and communication to provide the best care possible.

Communicating effectively with seriously ill patients and their families is an essential part of all clinicians' professional practice. A variety of reports have found that patients and their families benefit from clear, compassionate discussion with their clinicians about their illness understanding, goals, and values.

A serious illness conversation is any clinician-led conversation about the future outcome of the illness and associated prognosis, often including a reflection of the patient's goals, values, and priorities. Such conversations may include discussing goals of care, decision-making around specific medical procedures or interventions,

Table 16.2 Proposed triggers for when to conduct serious illness conversations with patients with renal disease [6]

Before dialysis	After beginning dialysis
Not surprised if the patient would die in the next 12 months	Not surprised if the patient would die in the next 12 months
Dialysis teaching or access referral	Access procedures
Transplant referral	Recurrent or prolonged hospitalization
Recurrent or prolonged hospitalization	Functional decline
Functional decline	Sentinel events (falls, weight loss, change in interdialytic weight gain, declining albumin, hemodynamic changes, etc.)
Sentinel events (falls, weight loss, declining albumin, etc.)	
Patient or family request	Patient or family request

delineating preferences for future medical care, discussing advance directives (including the identification of a surrogate decision-maker in the event of future decisional incapacity), and/or discussing end-of-life care and preferences [6].

Given the high morbidity and mortality associated with dialysis, patients' desire to discuss the future with their clinicians, and high rates of decisional regret over pursuing dialysis, serious illness conversations should be conducted with all patients with advanced CKD who are considering dialysis and at regular intervals thereafter [6]. For patients already on dialysis, various screening tools to identify high-risk patients who would benefit from ongoing conversations have been proposed, including age cutoffs, evidence of functional decline, the surprise question (e.g., "Would you be surprised if your patient died in the next 12 months?"), and validated mortality predictors [6]. Table 16.2 includes several proposed triggers for when to initiate or continue serious illness conversations in CKD and ESRD.

Serious illness conversations can be difficult for both patients and clinicians. Table 16.3 highlights several key serious illness conversation domains and sample language to lead such discussions effectively and empathically. For clinicians seeking further training to hone their communication skills, there are several dedicated communication training programs including VitalTalk [7], NephroTalk [8], Ariadne Labs' Serious Illness Care resources [9], and the "best case/worst case" tool [10].

Recommendation

- All medical professionals caring for patients with CKD stages 4 and 5 should be regularly engaging with their patients about disease trajectory and prognosis while also eliciting patients' illness understanding and goals.

Table 16.3 Serious illness conversation domains and example language

Conversation domain	Sample language and questions
Assessing illness understanding, expectations, information preferences	What is your understanding of your kidney disease? [6, 9] How have things been going lately with your health? What have your medical providers told you about… [7]: what to expect with your renal failure? your treatment options? dialysis? What is your understanding of what dialysis would provide in terms of survival and quality of life? What have you heard about the logistics and potential burdens of dialysis? What do you understand about what to expect if you cannot or choose not to receive dialysis? As you think about what lies ahead, what are you hoping for? What worries do you have? [7, 9]
Disclosing serious news and discussing prognosis	Pair hope/worry statements [6, 7, 9]: "I am hoping you have a long time to live with your kidney disease and I am also worried that time may be as short as a few years." We're in a different place now… [7]
Responding to emotions (appropriate throughout the conversation)	NURSE [7]: Name: It sounds like you are frustrated. Understand: This helps me understand what you're thinking. Respect: You've been a great advocate for your mom. Support: I will do my best to make sure you have what you need. Explore: Could you tell me more about that?
Assessing functional status and psychosocial support	What does a typical day look like for you? [8] What do you enjoy doing? How has your ability to do the things you want to do changed in the past year? [8] Who do you consider part of your support system? Can they help with medical follow-up? Transportation to dialysis if you need help with this? Are there personal factors that you think will lead to the success of dialysis? Anything that might make dialysis difficult?
Assessing quality of life and coping	What helps you live well despite your renal failure? [9] What gives you strength and gets you through difficult times? [6, 9] What is the role of religion or spirituality in your life?
Initiating advance care planning discussions (includes reviewing priorities, trade-offs, end-of-life planning, advance directives)	Given this situation, what's more important to you? [7] What are your most important goals? [7, 9] If you were to become sicker, how much are you willing to go through for the possibility of more time? [6, 9] Are there situations in which you would no longer want to continue dialysis? Are you aware that dialysis can be stopped if you were ever in a clinical situation in which your quality of life was not acceptable to you? What would be most important to you if/when you are nearing the end of your life? Who should make medical decisions for you if there ever comes a time when you cannot? How much do they know about your priorities and wishes? [6, 9]
Making recommendations that align with patients' goals and values	Given what is most important to you, I recommend… [6, 8, 9] Here is what we can do now to help you achieve these things…. What do you think? [7]

16.5 How to Approach Patients with CKD Stages 4 and 5 and Who Are Contemplating Initiating or Discontinuing Dialysis

The model for shared decision-making involves clinician expertise regarding medical options and prognosis and the patient's goals, values, and priorities (Fig. 16.2). Patients with ESRD have four options in managing their advanced kidney disease: (a) pursue an appropriate dialysis modality, (b) forgo any initiation of dialysis and continue conservative medical management, (c) pursue a time-limited trial of dialysis with reassessment of goals at the end of the trial, or (d) stop ongoing dialysis and receive end-of-life care. Patients who pursue dialysis most often hope to extend their life expectancy, though median survival after initiating dialysis is 15.6 months for patients aged 80–84 years, 11.6 months for patients aged 85–89 years, and 8.4 months for patients aged 90 years and older [11]. A discussion of prognosis should also review how functional status, care needs, and patient symptoms may evolve over time in the setting of progressive disease and multiple comorbidities.

There are two common scenarios in which patients may not pursue dialysis: a decisionally intact patient or their surrogate decision-maker declines this intervention, or the patient's poor prognosis and comorbidities limit the safe administration of treatment such that the physician does not offer it. The Renal Physicians Association recommends conservative management for patients older than 75 years with impaired functional status, severe malnutrition, and a terminal illness from non-renal causes or those whose clinicians answer "no" to the surprise question [12]. The median survival of nondialytic management in the older adult population ranges from 6 to 24 months [13]. Patients conservatively managed need support around common CKD complications and symptoms, continued advance care

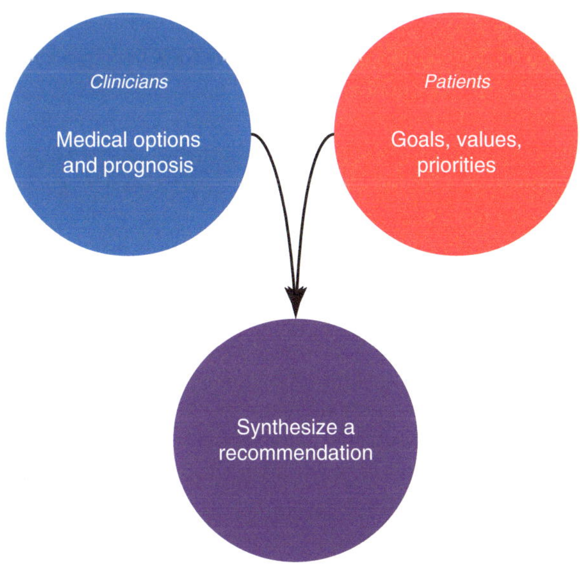

Fig. 16.2 A model for shared decision-making based on patients' goals

Table 16.4 Symptoms commonly seen in patients receiving conservative medical management [4, 13, 14]

Pain
Nausea and vomiting
Breathlessness
Anxiety
Pruritus
Fatigue
Depression
Cognitive dysfunction
Anorexia
Sleep disturbances
Restless legs syndrome

planning, and coordinated care for crises and end of life. Table 16.4 lists common symptoms necessitating aggressive symptom management in patients opting for conservative medical management [4, 13, 14].

Recommendation

– Patients not pursuing dialysis should be frequently assessed for symptoms related to uremia, anemia, and volume overload.

A time-limited trial of dialysis can be considered when patients have an uncertain prognosis or there is no consensus around goals of care about providing dialysis [12, 15]. In critical illness, short-term goals that outline both clinical milestones and quality of life goals need to be established. Goals in this situation may need to be reassessed within several days given the dynamic situation of critical illness, particularly if initial prognostic uncertainty becomes more certain over time. A trial period allows patients and their families to experience firsthand the benefits and burdens of treatment and in some cases provides time to cope with an overall poor prognosis. For patients who stabilize or improve, discussions can shift to focusing on long-term goals and examining how dialysis can optimize a patient's quality of life.

For patients wishing to stop dialysis, an exploration of the patient's motivation is necessary. The desire to stop dialysis could be interpreted as a patient: (a) emotionally responding to their current situation, (b) expressing distress and suffering, or desiring to relieve this, (c) seeking information about suicide or physician-assisted death, or (d) actively planning to end one's life [16]. A patient's request for hastened death is an opportunity for the medical team to readdress unresolved physical symptoms and/or psychological distress. Other disciplines such as social work, psychology, and spiritual care/chaplaincy can play a valuable role in identifying and addressing emotional, social, and existential distress.

Patients who achieve a level of equanimity related to their illness require counselling on what to expect, including preparing for end-of-life care and accessing

Table 16.5 Hospice eligibility criteria by country

Hospice eligibility criteria	United States (paid by Medicare)	Canada (varies by province and programs)	Europe
	Patient with advanced CKD and is expected to die within 6 months agrees to forgo dialysis Patient on dialysis agrees to withdraw from dialysis Patient has another terminal illness not related to ESRD while wishing to continue dialysis[a]	Patient has a life-limiting illness with a prognosis of 6 months or less A decision has been made to focus on comfort rather than cure Resuscitation will not be used when the illness brings a natural death	Varies by country

[a]Because the cost of dialysis is prohibitive for most hospice programs, access to this care is largely limited to the final days to weeks of life after dialysis withdrawal

hospice care (Table 16.5). Hospice is a palliative care delivery model intended for patients approaching the end of life when curative or disease-prolonging therapies are no longer beneficial or desired.

Recommendation

– A desire to stop dialysis or patterns of missing dialysis sessions warrants further exploration of patient goals and a psychosocial evaluation.

16.6 Identifying Psychiatric Disorders in the Palliative Care Setting

Patients faced with a life-limiting illness may experience a spectrum of emotions and find ways to adapt at each transition point of their disease. Some coping mechanisms and feelings of sadness, anger, and worries can be adaptive and a normal part of living with illness. In cases where coping becomes maladaptive and potentially impairs patient functioning and receipt of care, or when mood disturbances become severe, clinicians should have a low threshold for assessing for diagnosable psychiatric illnesses.

16.6.1 Major Depression

The prevalence of depressive disorders in patients receiving palliative care ranges from 3 to 38% [17]. Evaluation of physical (e.g., intractable symptoms, medications causing mood symptoms, delirium), psychological (e.g., grief, loss of dignity, worries about symptoms and disability, financial distress, hopelessness), and spiritual (e.g., existential distress, doubts or loss of religious beliefs or faith) etiologies and risk factors (e.g., history of major depression, substance use, poor social support) commonly associated with major depressive disorder should be explored [17, 18, 26]. Determining if a patient's symptoms are due to advanced kidney disease or a comorbid psychiatric disorder can be challenging. Advanced kidney disease (especially uremia) can mimic signs of depressive disorder including fatigue, anorexia, sleep disturbance, and cognitive changes. A useful framework to identify depression emphasizes psychological symptoms such as dysphoria, depressed mood, hopelessness, helplessness, worthlessness, and suicidal ideation over somatic signs and symptoms such as weight loss, fatigue, or difficulty concentrating [18]. A two-item screening questionnaire for depression has been validated in the palliative care population [19]: "Over the past 2 weeks, how often have you been bothered by (1) little interest or pleasure in doing things and (2) feeling down, depressed, or hopeless?" A positive screen using this tool is answering "yes" to one or both questions.

Another common diagnostic challenge in the palliative care setting is to distinguish depressive disorder from grief, though they can occur concurrently. Patients living with advanced illness may grieve the loss of independence and increasing reliance on others for caregiving, changes in physical appearance, and/or loss of control and dignity. Grief is a normal and expected response to loss or anticipated loss. Whereas patients with depressive disorder have a pervasive quality marked by a lack of self-worth, grieving patients can experience pleasure and hope with symptom intensity diminishing over time [20].

Goals of care and prognosis should guide the management of depressive disorder. Patients with good functional status and goals focused on extending as much quality of life as possible may wish to pursue a more aggressive workup to identify reversible causes. On the other hand, patients who are bedbound with a survival prognosis of days to weeks may wish to avoid further workup and opt instead on symptom management. Prognosis also guides the selection of pharmacologic management. While there are mixed outcomes in the use of stimulants to treat major depression [21, 22], agents such as methylphenidate potentially have a role in the treatment of depressive disorder in the seriously ill population given their rapid onset. A trial period of methylphenidate titrated upward until side effects (e.g., insomnia, anorexia) are reached may be reasonable for patients with a prognosis of less than 3 months. Patients who are expected to live for months to years usually tolerate standard antidepressants such as selective serotonin reuptake inhibitors (SSRIs) and serotonin-norepinephrine reuptake inhibitors (SNRIs) well, though there is insufficient evidence to recommend a specific antidepressant for use in palliative care [23]. In addition to medication management, several evidence-based, semi-structured psychotherapies have demonstrated improvements in depression and anxiety scores in the palliative care population [24, 25].

Clinical Pearl

- Depressive disorder is not a "normal part of living with a life-limiting illness" and needs to be distinguished from a normative depressed reaction and grief.
- A focus on the psychological aspects of depressive disorder can help distinguish it from overlapping somatic symptoms that commonly manifest in advanced illness.

Recommendation

- Patients with depressive disorder and a survival prognosis of less than 3 months may benefit from stimulants (e.g., methylphenidate); patients with a prognosis greater than 3 months benefit from standard antidepressant treatment.

16.6.2 Anxiety

The prevalence of anxiety disorders ranges from 7 to 14% in the palliative care setting [26]. Feelings of being overwhelmed, anxious, and worried can be a normal response to living with advanced illness, while *persisting* anxiety that *disables* a patient from caring out their daily functions should alert providers to assess for an anxiety disorder. Common causes for anxiety can be divided into physical (e.g., uncontrolled symptoms, medication withdrawal, dyspnea), psychological (e.g., uncertainty about disease progression or disease trajectory, effects of illness on caregiving burden on families, social isolation), or existential/spiritual concerns (e.g., loss of control or dignity) [26, 27]. The language patients use to describe anxiety may include "worried," "tense," "insecure," or "scared" rather than "anxious" [27]. The screening tool to assess for anxiety in the palliative care population is the Hospital Anxiety and Depression Scale, though it does not distinguish between the various types of anxiety disorders, including panic disorder, generalized anxiety disorder, trauma- and stressor-related disorders, and phobias.

Treatment of anxiety depends on goals of care and prognosis and is ideally managed by an interdisciplinary team that can address both physical and nonphysical needs. Standard medication treatments such as SSRIs and SNRIs are indicated when survival prognosis is months to years. Patients with a shorter survival prognosis of hours to days or weeks benefit from faster-acting medications including benzodiazepines and off-label medications that have anxiolytic properties (e.g., propranolol, trazodone, gabapentin, antipsychotics). The benefits of using benzodiazepines in the palliative care setting need to be weighed against the risks among medically frail patients whose status may already be partially impaired or have higher fall risks. Non-pharmacologic therapies such as relaxation strategies, cognitive behavioral psychotherapy, and meaning-centered psychotherapy can be utilized in patients with intact cognition who are not imminently dying.

Recommendation

- The risks and benefits of using benzodiazepines in seriously ill patients should be weighed; otherwise off-label use of other anxiolytic medications may be considered.

16.6.3 Delirium

Many dying patients will experience delirium, which can manifest as hypoactive, hyperactive, or mixed subtypes, with prevalence ranging from 20 to 88% [28]. The hallmarks of delirium include an abrupt change in attention and awareness of one's environment that is also associated with a change in cognition. Hyperactive delirium is characterized by symptoms of restlessness, paranoia, hallucinations, and agitation. More commonly missed and more prevalent in the palliative care setting, hypoactive delirium often manifests as lethargy, sedation, and decreased awareness. It can be difficult to distinguish among delirium, dementia (major neurocognitive disorder), and depression ("the three Ds"); for example, psychiatric symptom presentation may represent a superimposed delirium commingled with dementia or an occurrence of an accelerated cognitive decline of the dementia itself [29].

Given that delirium is reversible in up to half of cases, even among terminally ill patients, an assessment looking for potentially correctable causes by means of a relatively noninvasive approach that reflects the patient's goals of care is indicated. Some causes of delirium may be reversible such as constipation, urinary retention, and medication side effects, whereas other causes are often irreversible such as strokes, dementia, and end-stage organ failure [27, 28]. The intensity of a diagnostic workup depends on the patient's disease trajectory, prognosis, (e.g., hours to days of life versus weeks to months), functional status, and the degree of distress patients and their families experience.

Recommendation

- Workup identifying causes of delirium should incorporate patient's goals of care and take into consideration functional status and prognosis.

16.7 End-of-Life Symptom Management

Basic symptom palliation is a fundamental skill for all clinicians who care for dying patients. Consideration of the underlying etiology of symptoms is *always* warranted, but additional exhaustive diagnostic testing (particularly invasive, high-risk procedures) *may not be*, particularly if the results will not change management or improve the patient's quality of life. The extent of the diagnostic workup should be tailored based on the patient's underlying disease, prognosis, goals, and values; if additional testing will be low yield, purely symptomatic approaches are appropriate in this context. Here, we offer evidence-based recommendations regarding the management of several commonly encountered symptoms that affect actively dying patients [30].

16.7.1 Pain

Pain is common in ESRD and can be from renal and non-renal causes, including musculoskeletal pain, dialysis-associated pain, peripheral neuropathy, ischemic pain from peripheral vascular disease, kidney-specific issues such as painful polycystic kidney disease, secondary hyperparathyroidism causing bone pain, or rare complications such as calciphylaxis.

Given their potency and rapid onset, opioid analgesics are the mainstay of managing end-of-life pain. The available routes of medication administration and the severity of pain need to be considered when evaluating a patient with pain. For actively dying patients who can no longer swallow, medications may need to be given sublingually, subcutaneously, or intravenously. Subcutaneously administered opioids have similar pharmacokinetic profiles to intravenous opioids, making this a commonly used route for hospice patients who may lack intravenous access. When pain is severe, the use of parenteral routes is favored due to rapidity of effect.

Historically, many clinicians often place patients on continuous hourly infusions of opioids at the end of life, so-called morphine drips. However, this may not be warranted and can result in unintentional overdose. More importantly, this is not an effective means of controlling acute symptoms because the dose of medication is spread out over the course of an hour. Given it takes many hours for a continuous infusion to reach steady state, patients may have uncontrolled symptoms and suffer in the meantime. Instead, the optimal management for treating acute pain is to provide *bolus* dosing, *repeating* doses as necessary to control symptoms (Fig. 16.3). Fentanyl and methadone are considered the safest opioids in patients with renal

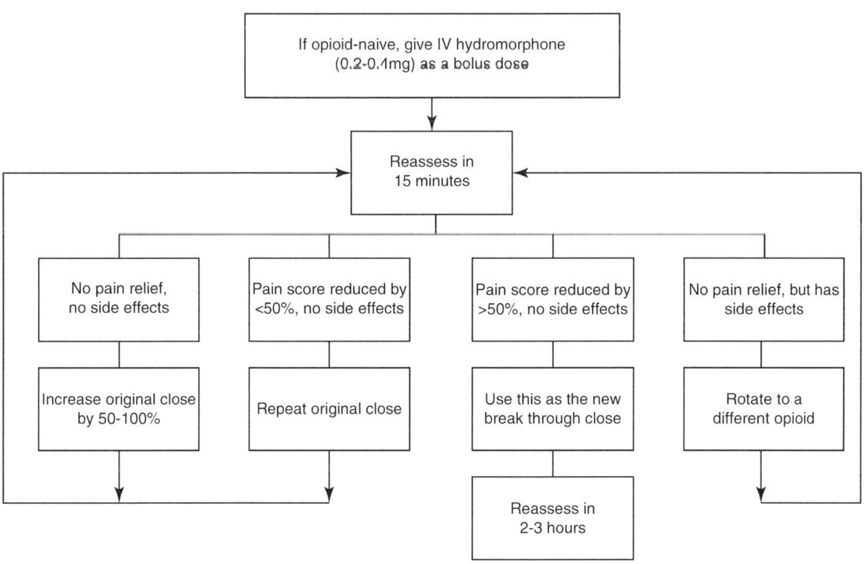

Fig. 16.3 Acute management of moderate to severe pain at the end of life

failure. Other opioids such as hydromorphone and oxycodone may be used with close monitoring and dose adjustment [31]. Morphine, codeine, hydrocodone, and meperidine should be avoided in renal failure unless death is imminent given their active, renally cleared metabolites can accumulate and cause delirium, myoclonus, or seizures [31].

Clinical Pearl

- Opiates such as fentanyl, methadone, hydromorphone, and oxycodone are preferred in renal failure to manage pain.

16.7.2 Dyspnea

Clinicians should watch for the presence of pulmonary edema and associated shortness of breath in renal failure patients, which can further be exacerbated by physical deconditioning and cachexia and worsen during the dying process. Notably, dyspnea does *not* always correlate with hypoxemia and can be highly distressing, often contributing to anxiety and more dyspnea, thus fueling a vicious cause-and-effect feedback loop. Recommended non-pharmacologic techniques include pursed-lip breathing or the use of a bedside fan. There are no data supporting the use of oxygen to alleviate dyspnea in the absence of hypoxemia, although simple air movement can help. Opioids are the gold standard for refractory dyspnea. Benzodiazepines are considered to be second-line agents since supporting their use to treat dyspnea is mixed. They can be helpful if there is significant anxiety present, but the risks of delirium and somnolence must be considered.

16.7.3 Delirium

Management of delirium in palliative care does not significantly differ from other settings except in the case of refractory delirium. Non-pharmacologic strategies for the prevention and treatment of delirium should be used for all patients, including frequent reorientation and cueing, correcting sensory deficits, normalizing sleep-wake cycles, and minimizing noise or other stimulating environmental factors. While no medications are US Food and Drug Administration-approved for the treatment of delirium, antipsychotic medications are often used to treat unsafe or distressing symptoms such as agitation and hallucinations (Table 16.6). There is little evidence to support treating hypoactive delirium pharmacologically.

Haloperidol has long been considered first-line therapy for hyperactive delirium due to its efficacy, relative safety, versatility, and low cost. Chlorpromazine is an effective alternative to haloperidol, especially for severe agitation, but has significant anticholinergic adverse effects, including potentiation of delirium. The second-generation antipsychotics olanzapine and risperidone have been shown to

Table 16.6 Pharmacologic management of delirium at the end of life [30]

Medication	Dose and frequency	Comments
Antipsychotics[a]		
Haloperidol	0.5–1 mg IV/SC/PO q1h PRN, then often scheduled q6–12h; titrate doses to 2 mg, then 4 mg if agitation continues	Preferred agent; often scheduled q6–12h in divided doses once effective daily dose is determined; may need 5 mg q6h for severe symptoms
Chlorpromazine	25–50 mg PO/IV q1h PRN, then often scheduled q6–12h	Often scheduled q6–12h; consider if more sedation is needed; can cause hypotension
Risperidone	0.25–0.5 mg PO q12h, titrate to 1.5 mg q12h	Limited to oral route; doses up to 4–6 mg/day have been used
Olanzapine	2.5–5 mg PO daily q8h	Dosages up to 20 mg daily have been used
Quetiapine	12.5–25 mg PO q6–12h	Dosages up to 300–400 mg daily have been used
Benzodiazepines		
Lorazepam	0.5–1 mg PO/SL/IV/SC/PR hourly until calm	Consider doses as low as 0.25 mg for geriatric patients; can paradoxically worsen delirium, so reserve if antipsychotics are contraindicated or already on board

[a]Antipsychotics have been shown to be associated with an increased risk of death and possibly stroke in elderly patients with dementia-related psychosis, resulting in a US Food and Drug Administration issued black box warning for these medications in 2005. This mortality risk has not been demonstrated in delirium. The use of these medications for this indication should be individualized, as the benefits of controlling agitated delirium among terminally ill patients usually outweighs the risk.

be equally effective to haloperidol and carry less risk of extrapyramidal symptoms but are more expensive and primarily limited to the oral route of administration (except in the case of olanzapine which is also available intramuscularly). Benzodiazepines can worsen delirium and generally are avoided unless there is history of alcohol or benzodiazepine withdrawal-related delirium. The addition of anticonvulsants to control behavioral symptoms of delirium when conventional therapy is inadequate may be considered. Physical restraints should be only used if behaviors are posing a safety risk to the patient or others and are unresponsive to the above therapies. In refractory cases, palliative sedation may be considered when delirium is determined to be irreversible and prognosis is less than 2 weeks [29]. Common medications used for sedation include midazolam, chlorpromazine, propofol, and dexmedetomidine. Sedation is an *outcome* rather than the *objective* of treatment in palliative sedation; when appropriately used, it does not hasten death.

Clinical Pearl

– Haloperidol is usually the medication of choice to pharmacologically manage hyperactive delirium.

Table 16.7 Prevention and treatment of constipation in seriously ill patients [30]

Medication	Dose and frequency	Comments
Stimulants		
Senna	1–2 tab PO daily; titrate up to 4 tabs BID	Can worsen colic, available over the counter
Bisacodyl	5 mg PO daily; titrate up to 3 tabs BID 10 mg PR daily PRN; titrate up to BID	Can worsen colic, available over the counter, use a suppository if swallow function is lost
Osmotic laxatives		
Lactulose (10 g/15 mL)	15–60 mL PO BID-QID	Can cause bloating
Polyethylene glycol	17 g powder dissolved in liquid PO daily; titrate up to TID	Tasteless, often well tolerated, available over the counter
Enemas		
Warm "tap" water	One PR administration; can repeat 1–2 times daily	Can soften stool before manual disimpaction or bisacodyl suppository attempt
Mineral oil	One PR administration	Can soften stool before manual disimpaction or bisacodyl suppository attempt
Milk and molasses	Added to a liter of water; 1 PRN administration	Combines osmotic and colonic stimulant, often used when all else fail

16.7.4 Constipation

Constipation is common and multifactorial at the end of life, resulting from dehydration, electrolyte disturbances, immobility, and medications. Both stimulants and osmotic laxatives have been shown to be effective for constipation and are considered first-line agents (Table 16.7). Bulk-forming laxatives such as psyllium and methylcellulose can worsen constipation without adequate fluid intake and are not routinely recommended. Milk of magnesia and magnesium citrate can cause significant cramping and are generally avoided in renal failure due to their high magnesium load. Docusate has not been shown to be more beneficial than placebo among terminally ill patients. When swallowing ability is lost or escalating oral laxatives fail, rectal-based therapies are often required, including stimulant suppositories or enemas. Saline or sodium phosphate enemas are not recommended given the high electrolyte load, risk of dehydration, and cause for worsening renal failure.

16.7.5 Secretions

Actively dying patients almost universally lose the ability to swallow and clear their secretions as their cough/gag reflex becomes impaired. The pooling of saliva in the posterior oropharynx and the retention of tracheobronchial secretions can lead to gurgling and noisy breathing that is often referred to as the "death rattle." While

Table 16.8 Anticholinergic medications to treat oral secretions at the end of life [30]

Medication	Dose, route, frequency	Comments
Atropine	1% ophthalmic drops, 1–2 drops SL q1–2h PRN	
Scopolamine	1–3 patches TD q3days	12 h to onset, so may be of limited utility for patients with a prognosis of hours More than one patch may be used, but given time to onset, other agents should be considered if secretions persist
Glycopyrrolate	0.2–0.4 mg IV or SC q4–8h PRN	Often preferred in the hospital setting given route, rapidity of onset, less deliriogenic potential compared to atropine or scopolamine
Hyoscyamine	0.125–0.25 mg PO or SL (orally disintegrating tabs) q4–6h PRN	Less deliriogenic potential compared to atropine or scopolamine

there is no evidence to suggest patients suffer from this, it can be highly distressing for families and caregivers to observe. Education and anticipatory guidance are imperative in preparing loved ones for this phenomenon. Repositioning the patient for postural drainage is first-line treatment. Deep suctioning should be avoided, as this can cause discomfort and often fails to reach inaccessible secretions located deeper in the respiratory tract. Anticholinergic medications are the pharmacologic agents of choice to treat copious secretions at the end of life and are considered equally efficacious (Table 16.8). Glycopyrrolate and hyoscyamine are often preferred over atropine or scopolamine due to their relatively reduced propensity to cause delirium and confusion.

16.8 Case Vignette Analysis

The case vignette previously presented highlights the importance of regularly engaging patients with advanced kidney disease about their goals of care, values, and preferences for treatment at different intervals of their disease. Based on the patient's goals, the nephrologist recommended hemodialysis earlier in the disease trajectory. Ms. X's mood symptoms prior to initiating hemodialysis could have represented a normal response to living with a life-limiting illness. Ms. X was able to continue experiencing a good quality of life until she developed heart failure that contributed to a functional decline and comorbid depressive disorder. Her refusal of medications and missed hemodialysis sessions raised concerns that depressive symptoms were interfering with her care and warranted further evaluation and treatment. It was important to explore if Ms. X was seeking to hasten her death by missing hemodialysis, if she was experiencing a grief response to her overall decline and illness, or if she had developed a comorbid depressive disorder. When Ms. X reached a point where the benefits of hemodialysis were minimal relative to the risks, the team was able to establish a trial period and define parameters for continuation versus cessation of this specific therapy. Palliative care offered recommendations for expert symptom management while supporting her and her family through complex decision-making and in transitioning to comfort-focused hospice care.

16.9 Key Takeaways

- Palliative care should be offered to all patients living with serious illness early in their disease course to support them with symptom management, disease understanding, and advanced care planning.
- Clinicians should engage patients with CKD stages 4 and 5 about their values and goals, especially in cases when patients show a functional decline, worsening medical comorbidities, or worsening renal function that pushes patients closer to ESRD.
- Patients forgoing dialysis need regular assessment and treatment of symptoms related to uremia. These patients also need support in planning for end-of-life care including hospice support.
- When patients already on dialysis develop complications that limit the safety of continuing treatment, a trial period that establishes goals and outcomes can be considered.
- There is a spectrum of normal responses and emotions to living with serious illness. Clinicians should have a low threshold for assessing for mood and anxiety symptoms if patients and families endorse such symptoms or changes in behaviors that compromise their care (e.g., skipping dialysis) are observed.
- Hypoactive delirium is commonly seen in the palliative care setting as opposed to hyperactive delirium.
- Oxycodone, fentanyl, methadone, and hydromorphone are the preferred opioids to manage pain and dyspnea in advanced kidney disease and at end of life.

References

1. Center to Advance Palliative Care: About Palliative Care. https://www.capc.org/about/palliative-care. Accessed 6 Feb 2021.
2. Lam DY, Scherer JS, Brown M, Grubbs V, Schell JO. A conceptual framework of palliative care across the continuum of advanced kidney disease. Clin J Am Soc Nephrol. 2019;14:635–41.
3. Gelfand SL, Scherer JS, Koncicki HM. Kidney supportive care: core curriculum 2020. Am J Kidney Dis. 2020;75:793–806.
4. Cohen LM, Moss AH, Weisbord SD, Germain MJ. Renal palliative care. J Palliat Med. 2006;9:977–92.
5. Davison SN. The ethics of end-of-life care for patients with ESRD. Clin J Am Soc Nephrol. 2012;7:2049–57.
6. Mandel EI, Bernacki RE, Block SD. Serious illness conversations in ESRD. Clin J Am Soc Nephrol. 2017;12:854–63.
7. VitalTalk. https://www.vitaltalk.org. Accessed 6 Feb 2021.

8. NephroTalk. http://nephro-talk.com. Accessed 6 Feb 2021.
9. Ariadne Labs Serious Illness Care Program. https://www.ariadnelabs.org/areas-of-work/serious-illness-care. Accessed 6 Feb 2021.
10. Best Case/Worst Case (BC/WC) Nephrologist Communication Tool – Whiteboard Video. https://www.youtube.com/watch?v=oXfXr7koz_A. [2019] Accessed 6 Feb 2021.
11. Tamura MK. Incidence, management, and outcomes of end-stage renal dialysis in the elderly. Curr Opin Nephrol Hyperten. 2009;18:252–7.
12. Renal Physicians Association. Shared decision-making in the appropriate initiation of and withdrawal from dialysis. 2nd ed. Rockville, MD: Renal Physicians Association; 2010.
13. O'Connor NR, Kumar P. Conservative management of end-stage renal disease without dialysis: a systematic review. J Palliat Med. 2012;15:228–35.
14. Davison SN, Tupala B, Wasylynuk BA. Recommendations for the care of patients receiving conservative kidney management: focus on management of CKD and symptoms. Clin J Am Soc Nephrol. 2019;14:626–34.
15. Scherer JS, Holley JL. The role of time-limited trials in dialysis decision-making in critically ill patients. Clin J Am Soc Nephrol. 2016;11:344–53.
16. Hudson PL, Kristjanson LJ, Ashby M, et al. Desire for hastened death in patients with advanced disease and the evidence base of clinical guidelines: a systemic review. Pall Med. 2006;20:693–701.
17. Block SD. Psychological issues in end-of-life care. J Pall Med. 2006;9:751–72.
18. Block SD. American College of Physicians-American Society of Internal Medicine End-of-Life Consensus Panel. Assessing and managing depression in the terminally ill patient. Ann Intern Med. 2000;132:209–18.
19. Payne A, Barry S, Creedon B, et al. Sensitivity and specificity of a two-question screening tool for depression in a specialist palliative care unit. Palliative Med. 2007;21:193–8.
20. Widera EW, Block SD. Managing grief and depression at the end of life. Am Fam Physician. 2012;86:259–64.
21. Hardy SE. Methylphenidate for the treatment of depressive symptoms, including fatigue and apathy, in medically ill older adults and terminally ill adults. Am J Geriatr Pharmacother. 2009;7:34–59.
22. Prommer E. Methylphenidate: established and expanding roles in symptom management. Am J Hosp Pall Med. 2012;29:483–90.
23. Rayner L, Price A, Evans A, et al. Antidepressants for the treatment of depression in palliative care: systemic review and meta-analysis. Palliat Med. 2011;25:36–51.
24. Martinez M, Arantzamendi M, Belar A, et al. "Dignity therapy," a promising intervention in palliative care: a comprehensive systemic literature review. Palliat Med. 2017;31:492–509.
25. Thomas LP, Meier EA, Irwin SA. Meaning-centered psychotherapy: a form of psychotherapy for patients with cancer. Curr Psychiatry Rep. 2014;16:488.
26. Fairman N, Hirst JM, Irwin SA. Clinical manual of palliative care psychiatry. Washington, DC: American Psychiatric Association Publishing; 2016.
27. Zweers D, de Graeff A, Duijin J, de Graaf E, Witteveen PO, Teunissen SCCM. Patients' needs regarding anxiety management in palliative cancer care: a qualitative study in hospice setting. Am J Hosp Palliat Care. 2019;36:947–54.
28. Breitbart W. Agitation and delirium at the end of life: "We couldn't manage him". JAMA. 2008;300:2898–910.
29. Bush SH, Tierney S, Lawlor PG. Clinical assessment and management of delirium in the palliative care setting. Drugs. 2017;77:1623–43.
30. Quill T, Bower K, Holloway R, et al. Primer of palliative care. 6th ed. Chicago: American Academy of Hospice and Palliative Medicine; 2014.
31. O'Connor NR, Corcoran AM. End-stage renal disease: symptom management and advanced care planning. Am Fam Physician. 2012;85:705–10.

Difficult Patient Encounters in Nephrology

17

Alan Eppel and Lynda Marfisi

17.1 Introduction

The term "difficult patient" is used throughout general and specialty medical practice to refer to difficult encounters with patients. The term does not apply to difficulties with diagnosis, treatment, or prognosis. The term is not attached to specific diagnoses but rather to the nature of the interaction between the patient and the physician and other healthcare professionals.

The phrase "difficult patient encounter" is more fitting and emphasizes the interactional nature of the difficulty. The physician or other clinician experiences uncomfortable emotions when anticipating the encounter with the patient. These emotions commonly include anxiety, dread, frustration, irritation, and even anger. These feelings may or may not be recognized by the healthcare professional. They may be accompanied by a pessimistic view of the prognosis.

This chapter does not address the impact of specific psychiatric disorders such as depressive disorder, anxiety disorder, posttraumatic stress disorder, substance abuse, and major neurocognitive disorder (dementia). For this, please refer to the relevant chapters in this volume.

A. Eppel (✉)
Department of Psychiatry & Behavioural Neurosciences, McMaster University, St. Joseph's Hospital, Hamilton, ON, Canada
e-mail: eppela@mcmaster.ca

L. Marfisi
Hemodialysis Program, Grand River Hospital, Kitchener, ON, Canada

A. Hategan et al. (eds.), *Psychonephrology*,
https://doi.org/10.1007/978-3-030-84740-1_17

Clinical Pearl
- Difficult patient encounters are the result of emotional and relational factors operating in the relationship between the healthcare professional and the patient.

Studies report that 15–20% of patient encounters in medical settings are viewed as "difficult" [1–3]. Physicians experience such patients as being demanding and emotionally draining. They require extra time often disrupting the physician's schedule. Specific patient and physician factors have been identified in a number of clinical settings [4–9]. These are described in relation to diagnosis, personality, physician experience, and disposition.

17.1.1 Case Vignette 1

Dr. Smithson, chief of nephrology, walked along the corridor toward the dialysis unit. He was hardly aware of a slight queasy feeling in the pit of his stomach. After checking in at the nursing station, he efficiently made his rounds of all his patients coming finally to Mr. Grabach's bed. The queasy feeling in Dr. Smithson's stomach intensified and he felt a tightening of the abdominal muscles.

"Good morning, Mr. Grabach; how are you today?" He offered his best upbeat voice. Mr. Grabach scowled, "you never got back to me about the side effects to the new medication."

"Well I don't have too much time to discuss this now so it will have to wait till next time." Mr. Grabach's face flushed, his voice now louder with anger: "you never seem to have any time for me. You just rush in and rush out after a quick glance at your patients."

Dr. Smithson, trying to contain his own anger but failing, told Mr. Grabach that he had a very large caseload of seriously ill patients and Mr. Grabach's problem could wait. Mr. Grabach began yelling and swearing. Dr. Smithson left the unit at a brisk walking pace while several of the nurses huddled around Mr. Grabach's bed in an effort to "talk him down."

17.2 Etiology

As in the case vignette 1, many nephrologists and team members will have had similar encounters. This was an encounter that broke down. This difficulty was not because of the patient's diagnosis. It was not because of treatment failure or deterioration in his condition. The difficulty here related to the interaction between the patient and the physician. Multiple factors converge to lead to this sort of difficult encounter, including the following factors described below:

- **Patient factors** are predominantly related to personality traits or personality disorder (e.g., narcissistic and borderline personality disorder). Social factors such as social isolation, lack of family support, unstable housing, and poor access to primary care and acute problems adapting to illness may contribute to the patient's behaviors.
- **Physician factors** may be similar to the patient factors and relate to the physician's own personality traits and level of anxiety, communication skills, and comfort in dealing with overt emotional expressions or conflict, as well as overwork, distraction, and burnout.

Additional factors include *organizational* aspects, which include the culture of the unit, the cohesion of the staff with regard to a consistent treatment plan and approach, leadership, staff morale, team collaboration, interdisciplinary conflict, excess productivity demands, and working conditions.

17.2.1 Patient Factors

17.2.1.1 Special Characteristics of Nephrology Patients

Nephrology patients are in it for the long haul. They frequently require dialysis for many years. Even in comparison to patients receiving chemotherapy, those with chronic kidney disease do not experience a period of remission. Dialysis patients depend on complex machinery to which they are attached several times a week without which they will die. Patients on dialysis face particular existential, psychosocial, and psychological and physical burdens.

They are dependent on medical technology and the competence and compassion of the treatment team to keep them alive. Both the illness and the treatment impose enormous restrictions on the day-to-day participation in personal, social, and work activities. Patients and the team have a long-term relationship. Those on dialysis spend a considerable amount of time each week in the dialysis unit.

Existential issues include the prospect of worsening of symptoms and the inevitability of illness progression without lifesaving interventions (e.g., transplant) that entail added fears. This may be unspoken but, nevertheless, an ongoing source of anxiety and fear. An explicit discussion with family or an empathic team member can attenuate this stress and counteract misconceptions about the prognosis.

The problems of patients with kidney disease are complex and may be stigmatized by clinicians in other specialties and services in the hospital. This can be due to a lack of understanding of how to address the patient's complex needs in other areas of the hospital. This can lead to avoidance by physicians and nurses. This can occur when a patient is asked to attend the emergency department or be transferred to another service. These clinicians may experience anxiety and self-doubt about their abilities to cope, which may manifest as rejection, stigmatization, or anger toward the patient.

From the treatment team's perspective, major patient issues include the following:

- Nonadherence to treatment; this includes nonadherence to medication, diet, or attendance for dialysis
- Special requests
- Verbal abuse of staff
- Verbal threats or acts of physical violence

Frequent problematic behaviors identified in a survey of 3000 randomly selected dialysis patients were [4]:

- Missing dialysis treatments (18%)
- Ending dialysis before completion (31%)
- Noncompliance (nonadherence) with medication (23/%)
- Noncompliance with recommended diet or fluid restriction (58%)

Arriving late to appointments and refusing procedures are additional factors that can lead to problematic behaviors. All these behaviors are likely to be associated with difficult patient encounters.

In common with all other patients and healthcare professionals, nephrology patients may exhibit troublesome personality traits or even definite personality disorders. The two major systems for formal diagnosis of patients with psychiatric disorders are the Diagnostic and Statistical Manual of Mental Disorders, 5th edition (DSM-5), and the International Classification of Diseases, 11th edition (ICD-11). The DSM-5 is produced and published by the American Psychiatric Association. The ICD-11 is produced by the World Health Organization. In this chapter, the authors use the ICD-11 terminology when discussing personality traits, as this is based on a dimensional rather than categorical approach and is more applicable to a range of clinical settings. When talking about specific personality disorders, the authors use the categorical nomenclature as found in ICD-11 and DSM-5, as these terms are widely used and recognizable at the present time.

It is estimated that approximately 12% of the population in the general community meet diagnostic criteria for personality disorder. This level increases to 25% of primary care patients and as many as 50% among psychiatric patients [10].

Clinical Pearl

- Among the population of nephrology patients, it is probable that the majority will not have a diagnosable personality disorder. A certain percentage of these patients will display some of the traits of personality disorder of mild, moderate, or severe levels of difficulty in domains such as sense of self, interpersonal relationships, and emotional expression.

Table 17.1 The five trait domain qualifiers that contribute to the expression of personality dysfunction [5]

Negative affectivity	Fear, anger, vulnerability, hostility, shame, depression, mistrust
Detachment	Avoidance of social interaction, limited expression of emotion, may appear aloof
Dissociality	Self-centeredness, entitlement, lack of empathy, denigrating of others, deceptive, exploitative, physically aggressive
Disinhibition	Impulsivity, recklessness, lack of planning
Anankastia	Perfectionism, overconcern with rules, orderliness, neatness, need for control of situations

17.2.1.2 Personality Trait Domains

The central features of personality disorders are impairments of self and interpersonal functioning. This can be mild, moderate, or severe. Some patients may not meet the diagnostic threshold for personality disorder and are described as having "personality difficulty." This is not considered to be a mental disorder but rather an accentuation of normal personality traits. In these cases the difficulties in functioning and relationships are of intermittent or low intensity and limited to specific situations.

These difficulties may manifest in the form of particular traits. The ICD-11 classification identifies the following five trait domain qualifiers (see also Table 17.1):

1. **Negative affectivity:** a tendency to experience a range of negative emotions with greater frequency and intensity. This is out of proportion to the situation and outside of the expected range of the population at large.
2. **Detachment:** a tendency to maintain interpersonal distance or emotional distance (avoidant attachment).
3. **Disinhibition:** a tendency to act on immediate external or internal stimuli (i.e., sensations, emotions, thoughts), without consideration of potential negative consequences.
4. **Dissociality:** disregard for the rights and feelings of others, encompassing both self-centeredness and lack of empathy.
5. **Anankastia (obsessionality):** a narrow focus with rigid standards of perfection and a rigid belief of right and wrong. It includes the attempt to control one's own and other people's behavior. This has an impact on the therapeutic alliance and adherence to treatment and to medical outcome.

As time goes on, chronic care patients may develop certain obsessional rituals regarding their "space" while they are on the units, including in the dialysis unit. This can result in some "territoriality." For example, patients may insist on one particular location in the unit. This may take on a dimension of superstition. Superstitions are irrational thoughts and/or behaviors that clinically are known as obsessions and compulsions. This is a form of magical thinking. It is similar to baseball players having to wear certain items of clothing or repeat ritualistic movements, "If I do this, nothing bad will happen and everything will turn out well."

17.2.1.3 Case Vignette 2

Mr. Charles, a 58-year-old retired police officer, arrived on the dialysis unit and quickly noticed that "his" blue recliner was not in the spot where he was to dialyze that day. He requested quite loudly that the chairs be "switched out," giving him his desired chair. Many of the patients had already arrived on the unit and had up their positions. Mr. Charles' chair was already occupied by another patient.

Regarding the case vignette 2, how should the nursing staff respond to this request? Should the nurse ask the other patient to get up from the recliner and wait while another chair is moved in for them? And, of course, this furniture must be cleaned before it can be used. Some nurses may immediately accede to the demand preferring to accommodate all requests in order to keep "the peace." Others may refuse and then be perceived by the patient as unsympathetic and unhelpful. This may then lead to discontent and even anger that remains unexpressed, simmering under the surface.

In response, the nursing staff may feel inconvenienced or even manipulated, further damaging the ongoing therapeutic relationship with that patient. Obsessional behaviors represent a way of coping with anxiety. By shifting the focus from underlying feelings of fear to apparently minor and inconsequential routines, the anxiety is kept at bay.

Physicians and nurses are quite familiar with obsessional defenses manifesting during their years of training at university or college, for example, spending too much time in the preparations for studying by buying notebooks and stationery supplies and drawing up lists and plans while avoiding the anxiety-provoking act of studying itself.

Another behavior exhibited by patients is loss of confidence in their own abilities resulting in increased dependency.

Examples of this may include asking a nurse to bring a cup of ice even though they have no difficulty going to the ice machine themselves. They may expect staff to notice when they have finished their coffee, at which time they would like the nurse to be immediately at hand to adjust their chair and blankets in a certain way. Patients may insist on having the tape applied to their arms in a very specific way, different from the standard approach. They may require that the TV remote control is placed "just so" in a specific spot. Patients may bring an assortment of things along and set up their "encampment" for the duration of their stay. All of these, and more, get repeated in many variations. Nurses may be viewed as either "good" or "bad" depending on how they respond to these requests. This may represent a defense mechanism known as "splitting." The nurse, on the other hand, is trying to get through her/his shift and complete the complex tasks that need to be attended to. Keeping the peace helps everything run more smoothly, in the short run.

Clinical Pearl

- Patient behavior is often attributed to a personality disorder. Unfortunately, this term is inherently pejorative as it implies that "you have a bad personality." In reality, personality disorders are on a continuum with what are considered normal personalities. They represent points on a continuum which at one end is adaptive and the other end is maladaptive.

Specific psychiatric diagnoses such as major depressive disorder, a range of anxiety disorders, psychotic disorders, substance misuse, posttraumatic stress disorder, and neurocognitive disorders can also impact the dynamics, whether in an inpatient or outpatient setting (see Chaps. 10, 11, 12, and 15 in this volume). Difficult patient encounters are not defined by these specific psychiatric diagnoses, but these diagnoses can help magnify the type of problems that may arise.

Clinical Pearl

- It should be apparent that members of the clinical team, physicians, nurses, social workers, and others can also manifest the same problems as the patients.

17.2.1.4 Categorical Personality Disorders

Personality disorders are characterized by problems in several areas of personality functioning including sense of self, difficulty in forming intimate relationships, and difficulties controlling impulses. These factors lead to impairment in personal, family, social, educational, occupational, or other important areas of functioning. Personality disorders are categorized as either mild, moderate, or severe in intensity. Individuals with personality disorders may manifest in combinations of the five specific trait domains (see Table 17.1).

Although the current trend is to move toward dimensional models when describing personality features, the authors have included the former ICD-10 and the current DSM-5 categorical terms, which may be more familiar to some readers. There are four particular categorical personality disorders that are most likely to be involved in difficult encounters as follows:

- Narcissistic personality disorder
- Borderline personality disorder
- Dissocial personality disorder (antisocial personality disorder, psychopathy)
- Obsessive-compulsive (anankastic) personality disorder

Narcissistic Personality Disorder

The following may be evident early on in the treatment relationship:

- Dissociality, which is a disregard for the rights and feelings of others encompassing self-centeredness, expectation of admiration, and lack of empathy.
- Lack of underlying self-esteem may lead to envy of other's success, including the physician or nurse. There may be a need to devalue the physician or demonstrate his or her incompetence by not getting better. They may react with a sense of justified anger in response to perceived slights.

On the surface, these patients may convey a sense of condescension and question the physician's competence or intelligence. They appear to want to be treated as "special." To this end, they may make demands and requests that are not routinely provided to other patients. Subconsciously, the patient's self-esteem is fragile and can only be sustained by constant external admiration and acknowledgment. This type of personality is very frequently observed among movie stars, CEOs, and other performers who cannot internally sustain a sense of self-esteem and require constant external applause and admiration. If the patient's desires to be treated as special are not acceded to, the patient's demeanor may switch to one of contempt, anger, personal derogation of the physician, or formal complaints. These patients are among the most difficult to work with.

Borderline Personality Disorder

Essential traits are negative affectivity, which is the experience of a broad range of emotions such as anxiety, anger, fear, vulnerability, shame, hostility, depression, and mistrustfulness.

The underlying difficulty is the combination of emotional dysregulation and insecure attachment. Both of these arise during childhood development as a result of early attachment experiences and their impact on neurodevelopment in relation to emotional regulation. This involves inadequate control by the prefrontal cortex on the emotional centers in the brain, particularly the amygdala.

Emotional dysregulation involves a deficit in top-down emotional control leading to more intense mood reactivity and a slower return to baseline. This leads to impulsivity, frequent self-harm, and thoughts of suicide. Angry confrontations with clinical staff are common. Physicians may feel anxious because of the high levels of emotional arousal and the fear that the patient may become violent, elope, or attempt to self-harm.

Dissocial Personality Disorder

These patients display a lack of empathy, callous, deceptive, manipulative, exploitative, and physically aggressive behavior. Characteristically, they lack guilt or remorse. These patients may have ulterior motives and try to manipulate the physician by flattery or threats.

Obsessive-Compulsive (Anankastic) Personality Disorder
These patients present with perfectionism, orderliness, risk avoidance, perseveration, and overcontrol of emotions. Therapeutic recommendations may become the focus of interpersonal battles for control.

17.2.2 Physician Factors

Physicians are motivated by the desire to help others and to get good treatment results.

The physician's own a sense of effectiveness or even omnipotence, and feeling of personal responsibility for treatment outcomes is undermined by difficult patient encounters. This can lead to a drop in self-esteem and mood, loss of enthusiasm, and "burnout." If the physician has narcissistic or perfectionistic traits, his or her response may be more acute.

Clinical Pearl
- Physicians who are less aware of emotional and psychological dimensions of patient care are more likely to experience difficult patient encounters [7].

Patients who meet the threshold for a definitive personality disorder are more likely to trigger more intense emotions in physicians and other clinicians. A particular form of response by a physician or other healthcare professional is known as "countertransference." This refers to those responses that are not proportionate to the real difficulty but result from subconscious feelings that derive from the physician's own personality and experiences of early relationships.

One of the major and most problematic responses made by physicians is that of avoidance, which provokes an amplifying feedback loop leading to increasing patient-physician conflict. The patient may feel disregarded or abandoned. Alternatively, physicians or nurses may respond with brusqueness and lack of empathy.

Another category of response is that of overzealous therapeutic interventions or investigations. This represents the defense of "reaction formation." The exaggerated solicitude conceals the subconscious angry feelings directed toward the patient. This is colloquially known as "killing with kindness."

17.2.3 Case Vignette 3

Dr. Clark sat across the desk from his patient, Ms. Margaret Jones, a 37-year-old single woman who worked at a retail grocery store. She was unhappy with her life and apparently had made a number of suicide attempts in the past. He noted a healed linear scar on her left wrist.

Dr. Clark was the director of the nephrology outpatient clinic at a well-known teaching hospital.

"Your blood pressure is still high. How are you finding the new blood pressure medication?"

"I stopped taking it" she replied casually.

"How long did you take it for and why did you stop it?" "Oh, I took it for about four or five days but then I was feeling tired and had a bit of a headache so I stopped it."

"You didn't give it much of a chance, did you?"

"Well, you've tried so many different drugs on me that I feel like a guinea pig. I really wonder if you know what you're doing!"

Now with an edge to his voice, Dr. Clark replied:

"Look, I'm not getting much cooperation from you. If you do not get your blood pressure under control, there could be serious complications."

"What makes you think I care about that? My life is a waste of time as it is and I don't really care what happens to me."

"Don't be ridiculous! If you don't comply with the treatment that I've ordered I will have to discharge you from the clinic."

With that, the patient got up from her chair and raised her voice telling the doctor that he was "arrogant" and "superior." She swore loudly, drawing the attention of other patients in the waiting room, and left the office slamming the door behind her.

Dr. Clark felt irritated, frustrated, and completely defeated.

17.3 Interventions

The clinical team should clearly and objectively define the problem behaviors and document them in the clinical record [5]. Specific effects of the medical condition such as metabolic changes, medication effects, and substance abuse should be ruled out [6]. Also the identification of specific psychiatric disorders in patients such as depression, psychosis, posttraumatic stress disorder, or cognitive impairment should be considered (see Chapters 10, 11, 12, and 15 in this volume). Consultation with the psychiatric consultation-liaison team can assist with diagnosis and management.

Recommendation

- Clinicians must be self-aware. They need to identify which types of patients "push their buttons" (i.e., triggering feelings of anxiety, discomfort, or irritation).
- It is important to understand the concept of countertransference and to be able to discuss the reactions to patients within the context of a supportive team.

17.3.1 Strategies

- First and foremost, "avoid avoidance" of patients. This only magnifies problems in the long run. It is recommended to have at least a focal encounter and to commit to arrange a longer meeting at a specific time as soon as possible.
- When discussing difficult encounters, arrange for adequate time and a private setting to discuss the difficulties with the patient. Prior to the meeting, review the clinical record paying particular attention to nursing notes and incident reports.
- Where the family is supportive and has a good relationship with the patient, they can be enlisted to problem-solve. They may have developed strategies to cope with the patient's problem behavior.
- The family physician may be able to play a role and represent a sense of continuity and support for the patient.
- Setting limits as to behavior that is not permissible and identifying potential consequences is essential. Matters of safety and acting out need to be addressed urgently.
- A written contract regarding mutual expectations of patient, physician, and team may be useful.

Recommendation
- Avoid avoidance of the patient (avoidance is one of the principal defensive behaviors).
- Arrange for adequate time and a private setting to discuss the difficulties with the patient.
- Family members and family physician can be enlisted to problem-solve and for support to the patient.
- Patient limit setting for unacceptable, unsafe behavior is essential.
- Written contract of mutual expectations of patient and medical team may be useful.

Because of the special difficulties recognized within dialysis treatment, a special task force developed a manual called "Decreasing Dialysis Patient-Provider Conflict" [11]. This involves a comprehensive educational program for both leadership and frontline staff. Topic areas are represented by the acronym CONFLICT, which is outlined below [11] (see Fig. 17.1).

Create a Calm Environment

- Use a private setting to address the conflict.
- Avoid discussing the issue in front of other patients, uninvolved staff, or visitors.
- Take the time needed to calm yourself and organize your thoughts before engaging the patient. If you are frustrated or angry, a successful resolution will be more difficult.
- Avoid a threatening presence, such as standing over the patient, pointing a finger, or placing your hands on your hips.

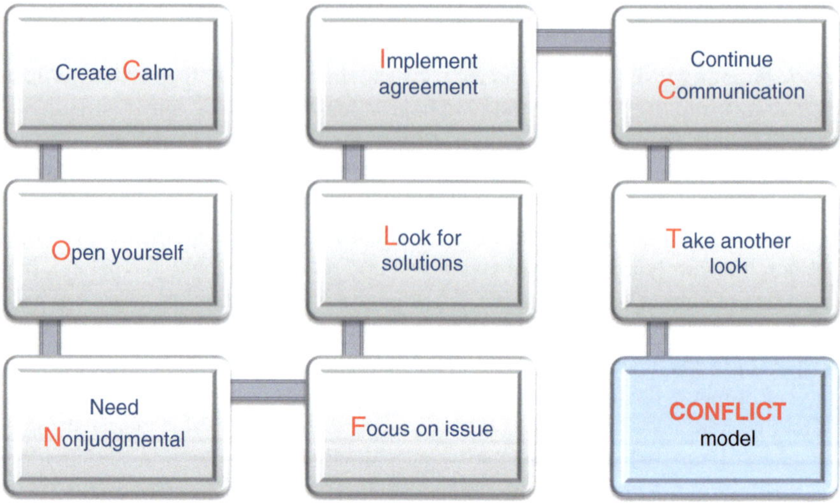

Fig. 17.1 Strategies for clinicians to manage difficult patient encounters based on the CONFLICT model. (Adapted from [11])

Open Yourself

- Acknowledge the perspective and feelings of the other individual(s) involved.
- Listen closely to what the person is telling you about the complaint or concern.
- Avoid being defensive.
- Show that you are trying to understand what the other individual is saying about the conflict.
- Ask questions and clarify with the patient what has been said.
- Recognize and accept that a patient has the right to disagree, question, or refuse a medical recommendation, even though you may believe that the patient is making a "poor" decision.

Need a Nonjudgmental Approach

- Be objective and "factual."
- Understand how you react to conflict. If conflict makes you uncomfortable, it becomes more difficult to maintain a professional approach.
- Avoid using remarks toward the patient that are blaming, threatening, or those that project guilt.
- Understand your values and beliefs about people who might be of a different race, age, gender, religion, or culture than you.
- Avoid using your authority as a healthcare professional to impose your beliefs on a patient. Rather, seek collaboration and shared decision-making with the patient.
- Make no assumptions about a patient's ability to understand or comprehend what you are trying to communicate.
- Get the patient to teach back by paraphrasing material.

Focus

- Maintain focus on the agreed upon issue. If other complaints enter the conversation, indicate to the patient you will address those issues at a later time once the initial complaint has been discussed.
- Repeat or clarify what has been said in an effort to understand what the conflict is about.
- Get patient agreement on what the conflict is about.
- Demonstrate a willingness to address the conflict because conflict is getting in the way of best care.
- Do this by ceasing any other activity, listening to what the patient is saying, and telling the patient that you are committed to addressing his or her concerns.
- Sit, at the level of eye contact, and turn off devices.

Look for Solutions

- Brainstorm possible solutions with the patient. Ask the patient what he or she hopes to accomplish.
- Hold a care conference and enlist family members, friends, staff, or others whom the patient trusts.
- Consider all available reasonable options to resolve the conflict.
- Let the patient know that even if the entire problem cannot be fixed, there are parts of the conflict that can be resolved.
- Only make promises you can keep.

Implement Agreement

- Use action statements to describe the agreement. For example, "In the future, I will tell you the name of the medication I am going to give you before giving it."
- Document and communicate to the necessary parties the agreement that has been reached.
- Be consistent with any agreements that are made. Agreeing to change some aspect of normal clinic operations and not following through will likely lead to more conflict. Set up a time to review with the patient later.

Continue to Communicate

- Effective resolution of a conflict requires follow-up communication.
- This will allow you to monitor the progress being made and will demonstrate to the patient your commitment to resolving the conflict.
- Set a specific timeframe (i.e., 1 week, 10 days, 30 days) to sit down with the patient again to look at the changes that were made and to evaluate the effectiveness of the changes.

- Be open and ready to deal with the fact that not all conflict is easily resolved and that you may have to repeat some of the steps in this model.
- Remember that not satisfying someone does not mean that your attempt to resolve the conflict has failed.
- If it is evident that the conflict is continuing, consider the use of an independent third party to help mediate the conflict.

Take another Look

- Review the steps used in addressing the conflict.
- Meet with other staff members to discuss other possible ways of responding to the conflict.
- Consider additional training in communication skills, crisis intervention, professionalism, boundary setting, or other topics you think will improve your ability to manage conflict.
- Take a close look at the role you played in the conflict. Ask yourself if you might have been able to defuse the conflict by responding in a different manner.
- Evaluate and understand the root of the conflict. It might be related to clinic policies or practices that could be changed to help prevent future conflicts.
- Ad hoc consultation from a psychiatrist, psychologist, or other members of the behavioral health team may add clear definition of the underlying problems. Brief psychotherapeutic interventions can be provided.
- Consider incorporating a psychiatrist or psychologist into the treatment team to provide regular assessment and consultation with regard to patient and team member interaction and dynamics. Group consultation in which physicians meet regularly with a psychiatric consultant to discuss difficult cases has been effective in general practice (Balint Groups) and has been used in the nephrology-dialysis department of Soroka Hospital in Israel [12].

17.4 Case Vignette Analyses

Based on the CONFLICT management model outlined previously, consider what your strategies of the patients presented in the three case vignettes would look like. The answers for some of those strategies are further presented in this section.

17.4.1 Case Vignette 1 Analysis

Clearly Dr. Smithson was anxious about meeting his patient Mr. Grabach. He displays a pattern of avoidance by leaving the patient to last and not getting back to him about side effects. He was unaware of his own feelings and oblivious to the patient's escalating anger. To resolve this pattern, Dr. Smithson needed to have a case conference with relevant team members to identify the underlying issues. He needed to reflect on his own responses and their meaning. The next step is to arrange adequate time for a meeting with the patient in a private and calm setting. This should include one of the nurses that has a relatively good relationship with the patient and other team members as required. The patient's prime family support person should also be present. Dr. Smithson should be objective, fact based, and nonjudgmental. He should listen attentively to the patient's understanding of the problem and try to be nonjudgmental and avoid blaming and making unilateral decisions. He must attempt to come to an agreed understanding of the issues and brainstorm possible solutions. The team needs to document the key points of the discussion and the agreed plan and set a date to follow-up to review the effectiveness of the plan. If necessary, they will need to renegotiate the plan.

17.4.2 Case Vignette 2 Analysis

Mr. Charles' insistence on having a specific recliner each time he comes to the dialysis unit created extra work, disruption, and stress for the nursing staff. This conflict needed to be addressed urgently. A care conference should be organized with the physician, team members, the patient, and one or more of his key supports. Mr. Charles' worries and concerns should be explored, including his motivation for insisting on a particular blue recliner. Questions should be raised, such as: "Is it based purely on comfort? Is it a way for him to reduce anxiety by returning to a familiar spot? Is it based on superstitious behavior (i.e., obsessive magical thinking)? Does he have a compulsion to always sit in the same chair because he is having obsessional thoughts telling him that he will not get well or that he will die if he does not do so? Alternatively, his behavior may be based on lack of understanding or empathy for the impact of this demand on other patients in the unit and staff. This may be based on feelings of entitlement due to narcissistic traits. Exploration about his beliefs and feelings will help to defuse the issue. If there are significant underlying obsessional thoughts leading to compulsive behaviors, cognitive behavioral therapy and/or consultation with a psychiatrist or psychologist may be helpful.

17.4.3 Case Vignette 3 Analysis

Ms. Jones does not appear to take her treatment very seriously. In fact she seems not to care whether she lives or dies. She is challenging toward Dr. Clark and critical of him. She exhibits negative affectivity and some disinhibition.

Dr. Clark is more used to being in control and normally receives great admiration and deference from his patients. He is not used to having his self-esteem attacked. When this does happen, he can become quite angry and take it out on his staff. Despite his external appearance of confidence and superiority, he is quite vulnerable under the surface.

Ms. Jones exhibits some of the traits that are found in patients diagnosed with borderline personality disorder. Dr. Clark displays traits associated with narcissistic personality type.

Dr. Clark would benefit from getting advice on how to handle such patients. This could be from colleagues or from the psychiatric consultation team. He would be advised not to get into power struggles over medication compliance. Rather he should present the risks and benefits objectively and let the patient make her own decision. He needs to be conscious of the patient's tendency to negative affectivity leading to emotional dysregulation. He also needs to reflect on his own views about himself and his need to achieve and to receive admiration on an ongoing basis in order to maintain his fluctuating self-esteem.

17.5 Key Takeaways

- "Difficult patients" are more effectively conceptualized as difficult patient encounters.
- Difficult patient encounters are the result of interacting factors, patient factors, physician/other clinician factors, and organizational factors.
- Difficult patient encounters can lead to anxiety and distress among healthcare professionals.
- The expectation of a difficult patient encounter can lead to defensive behaviors by the healthcare professional.
- Avoidance is one of the principal defensive behaviors.
- Clinician self-awareness and reflection is required.
- Patient factors include habitual interpersonal patterns, specific personality traits, or specific personality disorders.
- The patient's social and family environment will also impact on how they relate with the treatment team.
- Organizational factors include team morale, leadership, appropriate facilities, and staff training.
- Interventions include avoiding avoidance, drawing on the CONFLICT model, making time to meet with the patient in a private setting, and listening objectively to the patient's point of view.

References

1. Hahn SR, Thompson KS, Wills TA, Stern V, Budner NS. The difficult doctor-patient relationship: somatization, personality and psychopathology. J Clin Epidemiol. 1994;47(6):647–57.
2. Hinchey SA, Jackson JL. A cohort study assessing difficult patient encounters in a walk-in primary care clinic, predictors and outcomes. J Gen Intern Med. 2011;26(6):588–94.
3. Mota P, Selby K, Gouveia A, et al. Difficult patient–doctor encounters in a Swiss university outpatient clinic: cross-sectional study. BMJ Open. 2019;9:e025569.

4. American Kidney Fund: Barriers to Treatment Adherence for Dialysis Patients – American Kidney Fund and Adherence Survey. http://www.kidneyfund.org/assets/pdf/akf-adherence-report.pdf, http://www.kidneyfund.org/assets/pdf/akf-adherence-report.pdf. 2018; Accessed 27 Jan 2021.
5. Sansone RA, Sansone LA. Personality disorders in the medical setting. In: Oldham JM, Skodol AE, Bender DS, editors. The American Psychiatric Publishing textbook of personality disorders. Washington, DC: American Psychiatric Publishing; 2014. p. 455–73.
6. Dhossche DM, Shevitz SA. Assessment and importance of personality disorders in medical patients: an update. South Med J. 1999;92:546–56.
7. Pare MF, Rosenbluth M. Personality disorders in primary care. Prim Care. 1999;26:243–78.
8. Meyer F, Block S. Personality disorders in the oncology setting. J Support Oncol. 2011;9:44–51.
9. Janosevic D, Wang AX, Wish JB. Difficult patient behavior in dialysis facilities. Blood Purif. 2019;47:254–8.
10. Bach B, First MB. Application of the ICD-11 classification of personality disorders. BMC Psychiatry. 2018;18:351.
11. Decreasing Dialysis Patient Provider Conflict. Forum of ESRD Networks: https://esrdnetworks.org/resources/special-projects/copy_of_DPPCProviderManual.pdf/view. Accessed 27 Jan 2021.
12. Shorer Y, Rabin S, Zlotnik M, Cohen N, Nadav M, Shiber A. Balint group as a-means for burnout prevention and improvement of therapist-patient relationship in a general hospital - the Soroka experience. Harefuah. 2016;155(2):115–118, 130. Hebrew

Part III

Special Issues in Psychonephrology

Chronic Kidney Disease and the Aging Population: Addressing Unmet Needs

18

Meera Joseph and Azim S. Gangji

18.1 Geriatric Syndromes in Patients with Chronic Kidney Disease

"Older adults" and "geriatric population" generally refer to those 65 years of age or older; however, in patients with chronic kidney disease (CKD) including end-stage kidney disease (ESKD), some younger patients will have worse functional impairment than certain octogenarians. The prevalence of geriatric syndromes, such as frailty, falls, cognitive impairment, and functional impairment, is increased in patients with renal disease including those who are younger than age 65 years [1].

18.1.1 Frailty

Frailty is a phenotype of decreased physiologic reserve resulting in a vulnerability to adverse health outcomes when facing stressors. The phenotype was originally defined and validated in older populations by Fried et al. as the presence of at least three of five components: exhaustion, unintentional weight loss, low physical activity, slow walking speed, and poor grip strength (Table 18.1) [2]. The presence of one or two of the criteria has been referred to as "pre-frailty."

Among ESKD patients, the prevalence of the Fried frailty phenotype is five- to seven-fold higher than in community-dwelling older adults, making the study of frailty among adults with kidney disease an important area of research [3].

In a cohort study of 2275 patients with ESKD on peritoneal dialysis and hemodialysis, it was found that two thirds of the study population met the study criteria

M. Joseph (✉) · A. S. Gangji
Division of Nephrology, Department of Medicine, McMaster University, St. Joseph's Healthcare Hamilton, Hamilton, ON, Canada
e-mail: meera.joseph@medportal.ca; gangji@mcmaster.ca

A. Hategan et al. (eds.), *Psychonephrology*,
https://doi.org/10.1007/978-3-030-84740-1_18

Table 18.1 Fried's criteria for frailty [2]

Frailty criteria		Indicators
1	Shrinking	10 lbs. of unintentional weight loss over the past year
2	Exhaustion	Self-reported exhaustion
3	Weakness	Maximal grip strength in kg using hydraulic handheld dynamometer; lowest 20% stratified by gender and BMI qualities
4	Slowness	Time in seconds to walk 15 feet at usual pace; slowest 20% stratified by gender and standing height
5	Low physical activity	Weighted score of kilocalories expended per week in physical activities that "you have done in the past 2 weeks": Males <383 kcal/week Females <270 kcal/week

Frailty = presence of three or more of the five criteria

for frailty [4]. What is notable about these results is that, although older age was related to frailty, a significant proportion of patients in younger age groups were also frail, including 44% of patients younger than age 40 and over half of patients between the ages of 40 and 50. Women more than men, and hemodialysis more than peritoneal dialysis patients, were more likely to be frail. Frailty was also associated with a history of diabetes mellitus or stroke and presence of lower serum albumin concentrations. Frail patients were more than three times as likely to die within 1 year (HR 3.42; 95% CI 2.45 to 4.76) and more likely to be hospitalized for any reason or to die (HR 1.90; 95% CI 1.67 to 2.17). In another prospective study of adults undergoing hemodialysis, frailty had a prevalence of 41.8% and was associated with a 2.6 times higher risk of mortality [5]. In addition to increased mortality and risk of hospitalization, frailty is also associated with increased falls, poor cognitive function, and poor health-related quality of life in patients with ESKD [3].

Recommendations to prevent frailty in the general population have largely focused on addressing drivers of functional decline, including lack of regular exercise, malnutrition, and cognitive impairment [6]. Frailty prevention should include monitoring of physiological reserve, performing regular exercise to prevent chronic loss, interventions to prevent acute and subacute loss (e.g., vaccinations), increasing physiological reserve prior to anticipated loss (e.g., pre-rehabilitation prior to an elective hospitalization), and removing obstacles to recovery [6]. For ESKD patients, interventions such as intradialytic activities and pre-rehabilitation have been proposed to reverse frailty [3].

Recommendation

- Clinicians must strive for early identification, targeting the pre-frailty period, and intervene in attempts to prevent frailty, thereby minimizing the risks associated with the frailty syndrome.

18.1.2 Case Vignette 1

Mrs. Peach was a 75-year-old female on hemodialysis three times weekly who functioned independently at home. She was admitted to the acute care ward with a right trochanteric hip fracture after a fall at home and underwent a right open reduction internal fixation of that hip shortly after admission. Postoperatively, she was transferred from the acute care ward to the rehabilitation ward with a plan to be discharged home within 2 weeks. On the rehabilitation ward, she sustained a second, unwitnessed fall and fractured her third metatarsal of the right foot. Her foot was placed in an air boot. With the prolonged admission and limited mobility, she became deconditioned. She was finally discharged home 2 months after her admission date, requiring family and home supports for dressing, bathing, shopping, housekeeping, and transportation.

18.1.2.1 Case Vignette 1 Analysis

Mrs. Peach had an increased risk of falling in hospital due to her history of a recent fall. Dialysis patients, like Mrs. Peach, are also at increased risk of fractures due to alterations in their bone-mineral metabolism. Mrs. Peach should have had high fall-risk alerts in place, strategies to prevent falls (e.g., bed alarms), and strategies to minimize injuries from falls (e.g., crash mats). The fall resulted in a longer stay in the hospital and loss of independence at home.

18.1.3 Case Vignette 2

Mr. Hayward was a 72-year-old male on hemodialysis three times weekly. His medications included three antihypertensives, gabapentin, and a low-dose aspirin. Post-hemodialysis 1 day, he complained of dizziness. His blood pressure post-dialysis was 145/98 mm Hg sitting and 121/75 mm Hg standing. He was told that his blood pressure was normal and was discharged to go home by the nursing staff. Before he exited the hemodialysis unit, he fell and sustained a head injury with an acute decline in his level of consciousness. He was transferred to the emergency department where CT of his head demonstrated a subarachnoid hemorrhage with a subdural hematoma. He was admitted to the hospital, and serial CT scans demonstrated a multi-compartmental intracranial hemorrhage with expansion of the bleed. There was no indication for neurosurgery. Mr. Hayward was managed with comfort measures only and died 2 days later. After his death, it was later learned that he experienced a fall at home 1 week prior.

18.1.3.1 Case Vignette 2 Analysis

Although Mr. Hayward had systolic and diastolic pressures that were within normal range, when he went from sitting to standing, he had symptomatic orthostatic hypotension that was not recognized and managed. This was likely the major contributing factor to his fall. Additionally, his history of recent falls put him at increased risk of falling, and aspirin put him at increased risk of bleeding from an injury.

18.1.4 Falls

It is estimated that 30% of patients over the age of 65 fall at least once per year, and it is known that falls predict hospitalization, functional decline, and need for long-term care [7, 8]. The incidence rate of falls in hemodialysis patients over the age of 65 in one Canadian center was 1.6 falls per person-year [9]. This incidence rate is much higher than what has been observed in the non-hemodialysis population (0.3 to 0.7 falls per person-year) and is much closer to what is observed in nursing homes at 1.6 falls per bed-year [10–13].

Falls often lead to serious consequences. Men and women with CKD are at an increased risk of fracture, and this risk increases further as kidney function deteriorates [14]. For those on hemodialysis who sustain a hip fracture resulting from a fall, the 1-year mortality is 50%, compared to less than 20% in the general population [15]. An association has also been demonstrated between accidental falls and increased mortality in older dialysis patients [16].

Risk factors for falls in renal patients include advanced age, frailty, a history of falls, increased comorbidities, recent initiation of hemodialysis, and a low mean pre-dialysis systolic blood pressure [16–18]. The odds of falling has also been shown to increase with a CES-D (Center for Epidemiological Studies - Depression Scale) score over 18 points, suggestive of depressive symptoms [19].

Very little research has been done in fall prevention in CKD including ESKD patients. One quality improvement study demonstrated positive results in the hemodialysis unit with the implementation of relatively simple interventions such as (i) staff and patient education about falls, (ii) assessment of fall risk, (iii) improved lighting, (iv) construction of an in-ground weight scale, and (v) installation of support bars in the patient restrooms [20].

Clinical Pearl

- A history of falls in patients should alert the care team that the patient is at higher risk of recurrent falls and frailty.

Recommendation

- Patients with ESKD should be screened for fall risk on a routine basis, and any modifiable risk factors should be addressed.
- Patients should be educated about their fall risk.

18.1.5 Cognitive Impairment

The prevalence of cognitive impairment in patients with ESKD has been shown to be 30–60%, which is much higher than what is seen in the age-matched general population [21, 22]. Prevalence of cognitive impairment is high in as early as stage 3–4 CKD and increases as patients progress to ESKD [22]. Although previous studies have suggested decreased prevalence in patients on peritoneal dialysis when compared to those on hemodialysis, some recent studies have shown no significant difference between the two modalities [23–26].

The spectrum of structural brain injury seen in patients with CKD and on dialysis includes classic strokes, silent cerebral infarcts, cerebral atrophy, and white matter hyperdensities (leukoaraiosis) [27–30]. The most significant finding in this patient population is leukoaraiosis, which is a subcortical injury that occurs in the vascular watershed area of the brain, where one would expect the effects of hypoperfusion to have a maximal effect [8, 11]. This is consistent with the finding that patients with ESKD tend to have relative preservation of language and memory (i.e., cortical functions) and show more significant impairment in executive functioning and decision-making (i.e., subcortical functions) [31].

Several risk factors have been proposed to explain the increased prevalence of cognitive impairment in renal disease, including traditional systemic vascular risk factors such as hypertension and diabetes mellitus; additional systemic vascular risk factors, such as anemia, oxidative stress, and inflammation; and dialysis-related risk factors such as cerebral hypoperfusion and microemboli (Table 18.2) [32]. Not all risk factors are fully understood regarding their contribution to cognitive impairment. The concept of "cerebral stunning," or reduced blood flow to the brain during hemodialysis sessions, has recently been shown to correlate with decrements in performance on cognitive function tests [33, 34]. Cerebral blood flow remains relatively stable in the first hour of dialysis and gradually decreases thereafter. This

Table 18.2 Risk factors and contributors to impaired cognition in renal disease patients [32]

Cerebrovascular disease risk factors	Hypertension, chronic hypotension, diabetes mellitus, hyperlipidemia, cardiovascular disease (including myocardial infarction, atrial fibrillation), cigarette smoking, microalbuminuria, elevated homocysteine, hemostatic abnormalities, hypercoagulation, oxidative stress, inflammation, acute stroke
Biologic intrinsic	Vascular changes in the brain, anemia, white matter lesions, cortical atrophy, hyperparathyroidism, microalbuminuria, subclinical atherosclerosis
Psychosocial/ treatment related	Syndromal depressive disorder, depressed mood and other psychosocial variables, polypharmacy, malnutrition
Dialysis related	Hypotensive episodes, chronic microemboli, subclinical increases in brain edema, acute stroke, silent and asymptomatic stroke, hemodynamic changes and fluid shifts, recurrent cerebral ischemia, acute dynamic cerebrovascular changes, lacunar infarcts, microbleeds

effect is sustained at least until 30 minutes after completion of the dialysis treatment [33]. Therefore, any cognitive evaluation and testing of hemodialysis patients should be done before or during the first hour of treatment, especially if cognitive impairment is detected. Evaluation of cognition should also include a screen for depression with its increased prevalence in the patient population (see Chap. 10) and ability to mimic cognitive impairment (see Chap. 12). (For more information on the cognitive ramifications of CKD, including risk for delirium, the reader is directed to Chap. 12.)

Clinical Pearl

- Cognitive impairment has many implications for patients with CKD including decreased adherence to treatment and medications, impact on dialysis modality selection (home dialysis versus in-center hemodialysis), increased risk of secondary iatrogenic hospitalizations, renal transplant candidacy, and death.
- By identifying those patients with cognitive impairment, care teams can (1) design treatment plans to supervise medication administration, (2) design diet care plans, (3) hold appropriate discussions regarding medical directives and initiating and withdrawing dialysis, and (4) provide goal-directed care.

18.2 Treatment Decisions in the Older Adult Patient

18.2.1 Life Expectancy of Older Adult Patients with ESKD

Survival of older dialysis patients is poor; hence, the decision to initiate dialysis in older adults is complicated by more challenges than in younger patients [1]. Beyond geriatric syndromes, older patients are more likely to have problems with nonmedical barriers to care such as limited transportation, family support, and income [35, 36]. Additionally, older adults have increased cardiovascular and comorbid conditions and reduced life expectancy compared with younger patients [35–37].

In the United States, median survival after dialysis initiation is 15.6 months for patients 80–84 years of age, 11.6 months for patients 85–89 years of age, and 8.4 months for patients 90 years of age and older [36]. In a comparison study of patients aged 75 and older attending multidisciplinary pre-dialysis clinic, 1- and 2-year survival rates in those who chose dialysis were 84% and 76%, respectively, versus 68% and 47%, respectively, in the conservative care group [37]. However, survival advantage was lost in those with high comorbidity scores, especially ones that included ischemic heart disease. It is also important to recognize that mortality is not constant over time for patients over the age of 80 years who have initiated dialysis. Approximately 20% of patients die within the first 3 months after dialysis

Table 18.3 Six-month prognostic risk score in patients aged 75 and older who commence dialysis [38]

Risk factors	Points
Total dependence for transfers	3
BMI < 18.5 kg/m^2	2
Peripheral vascular disease stage 3 or 4	2
Congestive heart failure stage 3 or 4	2
Severe behavioral disorder	2
Unplanned dialysis initiation	2
Active malignancy	1
Diabetes mellitus	1
Dysrhythmia	1

Total score	6-month mortality rate
0	8%
1	8-10%
2	14-17%
3-4	21-26%
5-6	33-35%
7-8	50-51%
9+	62-70%

initiation, whereas 10% of patients between the ages of 65 and 79 years die within the first 3 months after dialysis starts [36]. Reasons for the high mortality rate in the first several months after dialysis initiation remain unclear, but may be related to severity of the underlying illness leading to dialysis initiation [36].

Whereas most older patients experience a reasonable amount of life expectancy on dialysis, a significant minority do not [3]. Couchoud et al. developed a prognostication tool to estimate 6-month mortality in patients over the age of 75 commencing dialysis (Table 18.3) [38]. Tools such as these can be used to assist patient and families in decision-making.

Clinical Pearl

- Age alone is not an adequate variable when considering dialysis as a treatment option for an older adult patient.

Recommendation

- The discussion around dialysis initiation must take into consideration the comorbidity burden, quality of life, functional status, and patient values, among other things, to predict whether the treatment will be life-prolonging, beneficial, and in alignment with the patient's values and preferences.

18.2.2 Hemodialysis vs. Peritoneal Dialysis

There are advantages and disadvantages to both hemodialysis and peritoneal dialysis in older adults. Hemodialysis may be appealing because it is done in a supervised setting and typically three times a week, 4 hours per session; however, barriers and challenges to in-center hemodialysis may be arranging transportation and successful vascular access creation [1]. Older patients also tend to be more sensitive to fluid shifts due to increased cardiac comorbidity, which may limit ultrafiltration [39, 40]. In contrast, peritoneal dialysis provides gentler ultrafiltration, can be performed at home, and eliminates the need for vascular access [1]. However, barriers such as functional limitations and insufficient social support are more frequent and problematic in older adults and may make peritoneal dialysis challenging [39, 41].

It is important to note that many patients will experience dialysis-related symptoms on hemodialysis, including headache, nausea, vomiting, cramping in the legs, pain, dizziness, restless legs, and fatigue. These can often be difficult to manage and cause significant distress for the patient and difficulty for the clinician. Some patients will report taking a full 48 hours to recover from their treatment – just in time for their next session. Often, these symptoms limit how well the patient does on dialysis, as they may be inclined to cut treatments short, decline fluid removal, or miss treatments altogether. For the older patient, these symptoms may result in a significant reduction in quality of life. Therefore, it is important to ask the patient about dialysis-related symptoms, validate their concerns, and do one's best to alleviate any discomfort. It is important for the patient to know that if at any point the symptoms become unbearable, dialysis discontinuation is an option (as discussed in Chap. 16).

Recommendation

– Dialysis modality choice in older patients should be multidisciplinary in nature and focused on personal/family values and goals.

18.2.3 Vascular Access Considerations for Hemodialysis

The Kidney Disease Outcomes Quality Initiative (KDOQI) recommends the "fistula first" approach for hemodialysis access, given the lower infection rate, prolonged access longevity, and lower mortality rate [42]. The KDOQI does not differentiate between younger and older patients, but does advise tailoring the vascular access options for the individual patient, which is particularly important for the older adult population. There are no randomized controlled trials to definitively answer whether fistulas confer the same benefits in the old as they do in the young. There are large cohort studies of vascular access in older hemodialysis patients that have demonstrated a mortality benefit in using arteriovenous fistulas over catheters [43–45]. However, when comparing fistulas to grafts, there may not be a significant mortality benefit in those aged 80 years and older [6]. It has also been shown that in those patients aged 75 years and older, the primary failure rate (an arteriovenous fistula that is never usable or fails within the first 3 months of its use) is higher for fistulas compared with grafts, and more fistulas require one or more interventions before their successful use compared with grafts [46]. The lack of prospective data makes it difficult to offer definitive practice guidelines, but it has been proposed that a "catheter last" and not "fistula first" approach be adopted in the older population [47].

18.2.4 Renal Transplant in Older Patients

Transplantation is the treatment of choice for patients with ESKD, and there is no age at which a patient should not be considered for transplantation, provided they are in otherwise good health and do not have significant comorbid conditions. However, several factors need to be considered when evaluating an older recipient for transplantation including recipient frailty and comorbidities, donor quality, immunosuppression, number of years on dialysis, and the strength of social support networks [48]. Furthermore, the impact of transplantation on quality of life and mortality is not equivalent in the older versus the younger patient [1]. Rao et al., who studied renal transplantation in patients older than age 70, showed that overall patients who received a kidney transplant had a 41% lower risk of death than similar patients who remained on the wait list (RR, 0.59; 95% CI, 0.53–0.65) [49]. However, in the first 45 days posttransplantation, the relative risk of death was 2.26 times higher than that of the wait-listed patients and remained higher until 125 days posttransplantation (time to equal risk). Survival was lower in the transplant group for almost 2 years (time to equal survival) and thereafter was greater than survival in the waiting list group.

Recommendation

- Patients should not be excluded from transplant based on age alone. However, older patients who are reasonable transplant candidates should be informed about the increased risk of mortality and time to equal survival of almost 2 years posttransplantation.

18.2.5 Comprehensive Conservative Care

Comprehensive conservative care is planned care for patients with ESKD that includes (i) interventions to delay the progression of kidney disease and minimize the risk of adverse events and complications, (ii) shared decision-making, (iii) active symptom management, (iv) detailed communication including advanced care planning, (v) psychological support, (vi) social and family support, and (vii) attention to cultural and spiritual domains of care. It does not include dialysis as a treatment modality [50].

There is limited evidence on the incidence or prevalence of conservative care of ESKD. In countries where resources, such as dialysis, are limited, conservative care may be more prevalent compared to others. Practices may also vary between centers. In an Australian cohort study of 721 patients with ESKD, 14% of patients were planned for conservative care, with a median age of 80; of those patients, 8% switched to dialysis, mainly for symptom control; of those who remained on conservative care, 18% were alive in 3 years [51].

Comparing survival of those who choose conservative care to those who choose dialysis is challenging due to the bias inherent in the decision pathway. Those who are more fit usually choose dialysis, and those who choose conservative care are often encouraged to do so because of comorbidity or other factors, which in themselves decrease survival. Without randomization to conservative care or dialysis, it is difficult to attribute survival differences to either treatment choice. Additionally, the conservative care group includes those suitable for dialysis who choose not to receive it. Older individuals with high comorbidity who are not offered dialysis and patients who lack decisional capacity may not always be offered dialysis; this heterogeneity adds another layer of complexity. However, there is observational literature suggesting that survival may not be significantly different in selected subgroups between those on chronic dialysis and patients with stage 5 CKD treated without renal replacement therapy [52].

What is important to recognize is that survival *alone* is not the most important value to be considered in decision-making. A comprehensive assessment should include symptoms, quality of life, and what the experience of the illness will be like if a conservative approach is chosen. Less hospitalizations and more patient bereavements at home may be possible with comprehensive conservative renal care, providing a more humane and dignified end-of-life experience for the patient and their family [52].

18.2.6 Case Vignette 3

Mrs. Sheer was an 86-year-old female who was attending her nephrologist appointment with her daughter. She lived at home with her husband but relied heavily on her daughter for support. She could dress and feed herself and used a telephone to call her daughter. She was sometimes incontinent of urine. She required assistance to shower. She used a cane or walker to mobilize and lately had been more unsteady on her feet. She relied on her daughter and husband for shopping, management of finances, transportation, and housekeeping. She had two recent hospital admissions for severe right-sided heart failure. The first admission was 3 weeks in length. She returned home and was readmitted to hospital 5 days later for an additional 10 days. She was now home and was very fatigued. She was bothered by the increased swelling in her legs and shortness of breath on exertion. She would like to feel better, but her daughter informed the nephrologist that the patient's biggest fear was being admitted to hospital once again. She would have liked to remain at home for as long as possible. On examination, she had evidence of volume overload with an elevated jugular venous pressure, crackles in the chest, and bilateral pitting edema in the legs. Her creatinine was 190 umol/L (normal, 60 to 110 umol/L) prior to her first admission. With increased doses of diuretics, her creatinine was now approaching 500 umol/L. The nephrologist broached the topic of dialysis. Mrs. Sheer and her daughter were very firm in not wanting to pursue dialysis, but were wondering what things would look like if she did not pursue that pathway.

18.2.6.1 Case Vignette 3 Analysis

Mrs. Sheer was an older patient with multiple organ failure (heart and kidneys). She was functionally dependent for all her instrumental activities of daily living and some basic activities of daily living. Despite being on higher doses of diuretics, she continued to be symptomatic, and her renal function was worsening. After two admissions to hospital, she did not wish be admitted a third time and was adamant about not wanting dialysis. With a patient like Mrs. Sheer, comprehensive conservative renal care is an appropriate treatment decision. The nephrologist should discuss expected survival, approaches to symptom management, and end-of-life care and preferences. Referrals should also be made to multidisciplinary professional services, such as home occupational therapy and palliative care.

Clinical Pearl

- Not all patients with ESKD benefit from dialysis.
- Comprehensive conservative care is a viable alternative to renal replacement therapy and should be considered for some patients.
- Comprehensive conservative care broadly includes maximizing renal survival and good symptom management, shared decision-making, and advance care planning.
- Patients with ESKD report as many symptoms as those with cancer, and symptom management must be a pillar of care.

18.3 Key Takeaways

- The incidence of geriatric syndromes such as frailty and falls is higher in patients with advanced CKD including ESKD and results in increased risk of hospitalization and death.
- Clinicians must strive for early identification of geriatric syndromes to minimize the associated risks.
- Options for renal replacement therapy in older patients is no different from options for younger patients. The modality choice must take into account the patient's comorbidities, functional status, goals, and values.

References

1. Berger JR, Hedayati SS. Renal replacement therapy in the elderly population. Clin J Am Soc Nephrol. 2012;7(6):1039–46.
2. Fried LP, Tangen CM, Walston J, et al. Frailty in older adults: evidence for a phenotype. J Gerontol A Biol Sci Med Sci. 2001;56(3):M146–56.
3. Rasmussen SV, Konel J, Warsame F, et al. Engaging clinicians and patients to assess and improve frailty measurement in adults with end stage renal disease. BMC Nephrol. 2018;19(1):1–8.
4. Johansen KL, Chertow GM, Jin C, Kutner NG. Significance of frailty among dialysis patients. J Am Soc Nephrol. 2007;18(11):2960–7.
5. McAdams-DeMarco MA, Law A, Salter ML, et al. Frailty as a novel predictor of mortality and hospitalization in individuals of all ages undergoing hemodialysis. J Am Geriatr Soc. 2013;61(6):896–901.

6. Walston J, Buta B, Xue QL. Frailty screening and interventions: considerations for clinical practice. Clin Geriatr Med. 2018;34(1):25–38.
7. Tinetti ME, Speechley M, Ginter SF. Risk factors for falls among elderly persons living in the community. N Engl J Med. 1988;319(26):1701–7.
8. Tinetti ME, Williams CS. Falls, injuries due to falls, and the risk of admission to a nursing home. N Engl J Med. 1997;337(18):1279–84.
9. Cook WL, Jassal SV. Prevalence of falls among seniors maintained on hemodialysis. Int Urol Nephrol. 2005;37(3):649–52.
10. O'Loughlin JL, Robitaille Y, Boivin JF, Suissa S. Incidence of and risk factors for falls and injurious falls among the community-dwelling elderly. Am J Epidemiol. 1993;137(3):342–54.
11. Day L, Fildes B, Gordon I, Fitzharris M, Flamer H, Lord S. Randomised factorial trial of falls prevention among older people living in their own homes. BMJ. 2002;325(7356):128.
12. Tinetti ME, Baker DI, McAvay G, et al. A multifactorial intervention to reduce the risk of falling among elderly people living in the community. N Engl J Med. 1994;331(13):821–7.
13. Rubenstein LZ, Powers CM, MacLean CH. Quality indicators for the management and prevention of falls and mobility problems in vulnerable elders. Ann Intern Med. 2001;135(8_Part_2):686–93.
14. West SL, Patel P, Jamal SA. How to predict and treat increased fracture risk in chronic kidney disease. J Intern Med. 2015;278(1):19–28.
15. Mittalhenkle A, Gillen DL, Stehman-Breen CO. Increased risk of mortality associated with hip fracture in the dialysis population. Am J Kidney Dis. 2004;44(4):672–9.
16. Li M, Tomlinson G, Naglie G, Cook WL, Jassal SV. Geriatric comorbidities, such as falls, confer an independent mortality risk to elderly dialysis patients. Nephrol Dial Transplant. 2008;23(4):1396–400.
17. McAdams-DeMarco MA, Suresh S, Law A, et al. Frailty and falls among adult patients undergoing chronic hemodialysis: a prospective cohort study. BMC Nephrol. 2013;14:224.
18. Cook WL, Tomlinson G, Donaldson M, et al. Falls and fall-related injuries in older dialysis patients. Clin J Am Soc Nephrol. 2006;1(6):1197–204.
19. Kutner NG, Zhang R, Huang Y, Wasse H. Falls among hemodialysis patients: potential opportunities for prevention? Clin Kidney J. 2014;7(3):257–63.
20. Heung M, Adamowski T, Segal JH, Malani PN. A successful approach to fall prevention in an outpatient hemodialysis center. Clin J Am Soc Nephrol. 2010;5(10):1775–9.
21. Sehgal AR, Grey SF, DeOreo PB, Whitehouse PJ. Prevalence, recognition, and implications of mental impairment among hemodialysis patients. Am J Kidney Dis. 1997;30(1):41–9.
22. Kurella M, Chertow GM, Luan J, Yaffe K. Cognitive impairment in chronic kidney disease. J Am Geriatr Soc. 2004;52(11):1863–9.
23. Wolcott DL, Wellisch DK, Marsh JT, Schaeffer J, Landsverk J, Nissenson AR. Relationship of dialysis modality and other factors to cognitive function in chronic dialysis patients. Am J Kidney Dis. 1988;12(4):275–84.
24. Buoncristiani U, Alberti A, Gubbiotti G, et al. Better preservation of cognitive faculty in continuous ambulatory peritoneal dialysis. Perit Dial Int. 1993;13(2_suppl):202–5.
25. Tilki HE, Akpolat T, Tunalı G, Kara A, Onar MK. Effects of haemodialysis and continuous ambulatory peritoneal dialysis on P300 cognitive potentials in uraemic patients. Ups J Med Sci. 2004;109(1):43–8.
26. Kalirao P, Pederson S, Foley RN, et al. Cognitive impairment in peritoneal dialysis patients. Am J Kidney Dis. 2011;57(4):612–20.
27. McIntyre CW, Goldsmith DJ. Ischemic brain injury in hemodialysis patients: which is more dangerous, hypertension or intradialytic hypotension? Kidney Int. 2015;87(6):1109–15.
28. Nakatani T, Naganuma T, Uchida J, et al. Silent cerebral infarction in hemodialysis patients. Am J Nephrol. 2003;23(2):86–90.
29. Kamata T, Hishida A, Takita T, et al. Morphologic abnormalities in the brain of chronically hemodialyzed patients without cerebrovascular disease. Am J Nephrol. 2000;20(1):27–31.
30. McIntyre CW. Recurrent circulatory stress: the dark side of dialysis. Semin Dial. 2010;23(5):449–51.

31. Pereira AA, Weiner DE, Scott T, et al. Subcortical cognitive impairment in dialysis patients. Hemodial Int. 2007;11(3):309–14.
32. Elias MF, Dore GA, Davey A. Kidney disease and cognitive function. Contrib Nephrol. 2013;179:42–57.
33. Findlay MD, Dawson J, Dickie DA, et al. Investigating the relationship between cerebral blood flow and cognitive function in hemodialysis patients. J Am Soc Nephrol. 2019;30(1):147–58.
34. Polinder-Bos HA, García DV, Kuipers J, et al. Hemodialysis induces an acute decline in cerebral blood flow in elderly patients. J Am Soc Nephrol. 2018;29(4):1317–25.
35. Buemi M, Lacquaniti A, Bolignano D, et al. Dialysis and the elderly: an underestimated problem. Kidney Blood Press Res. 2008;31(5):330–6.
36. Tamura MK. Incidence, management, and outcomes of end-stage renal disease in the elderly. Curr Opin Nephrol Hypertens. 2009;18(3):252–7.
37. Murtagh FE, Marsh JE, Donohoe P, Ekbal NJ, Sheerin NS, Harris FE. Dialysis or not? A comparative survival study of patients over 75 years with chronic kidney disease stage 5. Nephrol Dial Transplant. 2007;22(7):1955–62.
38. Couchoud C, Labeeuw M, Moranne O, Allot V, Esnault V, Frimat L, Stengel B; French renal epidemiology and information network (REIN) registry. A clinical score to predict 6-month prognosis in elderly patients starting dialysis for end-stage renal disease. Nephrol Dial Transplant. 2009;24(5):1553–61.
39. Brown EA, Johansson L, Farrington K, et al. Broadening options for long-term dialysis in the elderly (BOLDE): differences in quality of life on peritoneal dialysis compared to haemodialysis for older patients. Nephrol Dial Transplant. 2010;25(11):3755–63.
40. Lindsay RM, Heidenheim PA, Nesrallah G, Garg AX, Suri R. Minutes to recovery after a hemodialysis session: a simple health related quality of life question that is reliable, valid, and sensitive to change. Clin J Am Soc Nephrol. 2006;1(5):952–9.
41. Finkelstein FO, Afolalu B, Wuerth D, Finkelstein SH. The elderly patient on CAPD: helping patients cope with peritoneal dialysis. Perit Dial Int. 2008;28(5):449–51.
42. Third NKF-K/DOQI Clinical practice guidelines for vascular access: update 2000. Am J Kidney Dis. 2001;37(1):S137–81.
43. Xue JL, Dahl D, Ebben JP, Collins AJ. The association of initial hemodialysis access type with mortality outcomes in elderly Medicare ESRD patients. Am J Kidney Dis. 2003;42(5):1013–9.
44. DeSilva RN, Sandhu GS, Garg J, Goldfarb-Rumyantzev AS. Association between initial type of hemodialysis access used in the elderly and mortality. Hemodial Int. 2012;16(2):233–41.
45. DeSilva RN, Patibandla BK, Vin Y, et al. Fistula first is not always the best strategy for the elderly. J Am Soc Nephrol. 2013;24(8):1297–304.
46. Cui J, Steele D, Wenger J, et al. Hemodialysis arteriovenous fistula as first option not necessary in elderly patients. J Vascular Surg. 2016;63(5):1326–32.
47. Combe C, Berard X. Dialysis: 'catheter last' not 'fistula first' in elderly patients. Nat Rev Nephrol. 2013;9(11):632–4.
48. Huang E, Segev DL, Rabb H. Kidney transplantation in the elderly. Semin Nephrol. 2009;29(6):621–35.
49. Rao PS, Merion RM, Ashby VB, Port FK, Wolfe RA, Kayler LK. Renal transplantation in elderly patients older than 70 years of age: results from the scientific registry of transplant recipients. Transplantation. 2007;83(8):1069–74.
50. Murtagh FE, Burns A, Moranne O, Morton RL, Naicker S. Supportive care: comprehensive conservative care in end-stage kidney disease. Clin J Am Soc Nephrol. 2016;11(10):1909–14.
51. Morton RL, Webster AC, McGeechan K, et al. Conservative management and end-of-life care in an Australian cohort with ESRD. Clin J Am Soc Nephrol. 2016;11(12):2195–203.
52. Swidler MA. Geriatric renal palliative care. J Gerontol A Biol Sci Med Sci. 2012;67(12):1400–9.

Physical Activity and Nutrition in Chronic Kidney Disease

19

Heather Waters and Michele MacDonald Werstuck

19.1 Introduction

Engaging patients to introduce and sustain healthy habits such as physical activity and balanced nutrition is potentially among the greatest clinical management challenges physicians and healthcare teams might face. Performing clinical assessments, managing investigations, and prescribing medications are all generally handled in less time, with less effort, and with more uptake than empowering patients to embrace healthy lifestyle modifications [1–3].

Although a chapter on lifestyle management strategies such as physical activity and nutrition might be tempting to skip since it is common sense to "eat right" and exercise, it is important to consider why only 16% of Canadian and 23% of US adults achieve the minimum recommended levels of physical activity defined in evidence-based national guidelines and less than 40% of Ontarians consume the recommended fruits and vegetables servings per day [4–6]. This reality looms in spite of clear evidence linking physical activity and a healthy diet to improved health outcomes, including decreased premature mortality [3, 7, 8]. How does one explain the disconnect between what is *known* and what is *done* by the majority of North Americans? Herein lies the art of medicine for the clinician, and this chapter includes practical tips for patient-centered care, motivational interviewing, and self-management related to physical activity and nutrition in chronic kidney disease (CKD).

H. Waters (✉)
Department of Family Medicine, McMaster University, Hamilton, ON, Canada
e-mail: watersh@mcmaster.ca

M. M. Werstuck
Nutrition Program Coordinator, Hamilton Family Health Team, Hamilton, ON, Canada

A. Hategan et al. (eds.), *Psychonephrology*,
https://doi.org/10.1007/978-3-030-84740-1_19

We begin by clarifying key terms and concepts related to physical activity and nutrition, followed by review of the associated health benefits described in the literature. We then focus more specifically on CKD with attention to its most common challenges and complications as related to exercise and dietary management. Recommendations for physical activity and dietary modifications in the context of CKD are outlined. Specific nutrients such as "the three Ps" (protein, potassium, phosphorus), sodium, fluid, and fibers are discussed. The importance of cardiovascular disease risk reduction is highlighted.

We promote a patient-centered approach to care and education and interprofessional team-based collaboration in the care of people with CKD. Key resources to aid patients and providers in lifestyle management strategies are provided, along with tips for motivational interviewing. We conclude by emphasizing the important role for physicians in advocating for people with CKD, such that healthy lifestyle choices are both available and accessible.

Recommendation

- Consider the following questions:
  - What factors enable *you* to make healthy lifestyle choices such as including physical activity and healthy nutrition in your regular routine?
  - What barriers do you face to including regular physical activity and healthy food choices in your day?
  - What are the barriers and enablers your patients with CKD face in trying to follow advice related to physical activity and healthy eating?

Clinical Pearl

- Empower patients to make healthy choices in the aspects of their health and wellness over which they have the opportunity for some control, including physical activity and dietary choices.

Let us begin by reviewing a case vignette that highlights a common challenge faced by some people living with CKD.

19.2 Case Vignette: "Samuel and Soccer"

Samuel was 45 years old and had played soccer since he could stand upright. Having emigrated from El Salvador to North America as a young adult, his continued involvement in soccer had supported his learning of English and his connection to a social group. He had enjoyed the sport so much that he had subsequently trained to become an official and refereed local youth matches. Samuel was married with three teenaged children. He worked as a custodian and did not have health benefits. He was barely able to make ends meet each month.

Samuel lived with CKD caused by a hereditary nephropathy. His kidney function progressively worsened to the point of nearing dialysis (stage 5 CKD). He noted increasing fatigue and decreasing stamina and was no longer able to keep up with his teammates during games. He shared how sad he felt when he had to stop playing and worried about how he would maintain his fitness level. Medical appointments became more frequent as his CKD progressed, and he wondered how dialysis would impact his desire to remain active. He wanted your advice about how to optimize his energy and maintain his exercise capacity.

19.3 Health, Wellness, and Quality of Life

Engaging patients with CKD in discussion about lifestyle management strategies such as physical activity and nutrition is informed by the related concepts of health, wellness, and quality of life. Whereas healthcare providers may at times focus on specific scientific details of health and disease, it is important as well to maintain perspective on broader patient experiences of health and wellness:

- **Health** "is a state of complete physical, mental and social well-being, and not merely the absence of disease or infirmity" [9].
- **Wellness** "is an active, dynamic and holistic process that is subjectively perceived and self-directed; it relates to decisions of intentional healthy living and optimizing potential" [10].
- **Health-related quality of life (HR-QOL)** "refers to individual's perception of their position in life in the context of the culture and value systems in which they live and in relation to their goals, expectations, standards and concerns. It is a broad-ranging concept affected in a complex way by the individual's physical health, psychological state, level of independence, social relationships, and their relationships to salient features of their environment" [11, 12].

HR-QOL may be considered on both the individual and community levels. As related to individuals, HR-QOL involves perceived physical and mental health, energy level, mood, health risks, medical conditions, functional ability, supports, and finances [11, 12]. As related to the community, HR-QOL includes resources, policies, and practices that impact health perceptions and function of those in the community [11, 12].

In caring for patients with CKD, clinicians discuss the pros and cons of treatment options, balancing patient preferences and future goals with options that enhance quality of life and support optimal health outcomes, including lifestyle choices such as physical activity and healthy nutrition.

19.4 Physical Activity, Exercise, and Fitness

19.4.1 Defining Key Terms

Before delving into what the health and exercise science literature reveals about the benefits of an active lifestyle, this section clarifies a few relevant terms:

- **Movement** refers to a change in position of the entire body or a part of the body [13].
- **Physical activity** refers to movement of the body produced by skeletal muscles and requiring energy expenditure [13].
- **Exercise** is physical activity undertaken to maintain or enhance fitness or health [13].

Note that while all exercise is physical activity, not all physical activity qualifies as exercise. In daily life, physical activity may occur in a variety of domains including household, occupational, transportation, sport, and leisure. Exercise, in contrast, is carried out with the *primary* intention to achieve health and/or fitness goals [13]. For the purposes of reviewing health and lifestyle management strategies in this chapter, the terms will be used interchangeably:

- **Physical fitness** is a set of physical performance attributes that can be measured and is categorized as health-related or skill-related [13]:
  - **Health-related fitness** attributes include [13]:
    - **Flexibility** – the range of motion through which a joint is able to move.
    - **Muscular endurance** – the ability to maintain muscle use repetitively over time.
    - **Cardiovascular endurance** – the ability of the cardiorespiratory system to supply oxygenated blood to body tissues during sustained activity.
    - **Muscular strength** – the amount of force exerted by a muscle against resistance.
    - **Body composition** – the body's relative percentages of muscle, bone, and adipose tissue.
  - **Skill-related fitness** attributes include [13]:
    - **Agility** – the ability to change the position of the body quickly and control the movement.
    - **Balance** – the ability to maintain the body's center of mass above the base of support.
    - **Coordination** – the ability to use two or more body parts together.
    - **Power** – the ability to perform strength-based activities quickly.
    - **Reaction time** – the time taken to respond to a stimulus.
    - **Speed** – the ability to move body parts quickly.

Both health- and skill-related fitness attributes can impact health, wellness, and HR-QOL [11, 12]. Consider, for example, the importance of agility and balance in the prevention of falls in older adults. This issue is of relevance to people with CKD,

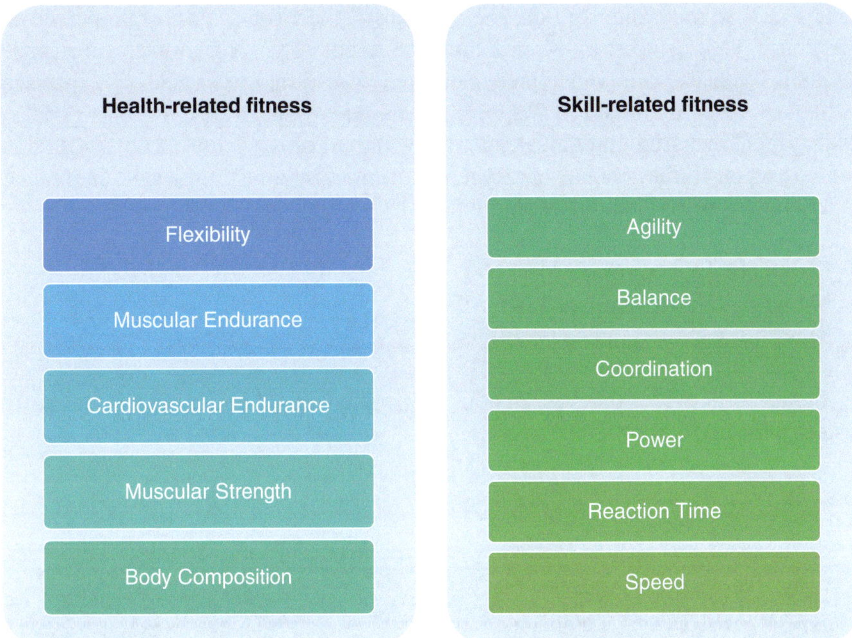

Fig. 19.1 Fitness attributes [13]

who are at increased risk for development of osteoporosis and fractures [14]. Another example is the need for coordination to prepare and inject insulin and to check blood glucose levels, for people with diabetes mellitus and CKD. Figure 19.1 summarizes the components of physical fitness.

Although all aspects of physical fitness have the potential to enhance HR-QOL for people with CKD, the literature highlights that in general, cardiovascular endurance offers the greatest potential health benefits as related to cardiovascular disease and CKD [3, 7, 8, 14–21]. Cardiovascular endurance activities are those in which physical exertion is sustained over time, resulting in increased heart rate, respiratory rate, and blood pressure, thereby creating potential to maintain or enhance cardiovascular health and decrease the risk of cardiovascular disease [3, 7, 8, 15, 17–19]. This will be further elaborated in subsequent sections of this chapter.

The degree to which physical activity impacts health and fitness depends on several factors related to the activity itself [22]:

- **Frequency –** how often the activity is performed.
- **Duration –** the amount of time spent doing the activity, measured per session or cumulatively over a day or week.
- **Intensity –** the amount of energy required to perform the activity over a unit of time.

The simplest means for one to measure the intensity of their own physical activity is by noting whether they are sweating and how hard they are breathing. Other means to determine intensity are the "talk test," the Borg scale to rate perceived exertion (RPE), or heart rate in relation to a target zone [22]. In exercise science research, intensity is most accurately measured by respiratory gas analysis expressed as liters of oxygen utilized by the body per minute. Metabolic equivalents (METs) define intensity based on equivalents to the amount of oxygen utilized at rest; one MET is equal to the amount of oxygen consumed by a resting, awake individual (3.5 ml O_2/kg of body weight/minute) [23]:

- Light activity requires <3 METs
- Moderate activity requires 3 to 6 METs
- Vigorous activity requires >6 METs

Table 19.1 provides practical options for people with CKD to gauge the intensity of their physical activity.

Table 19.1 A comparison of the talk test, level of exertion, the BORG/rate of perceived exertion (RPE) scale, and intensity of exertion

Talk Test	*Level of Exertion*	*BORG/RPE scale/10 (modified)*	*Intensity of Exertion*
Normal breathing. Can talk normally and sing.	Sleeping, Sitting	0–1	Sedentary (sitting, reading, watching TV, driving).
Easy to breathe and speak easily for a sentence or two, light breathing, can be maintained for an hour or more.	Casual walk	2–3	Light (slow walking, cooking, washing dishes, playing an instrument).
Can converse. Moderate to heavy breathing, can be maintained 30–60 minutes.	Fast to very fast walk/slow jog	4–5	Moderate (brisk walk, limited movement racquet games [tennis doubles, recreational badminton], water aerobics, resistancetraining).
From 1–2 sentences to broken sentences to only words, heavier to very heavy breathing, can be maintained up to 30 minutes.	Jogging, vigorous hiking	6–8	Vigorous (swimming with effort, more vigorous racquet games [singles tennis, squash]).
Can't talk, very heavy breathing.	Race pace	9	Vigorous (cross-country skiing with effort, shovelling snow,field games [soccer, basketball]).
Gasping for breath, feels as if giving 100%.	Racing to win	10	Vigorous –Training/competing in most competitive sports, any all-out activity.

Sources: 1) Thornton JS, Fremont P, Khan K, et al. Physical activity prescription: a critical opportunity to address a modifiable risk factor for the prevention and management of chronic disease: a position statement by the Canadian Academy of Sport and Exercise Medicine. Br J Sports Med. 2016;50(18):1109–14. 2) Reed JL, Pipe AL. The talk test: a useful tool for prescribing and monitoring exercise intensity. Curr Opin Cardiol. 2014;29(5):475–80. 3) Woltmann ML, Foster C, Porcari JP, et al. Evidence that the talk test can be used to regulate exercise intensity. J Strength Cond Res. 2015;29(5):1248–54. 4) Lyon E, Menke M, Foster C, Porcari JP, Gibson M, Bubbers T. Translation of incremental talk test responses to steady-state exercise training intensity. J Cardiopulm Rehabil Prev. 2014;34(4):271–5.
Reprinted with permission from the Foundation for Medical Practice Education [22]

Patient and Disease Factors also influence the degree to which physical activity impacts health and wellness in CKD (and other chronic diseases), including:

- **Baseline physical activity and fitness level** – patients who are sedentary and have lower levels of fitness have the relatively greatest potential for health and fitness gains when starting or increasing physical activity [7, 15, 19].
- **Baseline health and severity/stage of disease** – the severity/stage of CKD and other comorbidities may affect the type and degree of benefit achievable through physical activity, although even patients with severe CKD can experience positive results from physical activity [18, 19, 24, 25].

19.4.2 Physical Health Benefits of Exercise

In a review of the literature, Warburton et al. outlined "irrefutable evidence" of the effectiveness of regular physical activity in the primary and secondary prevention of several chronic diseases and of premature death [7]. The list of diseases preventable by regular physical activity includes cardiovascular disease, diabetes mellitus, hypertension, obesity, depression, osteoporosis, and certain cancers [7, 8, 15, 16, 19]. The review proceeded to endorse a linear association between physical activity and health status, such that a further increase in physical activity and fitness will lead to additional improvements in health status [7]. Research has confirmed that even short bursts of physical activity "count," as health benefits can be achieved through physical activity accumulated throughout the day, even in 10-minute bouts, when performed over most days of the week [7, 8, 19].

Scientific understanding of the impact of sedentary behavior, physical activity, and fitness on health and well-being has continued to evolve. The Canadian Society for Exercise Physiology (CSEP) recently updated and expanded its prior Physical Activity Guidelines to develop the Canadian 24-Hour Movement Guidelines for Adults; this document provides evidence-informed recommendations for the health-related behaviors of physical activity, sleep, and sedentary time [19]. Of note is the addition of recommendations based on recent evidence linking time spent sitting and in sedentary pursuits to elevated health risks and premature mortality, in spite of the amount and intensity of exercise performed at other times [19, 26, 27]. These revelations spurred the phrase "sitting is the new smoking," along with a renewed appreciation for movement in general. As a result, it is now more common for workplaces to promote standing desks, walking meetings, and treadmill boardrooms.

Table 19.2 provides a summary of the 2020 "Canadian 24-Hour Movement Guidelines for Adults" [19].

Table 19.2 Summary of Canadian 2020 Movement Guideline Recommendations [17]

For adults aged 18–64[a]
Participate in diverse physical activities across various environments, contexts, seasons
Limit long periods of sedentary behavior (≤ 8 hours/day total, break up periods of prolonged sitting, limit recreational screen time to ≤3 hours/day)
Practice healthy sleep habits including 7–9 hours of sleep/night; regular routine for bedtime and waking
Following these guidelines may be challenging at times
Any degree of progress will result in some health benefit over time
Include at least 150 min of cumulative moderate to vigorous physical activity per week
Include some physical activity in each day
Include muscle strengthening activity of major muscle groups at least two times/week
Include several hours of light physical activity/day, including standing
For adults aged ≥65[a] as above, with addition of physical activities that challenge balance

[a]May require modification during pregnancy and disability and in certain medical conditions

Clinical Pearl

- Encourage patients to consider all of the ways they can trade sitting for standing and moving [19].
- Small steps toward a more active lifestyle add up when sustained over time [19].

Recommendation

- Any movement is better than no movement, even in increments as short as 10 minutes [8, 19]!
- Standing has health benefits over sitting [19, 26, 27].

19.4.3 Mental Health Benefits of Exercise

Physical activity has well-established beneficial effects for mental health, as does decreased time spent in sedentary pursuits [19, 26, 28–31]:

- **Depression:** regular physical activity is consistently associated with improved mood and decreased risk of depression [28–31].
- **Anxiety:** regular physical activity is associated in some studies with improved stress and anxiety, although the trends have not been as consistent as in depression [28, 31].
- **Sleep:** regular physical activity is associated with improved quality and duration of sleep, although best avoided close to bedtime due to stimulation of the sympathetic nervous system [32].

Interestingly, a recent meta-analysis examined the various life domains in which physical activity occurs, to determine any influence on the relationship between physical activity and mental health or mental ill-health. Of note, physical activity during leisure and transportation time correlated positively with mental health, while work-related physical activity correlated with mental ill-health; household physical activity showed no correlation [33].

19.4.4 Physical Activity in Chronic Kidney Disease

Kidney Disease: Improving Global Outcomes (KDIGO) points out that in general, people with CKD have reduced exercise capacity and impaired physical functioning compared to age-matched controls; differences include lesser muscular strength and cardiovascular capacity [17, 18, 21]. Of note, research also highlights a correlation between low levels of physical activity, increased mortality, and poor quality of life in people with CKD [17, 18, 21].

While cardiovascular disease poses the greatest risk of morbidity and mortality for people with CKD, regular exercise is effective at reducing cardiovascular risk, possibly related to its beneficial effects on blood pressure, triglycerides, cholesterol, insulin resistance, and glycemic control [3, 18, 20, 21].

Cardiovascular disease risk and mortality are dependent on the number of uncontrolled cardiovascular risk factors, and as such, according to KDIGO practice guideline, multifactorial intervention is needed to target these risk factors with lifestyle modification, including smoking cessation support, dietary counseling, physical activity, and pharmacologic intervention [18]. In people with diabetes mellitus and early CKD, such multifactorial lifestyle interventions have shown long-term benefits for microvascular and macrovascular complications and mortality [18].

Through modification of cardiovascular risk factors, regular physical activity decreases the risk of developing CKD (primary prevention), in addition to slowing disease progression in those who have been already diagnosed with CKD [18, 20, 21]. For people with CKD, regular exercise leads to increased exercise capacity, improved blood pressure, improved overall functional capacity, decreased morbidity, and better HR-QOL [18, 20, 21]. Even for people with end-stage renal disease (ESRD), exercise has been shown to improve various health parameters such as arterial stiffness, blood pressure, cardiovascular fitness, and HR-QOL [18, 21, 24, 25]. In fact, even those who have received kidney transplantation benefit from physical activity, which has been shown to improve postoperative renal function and recovery [21, 34].

Beyond cardiovascular endurance exercise, weight-bearing and resistance-type physical activities positively impact bone and muscle mass, thereby decreasing the risk of osteoporosis and fractures in people with CKD, as well as increasing overall functional capacity [14].

Recommendation

- Patients with diabetes mellitus and CKD benefit from a comprehensive treatment strategy to reduce the risks of both kidney disease progression and cardiovascular disease [20].
- KDIGO, in its 2012 guideline, recommended that people with CKD undertake physical activity compatible with their cardiovascular health and tolerance, aiming for at least 30 minutes, at least five times per week [18].
- As research and guidelines in exercise science have since advanced, the more recent 2020 guideline for people with both diabetes mellitus and CKD advises moderate-intensity physical activity for a cumulative duration of at least 150 minutes per week, or to a level compatible with one's cardiovascular and physical tolerance [20].

Clinical Pearl

- Cardiovascular disease is the number one cause of morbidity and mortality for patients living with CKD.
- Cardiovascular risk factor prevention and modification are of paramount importance.
- Lifestyle strategies such as physical activity and dietary management are key components of the treatment plan [18, 20].

19.4.5 Mitigating Health Risk in Exercise

People with CKD who are sedentary are encouraged to initiate *low- to moderate-intensity* physical activity, gradually increasing duration and intensity over time [18, 20]. Prior to engaging in *strenuous, high-intensity* exercise, patients with known cardiovascular disease or at high risk for cardiovascular disease should undergo medical evaluation with possible exercise stress testing, particularly if they are experiencing cardiac symptoms. Although patients with CKD are at higher risk for cardiovascular disease, the recommendation for medical assessment and/or exercise stress testing does not apply routinely if initiating *low- to moderate-intensity* activity, particularly in the absence of any symptoms of cardiovascular disease [18, 20, 35]. For patients at high risk of cardiovascular disease (e.g., those who have recently experienced a cardiac event), supervised exercise programs may be of benefit and have been shown to enhance motivation [18, 20, 35].

For people who are uncertain about the medical safety of initiating exercise, the Physical Activity Readiness Questionnaire for Everyone (PAR-Q+) is a free online evidence-informed pre-participation risk stratification tool [35]. For those with chronic medical conditions, a further tool, the Physical Activity Readiness Medical

Examination (ePARmed-X+), is available for clinician use to guide advice around exercise participation [35]. These evidence-informed tools were designed to reduce unnecessary barriers to participation in physical activity for patients with chronic medical conditions, while supporting safety and defining the role of exercise professionals [35]. When employed, only 1% of individuals are further recommended for formal medical assessment and approval prior to engaging in physical activity [35]. Appropriate and gradual progression of exercise intensity is important, regardless of cardiovascular disease risk [6, 7, 18, 19].

During exercise, people with CKD may utilize various personal equipment options to monitor their blood pressure, heart rate, and glucose before, during, and after exercise [20]. Establishing a regular routine of physical activity and nutrition may allow some degree of predictability to how one's body is likely to respond to an exercise session. Patients should be encouraged to pay attention to how they are feeling during exercise and to respect the limits of their bodies with regard to intensity and duration of activity; this may vary depending on the stage of CKD and other comorbid conditions. It is normal to experience an ebb and flow to levels of motivation and exercise capacity, especially during times of illness, high heat, and humidity and around times of dialysis [20]. KDIGO describes exercise training as "imperative" for people with CKD to mitigate cardiovascular risk, promoting access to programs that support education, self-monitoring, verbal reinforcement, and motivation [18, 20].

Hypoglycemia is a potential risk for people with diabetes mellitus, especially those on insulin; blood glucose levels should be tested before and after strenuous exercise, in addition to times when feeling unwell. For low- to moderate-intensity exercise, timing exercise sessions to be following a meal lessens hypoglycemia risk. Maintaining adequate hydration is important during exercise; patients who are immediately post-dialysis treatment are at increased risk of dehydration and hypotension during exercise. Exercise in hot and humid environments exacerbates dehydration and heat-related illness risks and should be avoided [20, 35].

Recommendation

- The PAR-Q+ and ePARmed-X+ are free online tools for patients and clinicians to use in health screening prior to the start of an exercise program and are available at https://eparmedx.com/.

19.4.6 Prescribing Physical Activity

There is evidence to support the effectiveness of a simple intervention to improve the uptake of physical activity: a medical prescription for exercise [22, 36]. When providing an exercise prescription to patients, consider advice specific to CKD and any other common chronic health conditions that they are managing. The organization "Exercise is Medicine" provides valuable resources in this regard. Their "Rx for Health" series, which is endorsed by the American College of Sports Medicine, is accessible at the following web link:

http://www.exerciseismedicine.org/support_page.php/your-rx-for-health-series/.

Of further interest in terms of lifestyle prescribing, recent research has been assessing for health and wellness benefits associated with time spent outdoors and the effectiveness of "nature prescriptions" or "park prescriptions" [37, 38]. Although outdoor time often involves some degree of physical activity, researchers are exploring potential mental health benefits from just *being* in "green space" [37, 38]. This is an area worthy of further study, especially as society in general has been transitioning toward indoor and sedentary pursuits. Nature may be more difficult to access in some urban environments, and environmental planning to promote physical activity and health is important.

Albeit a relatively simple concept, the power of a formal, written recommendation from a physician (or other healthcare team member) is not to be underestimated [22, 36].

Recommendation

- Provide patients with medical prescriptions for physical activity and time spent in nature [22, 36–38].

19.5 Case Vignette: "Ana and Getting Going"

Ana worked long shifts in a local canning factory where she was on her feet all day. She was married with two adult children who lived independently. Spanish was her first language, although she could also read and write in English, and she had almost completed a secondary school diploma. In addition to CKD, Ana lived with type 2 diabetes mellitus, hypertension, dyslipidemia, and obesity. She was preparing for hemodialysis and had recently had a fistula created.

Ana was sedentary and valued time off her feet to relax when not at work. Lower extremity edema caused discomfort toward the end of her work shifts, and she had difficulty managing the compression stockings that had been prescribed. She had attended appointments with a dietician, although admitted that she was not watching her diet as carefully as she knew she should. She found it complicated to make food choices that she enjoyed and was able to afford. She had not been checking her blood sugars regularly due to fatigue. She endorsed low energy and lack of motivation.

As her healthcare provider, what are you able to offer to support her health and wellness?

19.6 Nutrition and Dietary Management

19.6.1 Nutrition Science Basics

At a basic level, food provides the body with nutrients to support healthy functioning (a source of energy and substrate for cellular structures). **Essential nutrients** are those that are required to sustain life, but that the body is not capable of producing on its own [39]. The six essential nutrients are illustrated in Fig. 19.2 and listed below:

Proteins – are metabolized into amino acids.
Carbohydrates – include monosaccharides, disaccharides, and polysaccharides, which are metabolized into glucose.
Fats – are categorized as *saturated* or trans-fatty acids or *unsaturated* (mono- and polyunsaturated fatty acids).
Vitamins – are categorized as water soluble (B1, B2, B3, B6, B9, B12, C) or fat soluble (A, D, E, K).
Minerals – include several relevant to CKD (e.g., sodium, potassium, iron, calcium, phosphorus).
Water – which decreases from approximately 75% of body composition in infancy to 55% in older adults [40].

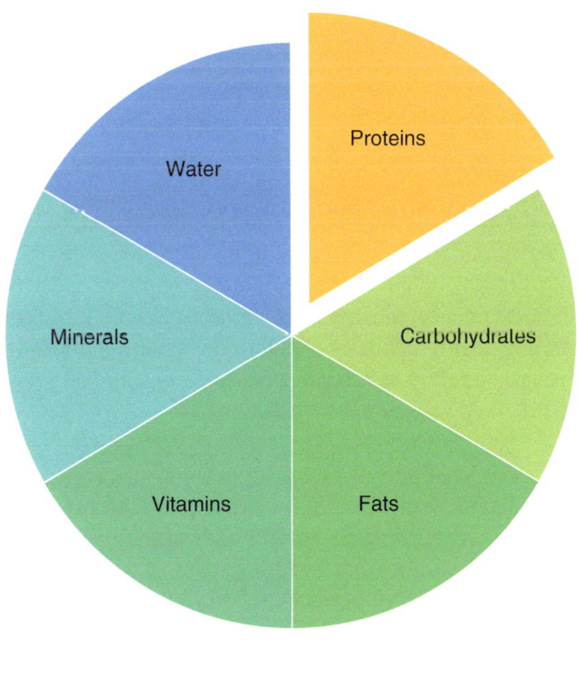

Fig. 19.2 Essential nutrients [39]

Macronutrients such as proteins, carbohydrates, and fats are required by the body in relatively large amounts to be converted into energy. The energy provided by food is measured in kilojoules or calories (4.2 kJ is equivalent to 1 calorie). Energy that is not used by the body is stored as fat, regardless of the food source; any of the macronutrients may be converted into fat if the energy is not needed for physical activity, growth, and metabolism. Fats (lipids) are the most energy-dense macronutrient, providing 9 kcal/g; protein provides 4 kcal/g; carbohydrates provide 4 kcal/g [39].

Micronutrients such as vitamins and minerals are required in relatively small amounts by the body, although they remain essential for optimal health [39]. You might be surprised to learn that micronutrient deficiencies are common particularly in patients living with obesity, including vitamin B12, vitamin D, magnesium, and iron [3].

Non-nutrients are components of food outside of the macro- and micronutrient categories; they may be natural (e.g., fiber) or synthetic (food preservatives); some may have beneficial effects, while others do not, and some may cause harm [39].

A well-balanced diet includes all the essential nutrients in the required amounts to optimize health and function [39]. Health conditions such as CKD impact nutrient requirements for optimization of health.

19.6.2 Nutrition for Physical and Mental Health

Health may be compromised when certain nutrients are consumed in excessive or insufficient amounts [39]. For example, excess intake of any of the macronutrients leads to unnecessary caloric energy which is converted into adipose tissue; insufficient iron intake can lead to the development of anemia, which is more common in those who follow a vegan diet and in those with CKD [18, 41]. In addition, scientific understanding of the important link between the human gut and brain, the impact of nutrition on mental health including cognition, continues to evolve [3, 42, 43].

It is well established that dietary choices lower the risk of developing many chronic health conditions, including diabetes mellitus, hypertension, cardiovascular disease, cerebrovascular disease, obesity, dementia, and certain types of cancer [3, 18, 20, 44]. Lifestyle interventions can:

- Lower HbA1c by 1–2% (like two diabetes mellitus medications) [45].
- Reduce risk of diabetes mellitus up to 70% [46].
- Lower blood pressure by 11 mmHg (like one blood pressure medication) [47].
- Reduce cardiovascular disease risk by 28–30% (like statin therapy) [48].
- Reduce risk of depression by 32% [49].
- Reduce risk of Alzheimer disease-related dementia by 53% [50].

For healthcare providers, consideration of patient preferences, cultural practices, food resources, budget, cooking skills, food intolerances, and comorbidities are key when recommending dietary options to patients and their families. It is not necessary for patients to entirely give up the foods that bring them pleasure, nor give up opportunities to eat at social outings, celebrations, or restaurants. With adaptability and flexibility, almost all foods can be worked into an acceptable dietary pattern. The goal of nutrition counseling is to help patients make changes in their food choices that improve their renal health and meet their personal needs and concerns while still allowing for food enjoyment [14, 18, 20, 53]. Offering acceptable alternatives and tailoring suggestions to budgetary and cooking skills considerations are essential in nutrition counseling and will improve patient quality of life, food enjoyment, and health outcomes. Encouraging homemade meals and purchasing locally grown foods can help reduce food costs and provide nutrient-rich meals [14, 18, 20, 53].

19.6.3 Nutrition and Cardiovascular Disease Risk

As noted earlier in this chapter, cardiovascular disease poses the greatest risk to health and life for people with CKD [18, 20]. Many patients with CKD either have or will develop cardiovascular disease and its associated risk factors such as diabetes mellitus, hypertension, obesity, and dyslipidemia. As such, dietary management to prevent and manage cardiovascular disease risk is key to reducing morbidity and mortality, as well as progression of CKD [18, 20, 53–55].

19.6.3.1 Diabetes Mellitus

Types 1 and 2 is the most common cause of CKD [18, 20]. Dietary strategies for diabetes mellitus encompass optimizing glycemic control, cardiovascular disease risk management, and renal health, all at once. The mainstay of the diabetic diet includes management of carbohydrates and lipids and minimizing hypertension risk. It includes considerations related to protein and fiber intake and choosing foods with a low glycemic index. In the presence of CKD, the need to regulate protein and specific vitamins and minerals is added, as will be elaborated in subsequent sections of this chapter. Improved glycemic control in diabetes mellitus has been shown to delay the onset and progression of CKD [18, 20, 53, 55].

19.6.3.2 Hypertension

According to Hypertension Canada, hypertension affects nearly a quarter of Canadian adults and represents a major risk factor for cardiovascular morbidity, chronic kidney disease, and death [44, 54]. Globally, nearly one third of adults have diagnosed hypertension [56]. Alongside diabetes mellitus, hypertension is a leading cause of CKD [18, 44, 54]. Blood pressure management has been shown

Table 19.3 Recommended diets to improve CVD risk factors and decrease CVD risk [18, 44, 46–48, 52, 53, 55, 57–60]

	DASH diet https://www.unlockfood.ca/en/Articles/Heart-Health/A-DASH-of-Healthy-Eating-Can-Help-Control-Blood-Pr.aspx	**Mediterranean diet** https://www.healthlinkbc.ca/health-topics/aa98646
Benefits	-decreases risk of hypertension -treats hypertension (lowers systolic BP by 11–15 mm hg, as much as one BP medication!) [46]	-decreases risk of CVD (lowers risk up to 30%) -associated with longer lifespan -associated with lower rates of depression, dementia, renal decline, and some types of cancer [47, 48, 52]
Key components	-plant-rich style of eating (vegetables and fruits and grains); high in fiber and potassium; lower in sodium, saturated fat, and added sugars -recommended daily servings include four servings of fruits and three to four servings of vegetables, six whole grain servings, two to three servings of low-fat dairy -recommended other servings include two servings of healthy fats, lean poultry, and fish two servings/week, nuts/seeds/beans three to four servings/week, and < 3 sweets each week	-plant-based diet rich in fruit, vegetables, whole grains, beans, peas, and other legumes -daily consumption of healthy fats including extra virgin olive oil, nuts, seeds -variety of both vegetable and animal proteins including fish/seafood eggs, poultry -moderate in meats and sweets
Cautions in CKD	-certain foods may be high in potassium and phosphates which may need to be limited in CKD -not for use if receiving dialysis treatments -assistance from a registered dietitian is recommended for people with CKD	-certain foods may be high in potassium and phosphates which may need to be limited in CKD -not for use if receiving dialysis treatments -assistance from a registered dietitian is recommended for people with CKD

BP blood pressure; *CVD* cardiovascular disease

to delay the onset and progression of both CKD and cardiovascular disease [18, 44, 54]. The Dietary Approaches to Stop Hypertension (DASH) diet, which limits its dietary salt thereby decreasing fluid retention, reduces the risk of developing hypertension and cardiovascular disease [44, 47, 54, 57, 58]. The adoption of DASH-like eating can lower systolic blood pressure by 11 points, irrespective of any change in weight [47].

Table 19.3 highlights key aspects of the DASH diet, as well as the Mediterranean diet, which will be discussed further in this chapter.

Recommendation

– To reduce the risk of hypertension, which subsequently reduces risk of CKD and cardiovascular disease, the Canadian hypertension guidelines recommend that clinicians prescribe [44, 54]:
  - 30–60 minutes of moderate-intensity dynamic exercise 4–7 days/week (e.g., swim, bike, walk).
  - A healthy BMI and waist circumference.
  - Weight loss if elevated BMI (≥25) or waist circumference (≥102 cm for men, ≥88 cm for women).
  - A multifaceted approach to weight loss, including education about dietary strategies, increased physical activity, and support for behavioral change.
  - Abstain from or limit alcohol (max two drinks/day).
  - Dietary strategies such as the DASH diet (high in vegetables, fruit, plant proteins, low-fat dairy, whole grains).
  - Limiting salt to 2000 mg/day.
  - Increasing dietary potassium, *except those with CKD and an eGFR < 60 who are at increased risk of hyperkalemia!*
  - Manage stress.

19.6.3.3 Obesity

Globally, obesity (BMI > 30) continues to increase in prevalence, contributing significantly to morbidity and mortality [3]. People with obesity are at increased risk for developing cardiovascular disease, diabetes mellitus, and hypertension, all of which elevate the potential for CKD [3]. Dietary advice in the context of obesity should include education to ensure adequate intake of nutrients, while avoiding excess calories, and attempting to improve body composition (increasing lean body mass, decreasing adiposity). Weight loss in people with CKD who are obese can reduce blood pressure and rate of CKD progression, although the current management focus has transitioned toward healthy lifestyle modifications as opposed to actual weight itself [3, 18]. Obesity is a complex condition, and our scientific understanding of its neurochemical and neurohormonal mechanisms continues to grow, including how the body defends *against* weight loss [3]. Viewing obesity management as simply a function of reducing excess calories and enhancing activity dramatically oversimplifies weight and neglects the complex key modulators of body size that are being discovered [3]. In fact, "obese malnutrition" is not uncommon in patients over 65 years, as well as those with multiple comorbidities, including CKD [61]. Current goals in the management of obesity are to focus on improving overall metabolic health, mental health, mechanical health, and monetary health, rather than weight loss alone [3].

Table 19.4 Patient resources for physical activity and nutrition in CKD

Resource	Organization	Web link
24-hour movement guidelines	Canadian Society for Exercise Physiology (CSEP)	https://csepguidelines.ca/
Physical activity guidelines	ParticipACTION	https://www.participaction.com/en-ca
Spice it up! Giving zest to your renal diet		https://www.myspiceitup.ca/
Resources for living with chronic kidney disease including lifestyle management	Ontario Renal Network (ORN)	https://www.ontariorenalnetwork.ca/en/kidney-care-resources/living-with-chronic-kidney-disease
Resources for living with CKD including lifestyle management	Kidney Foundation of Canada	https://kidney.ca/Support https://kidney.ca/Kidney-Health/Living-With-Kidney-Disease
Kidney kitchen- dietary guidance and menus	American Kidney Fund	https://kitchen.kidneyfund.org/?_ga=2.81859734.1617958351.1617369176-915828241.1616354735
Resources for living with CKD Including lifestyle management	National Institute of Diabetes and Digestive and Kidney Diseases (NIDDK)	https://www.niddk.nih.gov/health-information/kidney-disease/chronic-kidney-disease-ckd
Resources for living with CKD including lifestyle management	National Kidney Foundation	https://www.kidney.org/treatment-support
Resources for living with CKD including lifestyle management	American Association of Kidney Patients (AAKP)	https://aakp.org/center-for-patient-research-and-education/educational-brochures-and-resources/
Unlock food	Dietitians of Canada	https://www.unlockfood.ca
Understanding food labels		https://www.unlockfood.ca/en/Articles/Nutrition-Labelling/
Calcium		https://www.unlockfood.ca/en/Articles/Bone-Health/Food-sources-of-calcium.aspx
Iron		https://www.unlockfood.ca/en/Articles/Vitamins-and-Minerals/How-to-get-more-iron.aspx
Protein		Articles/protein/
Phosphorus		https://www.unlockfood.ca/en/Articles/Vitamins-and-Minerals/Food-Sources-of-Phosphorus.aspx
Potassium		https://www.unlockfood.ca/en/Articles/Vitamins-and-Minerals/What-You-Need-to-Know-About-Potassium.aspx
Sodium		https://www.unlockfood.ca/en/Articles/Heart-Health/Cut-out-the-Salt.aspx

19.6.3.4 Lipids

Dyslipidemia is a risk factor for the development of cardiovascular disease and may be improved through dietary strategies. For example, the Mediterranean diet has been associated with a decreased risk of dyslipidemia, obesity, CKD, cardiovascular disease, hypertension, and cancer [51, 57, 62]. The Mediterranean diet includes healthy fats such as those found in olive oil and fish and is high in fruits, vegetables, and whole grains. Intake of foods high in saturated fats and trans fats is limited, as is alcohol and sugar (refined carbohydrates) [60]. For people with CKD and elevated triglycerides, KDIGO recommends lifestyle management including dietary modification, weight reduction, increased physical activity, limited alcohol intake, and treatment of hyperglycemia in those with diabetes mellitus [62]. The KDIGO guideline notes specific dietary changes that may reduce serum triglycerides: a low-fat diet (< 15% total calories), reducing simple sugars and total carbohydrates, and including fish oils [62]. Through dietary strategies, increased physical activity, and at times the addition of pharmacologic management, cardiovascular disease and its related risk factors can be prevented, managed, and at times reversed, thereby decreasing the risk and progression of CKD.

19.6.4 Nutrition and Chronic Kidney Disease

Nutrition therapy is recommended for people with CKD to delay progression of CKD and to reduce mortality [18, 51, 53, 55, 58, 59]. Dietary adjustments reduce the risk of developing certain complications of CKD and help to manage existing complications. The appropriate dietary management strategy varies with the stage of kidney disease (1– 5) and type of dialysis. It is also influenced by comorbid health conditions and medications [18, 20, 53, 55]. Evidence supports early intervention for people with CKD stages 1 or 2; nutrition counseling from a registered dietician can reduce the rate of eGFR decline and transition to advanced stages [18, 53, 55]. In more advanced stages of kidney disease, the expertise of a registered dietician specializing in the care of patients with kidney disease is required [18, 20, 53, 55]. Benefits of pre-dialysis medical nutrition therapy counseling in stages 2 and 3 have been shown to delay progression to stage 5 and decrease first-year mortality after initiation of hemodialysis [53, 55].

Even for healthcare professionals, the dietary recommendations for CKD management can seem complex and confusing. Imagine, then, how challenging this aspect of care can be for patients without a background in science or with limited education. Nutrient deficiencies are very common for people with CKD, and even more so for those managing comorbidities, given the numerous and at times conflicting dietary restrictions recommended. Thankfully, there are accessible online patient education materials about dietary modifications in CKD, many of which include sample menus and meal plans and which come in various languages. Table 19.4 introduces several online resources for people with CKD and those involved in grocery shopping and meal preparation with them. This information should always be accompanied by consultation with a registered dietician and a specialized renal registered dietician for those patients with advanced CKD and receiving dialysis. Often, advanced CDK requires dietary changes that will be in contradiction to those recommended earlier in the disease. Key roles of the registered dietician are to personalize and simplify the multiple dietary recommendations [18, 20, 53, 55].

Scientific understanding of dietary management for people with CKD has continued to evolve, and it is important to note that plant-based eating is compatible with renal disease; the National Kidney Foundation supports "Meatless Mondays" and provides several resources to support adequate protein from plant-based sources, while monitoring the balance of other minerals [55, 63]. As always, the expert consultation of a renal registered dietician is recommended.

It is important that healthcare providers take time and care to avoid overwhelming patients with too much education and advice at once and that dialogue is supported to respect patient and caregiver capacity to understand and manage information. Repetition through follow-up sessions and resources for asynchronous reference are of benefit [14, 18, 20].

Recommendation

- KDIGO recommends that people with CKD receive expert dietary advice and information in an education program.
- Education and advice should be tailored to the individual's stage of CKD.
- Education should include modifications related to salt, phosphate, potassium, and protein as indicated based on the individual situation [14, 18, 20, 55].

Clinical Pearl

- Although the DASH and Mediterranean diets are beneficial in preventing and decreasing the progression of CKD, they are not adequate for patients with advanced CKD and those receiving dialysis treatment, who require additional specific nutrient modifications [18, 20].

An approach to dietary management of specific nutrients in CKD is to focus on "the three Ps" (protein, potassium, phosphorus), as well as sodium, fiber, fluids, iron, vitamin D, and calcium.

19.6.4.1 Protein

Protein is a major nutrient essential to body health for its use in production of amino acids required by all body cells and structures. Protein is retained by the kidney, and as CKD progresses, the kidneys become less able to optimally meet the body's protein requirements. As a result, patients with advanced CKD are at risk for loss of muscle mass and strength. Patients with advanced stages of CKD and on dialysis may require augmented protein sources. Since meat and animal products are common protein sources in some countries, attention must be paid to managing other nutrients which are found in high levels in animal products, such as phosphorus and saturated fats [14]. KDIGO highlights that "efforts to restrict dietary phosphate must not compromise adequate protein intake" [14].

19.6.4.2 Potassium

Although having increased levels of dietary potassium decreases the risk of developing hypertension and CKD, once CKD is diagnosed and has progressed to more advanced stages, there is potential for development of hyperkalemia [18, 55]. Potassium is an important mineral for maintenance of normal muscular and cardiac function; if severely elevated, it is associated with risk of sudden cardiac death. It is important for patients with advanced CKD to limit the amount of potassium in their diet to maintain serum levels within a normal range (3.5–5.0 mmol/L). Risk of hyperkalemia is higher for patients at more advanced stages of CKD and for those with comorbidities such as congestive heart failure, cardiovascular disease, and diabetes mellitus [18, 44, 53]. Medications such as angiotensin-converting enzyme inhibitors and certain foods also contribute to potassium levels. As such, potassium levels require close monitoring and may require adjustments to diet, medications, and dialysis treatments [18, 20, 53].

19.6.4.3 Phosphorus

The body's ability to manage phosphorus differs at various stages of CKD, and as such, the importance of dietary management of this mineral changes as well. In later stages of CKD, patients are at risk of elevated phosphorus levels which is a concern due its impact on other body hormones (e.g., PTH) and minerals (e.g., calcium). When phosphorus levels remain elevated, PTH and calcium abnormalities develop, and bone health is negatively impacted; patients become at increased risk of bone disease and fractures [14]. Elevated phosphorus contributes to hypercalcemia, as calcium is released from bone into the bloodstream; this can lead to calcium deposits in blood vessels and the heart, increasing risk of cardiovascular disease. A safe level of phosphorus is between 0.8 and 1.45 (Canada) or 2.5 and 4.5 mg/dL (USA). It is important for people with CKD to choose foods lower in phosphorus to bring serum phosphorus levels back to normal. In addition, phosphate binders may be used [14, 18, 20, 53, 55].

Phosphorus is mainly found in protein-rich foods such as meat and cheese and in commercially prepared foods. An important consideration related to dietary phosphate management is the "bioavailability" of phosphorus sources. Organic forms of phosphate are found in animal- and plant-based sources; inorganic phosphate is found in food additives. Whereas approximately 40%–60% of animal-based phosphate is absorbed, plant-based phosphate is generally less absorbable at 20%–50% [14, 53, 55, 63]. And inorganic phosphate's bioavailability is higher than both organic sources [14, 53, 55, 63]. People with CKD should be encouraged to choose fresh and homemade foods rather than processed foods in order to avoid additives [14]. Healthcare providers should consider the source of phosphate and its bioavailability in their counseling; for example, beans and nuts are listed as being very high in phosphorus, but in considering their lower bioavailability, they may be considered acceptable protein sources [14, 53, 55].

KDIGO recommends that hyperphosphatemia treatment include reduction of dietary phosphates either with or without phosphate binders, depending on individual circumstances, and that the source of dietary phosphate be considered (e.g., plant, animal, food additive) [14]. The expert input of a registered dietician is key!

19.6.4.4 Sodium

Sodium is an electrolyte that causes the body to retain fluid, thus increasing circulating fluid volume and increasing blood pressure. Limiting salt intake is an important aspect of the CKD diet, such that fluid balance and blood pressure are optimized, thereby limiting the progression of CKD [44, 54]. This can be challenging, as sodium is found in most prepared and packaged foods and drinks. Sodium is also used to flavor foods to enhance taste and enjoyment. Approaching sodium restriction for patients with CKD requires some creativity and adaptability, for example, using herbs and spices to season foods to add flavor and enjoyment to meals [18, 20, 44, 55]. Patients with CKD need to be cautious with salt substitutes, however, as these may contain high amounts of phosphorus [18, 20, 55].

19.6.4.5 Fluid

Adequate fluids and hydration status are important for healthy kidney function. Early stages of renal disease do not require adjustment to fluid intake. In more severe CKD and when patient management includes dialysis, limiting fluid intake is an important component of nutritional management to avoid edema and elevated blood pressure [18, 20, 55].

19.6.4.6 Iron

CKD is associated with an increased risk of anemia and iron deficiency; as such, maintaining adequate dietary iron is an important component of CKD management [41]. People with anemia may experience fatigue, effort intolerance, decreased stamina, loss of appetite, restless legs, and pica. More severe anemia may result in dyspnea, presyncope, chest pain, palpitations, and delirium. Even when iron stores are replete, anemia may still occur in patients with CKD due to impairment of the hormonal pathways related to erythropoietin (EPO) [41]. EPO is produced in the kidney and stimulates the bone marrow to produce red blood cells. In CKD, less EPO is produced, and there is a subsequent decrease in production of red blood cells, resulting in a decrease in hemoglobin. Many patients with advanced CKD require not only iron supplementation but also erythropoiesis-stimulating agents (ESAs) [41]. Supplementation with iron supports adequate stores for erythropoiesis and can prevent iron deficiency. Iron supplementation can be provided by either oral or intravenous routes. The advantages of oral iron therapy are its low cost, availability, and ease of administration; gastrointestinal side effects are common [41]. Intravenous iron is more effective, although it has the potential for uncommon but significant adverse reactions and is less convenient for some patients [41]. The approach taken may depend on the severity of anemia and iron deficiency, response to previous treatments, cost, and venous access considerations [41].

19.6.4.7 Vitamin D

A key vitamin for many aspects of health for all individuals, vitamin D is especially important for people with CKD as related to the prevention of mineral and bone disorder (CKD-MBD). Deficiency of vitamin D is very common in northern countries, as well as in individuals living with CKD, obesity, and other comorbidities [14]. Vitamin D is limited in our food supply, found only in fish, fortified milk, and shitake mushrooms. With limited sun exposure in northern climates between September and May, supplementation is required to meet daily nutrient needs, a minimum of 1000 IU vitamin D3 daily [64]. Adequate stores of vitamin D are required for calcium uptake into bone, and inadequate levels can lead to weakening of bone as calcium is unable to be deposited. KDIGO recommends that vitamin D deficiency and insufficiency be corrected with the same oral treatment as for people without CKD [14, 18].

19.6.4.8 Calcium

An important mineral for bone, muscular, and cardiac function, calcium is a key consideration for people with CKD, especially at more advanced stages. When phosphorus levels are elevated, calcium is unable to be taken effectively into bone and, instead, is released to accumulate in the blood and other tissues. This results in complications such as MBD and vascular disease, along with calcium deposition in other tissues [14]. It is well established that patients with CKD have increased fracture rates compared with the general population, and moreover, incident hip fractures are associated with substantial morbidity and mortality [14].

At times, patients with CKD might also develop hypocalcemia, in relation to abnormal PTH and phosphorus levels. In such cases, KDIGO recommends individualizing the approach to instead of routinely correcting hypocalcemia in *all* patients, given the potential risks associated with elevated calcium levels and a lack of compelling evidence on benefits to overall health and mortality with correction [14].

19.6.4.9 Calories

Caloric intake is the measure of energy potential consumed through dietary macronutrients. Excess caloric intake and complex metabolic and neurohormonal factors can increase the risk of obesity [3]. Insufficient caloric intake is a particular risk for those on restrictive diets and with advanced disease. It can also result from iron deficiency anemia which leads to decreased appetite. Insufficient caloric intake can lead to fatigue, weight loss, and loss of lean body mass due to protein catabolism. In people with CKD, it is essential that the body's energy requirements are met to prevent malnutrition and to optimize health outcomes, in consideration of the various dietary restrictions advised [14, 18, 20, 53, 55]. Again, the value of the registered dietician's expertise is not to be understated.

Table 19.5 summarizes key nutrient considerations for patients with CKD.

Table 19.5 Key nutrient considerations in adult renal disease [14, 18, 20, 41, 53, 55]

Nutrient	Adult RDI no CKD	Adjustment in CKD	Common sources
Sodium	1.5 g	Limit to <90 mmol/d (< 2 g/d) (equivalent to 5 mg sodium chloride)	Table salt, cooking salt, sauces, canned foods, preserves (e.g., pickles), prepared foods, restaurant foods, deli meats, cheese, salty snacks Practical tip: Read food labels and choose foods <400 mg sodium per serving
Potassium	4.7 g	Varies with stage of CKD, medications, and comorbidities	Some fruits and vegetables, lentils, beans, dairy products Practical tip: Limit/moderate intake of potato, banana, citrus (e.g., 1–2/week) Practical tip: Double boil potato
Phosphorus	4.0 g	Varies with stage of CKD, medications, and comorbidities; should be limited for most patients in advanced stages	Milk and dairy products, meat, eggs, lentils, beans, nuts, whole grains
Iron	8–18 mg Varies based on age, gender, menstrual status	Maintain an iron-rich diet while being attentive to avoiding excesses of other nutrients highlighted above, as iron deficiency and anemia are a risk for patients with CKD	Fortified grains/cereals, meat, seafood, fish, eggs, tofu, legumes, nuts, seeds, fortified grains, fortified soy, leafy green vegetables, molasses
Protein	0.8 g/kg 1.0 g/kg (seniors if malnourished as may occur in CKD)	Limit to 0.8 g/kg/d if diabetes mellitus or stages 4–5 Avoid high protein (> 1.3 g/kg/d) if risk of CKD progression in earlier stages	Meat, fish, eggs, tofu, nuts, seeds, legumes, milk, dairy products, soy products
Vitamin D3	600–1000 IU	Risk of deficiency if PTH elevated, stages 3–5; maintain dietary sources; supplement if deficient (supplementation required for adults living in northern climates from September to May as dietary sources are insufficient and sun exposure inadequate for vitamin D production)	Fatty fish (salmon, sardines), egg yolk, milk, fortified milks (soy, rice, nut), fortified juices
Calcium	1000 mg men, 1200 mg women	Individualized management in stages 3–5 (considered with levels of PTH, vitamin D, phosphorus)	Milk, cheese, yogurt, fortified beverages (soy, rice, nut, orange juice), tofu, fatty fish, nuts, beans, leafy greens

RDI, recommended dietary intake; *RDI values indicated apply to nonpregnant adults*

Clinical Pearl

- The Ontario Renal Network provides helpful Nutrition Fact Sheets for patients on phosphorus, potassium, sodium, and diabetes mellitus, which can be accessed at the following web link:

  https://www.ontariorenalnetwork.ca/en/kidney-care-resources/clinical-tools/home-dialysis/nutrition-fact-sheets.

For those living with advanced CKD and receiving dialysis, supplements and medications are usually required to maintain optimal balance of nutrients to prevent or minimize risk of complications [14, 18, 20, 41, 53, 55].

Table 19.6 lists a few of the common nutritional supplements and medications in patients with advanced CKD.

Recommendation

- All patients with CKD should be referred to a dietician for nutritional assessment and education on strategies to reduce risk of CKD progression and comorbidities that contribute to cardiovascular risk.
- Patients with more advanced stages of CKD should receive care from a specialized renal dietician [14, 18, 20, 53, 55].

19.7 Lifestyle Modification

19.7.1 Stages of Change

In counseling patients about physical activity and dietary management for CKD, it helps at the outset to assess their readiness to engage in lifestyle changes. Importantly, the role for the healthcare provider varies with each of the stages of change, according to patient needs. As presented earlier in Chap. 11 on "Substance Use Disorders and the Kidney," Table 19.7 reviews the stages of change according to the transtheoretical model, including corresponding roles for the healthcare provider [65, 66].

Clinical Pearl

- Limit to one or a small number of lifestyle goals at a time, to increase the likelihood of success and build confidence.
- Consider asking, "What is one thing you could do this week to improve your eating pattern? What is one thing you could do to increase your movement this week?"

Table 19.6 Common nutritional supplements and medications in CKD

Supplement/medication	Indication	Common side effects
Vitamin D3 Recommend vitamin D supplementation in northern climates to meet nutrient needs as food sources are limited (e.g., fortified milk, fish) and sun exposure is limited in fall and winter months RDI: 600 IU vitamin D3 daily 9–50 years RDI: 800 IU vitamin D3 daily >51 years Information about vitamin D: https://www.unlockfood.ca/en/Articles/Vitamins-and-Minerals/What-you-need-to-know-about-Vitamin-D.aspx	Documented vitamin D deficiency or living in northern climate where deficiency is presumed Hypocalcemia with elevated PTH	-usually none
Vitamin D analog (calcitriol)	Documented vitamin D deficiency Hypocalcemia with elevated PTH	-GI upset is most common including gas, bloating, nausea; dry mouth, headache, palpitations
Calcium Recommend calcium-rich diet +500 mg calcium citrate 1–2x/day, depending on dietary intake RDI = 1000 mg calcium daily for men RDI = 1200 mg calcium daily for women Food sources of calcium: https://www.unlockfood.ca/en/Articles/Bone-Health/Food-Sources-of-Calcium.aspx	Hypocalcemia	-GI upset including nausea, diarrhea, constipation -excess may lead to stone formation, soft tissue deposition, cardiac abnormalities
Phosphate binders	Hyperphosphatemia	-GI upset including nausea, vomiting, diarrhea, constipation, anorexia, abdominal pain
Iron Recommend iron-rich diet + ferrous sulfate 45–60 mg *elemental* iron once or twice daily if needed based on low MCV <80 and low ferritin <30 RDI = 8 mg daily males + females >51 years RDI = 18 mg daily menstruating females How to get more iron from foods: https://www.unlockfood.ca/en/Articles/Vitamins-and-Minerals/How-to-get-more-iron.aspx	Iron deficiency with or without anemia	-GI upset including nausea, vomiting, constipation -practical tip: less GI upset with ferrous sulfate or taking iron supplement after eating

Table 19.6 (continued)

Supplement/medication	Indication	Common side effects
Erythropoietin-stimulating agents (ESAs)	Anemia (with or without iron deficiency), to stimulate the bone marrow to produce red blood cells	-hypertension, edema, nausea, fever, dizziness, pain at injection site -uncommon but severe: polycythemia and associated complications, DVT and associated complications -promotion of malignancy, if present

Data derived from [14, 18, 20, 41, 53, 55]

19.7.2 Patient- and Person-Centered Care

In the large, busy, and complex healthcare system, there is risk of losing sight of the patient as "person," an autonomous individual with a broad life context outside of healthcare [76]. Patient-centered care has been demonstrated to improve patient satisfaction, engagement with treatment recommendations, health outcomes, and quality of life [10, 14, 20, 67]:

- **Patient-centered care** is respectful of and responsive to individual patient preferences, needs, and values, ensuring that clinical decisions are guided by patient values [10, 67].
- **Humanism in medicine** is the application of scientific knowledge and skills with respectful, compassionate care that is sensitive to the values, autonomy, and cultural needs of individual patients and their families [10].

Table 19.8 outlines key elements of patient-centered care.

Recommendation

- Consider this context for each individual patient:
  - What do they value?
  - What gives meaning to their life?
  - How do they spend their time?
  - What do they enjoy?
  - Who are their key people?

KDIGO acknowledges shared decision-making as a key component of patient-centered nutrition management. The process of adapting diet to manage CKD and comorbid conditions is a long and complex process that requires repeated

Table 19.7 The six stages of behavior change according to transtheoretical model [65, 66]

	Stage of change	Description of stage	Clinician role
1	Precontemplation	Individual does not intend to make changes or may not be aware that they have a behavior that needs changing	Be curious. Ask questions to understand. Empathize. Reflect what you have heard. make a brief recommendation. Offer support and opportunity to revisit topic.
2	Contemplation	Individual is considering change and possibly weighing the pros and cons; however, ambivalence about change may persist	As above. Inquire as to future goals; acknowledge potential gains and losses. Identify current barriers, what it would take to initiate change.
3	Preparation	Individual is ready to change behavior and taking small steps toward change	As above. Provide education. Support setting SMART goals. Plan for managing barriers and challenges. Assess supports. Ensure follow-up.
4	Action	Individual has changed behavior and building new healthier habits	As above. Provide encouragement. Assess noted gains. Support focus on learning and stepwise approach toward goals. Ensure follow-up.
5	Maintenance	Individual is sustaining behavior change	As above. Reinforce gains. Assess supports. Reflect on learning, challenges, enablers. Ensure follow-up.
6	Termination (or relapse)	The ultimate goal is ongoing integration of healthy lifestyle behaviors although maintenance over the long term can be difficult and fluctuation in choices and behaviors is commonly part of the cycle and should not be viewed as failure	Promote self-compassion, learning, perseverance, ongoing goal setting, stepwise approach, future focus. Offer ongoing support.

Table 19.8 Elements of patient-centered care [67]

Engage the patient as a whole person
Recognize and respond to emotions
Foster a therapeutic alliance
Promote an exchange of information
Share decision-making
Enable continuity of care, self-management, patient navigation

adjustments over time [14, 18, 20, 53]. KDIGO promotes patient-centered solutions, including recognition of differences in individuals such as age, dentition, cultural food preferences, finances, and patient goals, while navigating dietary requirements that may at times be conflicting [20]. Working together with patients to set small, realistic achievable (SMART) goals is an effective strategy to facilitate sustainable behavioral change. SMART goals are [68]:

- Specific
- Measurable
- Achievable
- Realistic
- Timely

Recommendation

- Ask patients about their own health priorities.
- Review your role and perspective.
- Negotiate what you will focus on together.

Patient-centered care models include patient problem-solving, allowing patients to select strategies they feel will be successful for them, supporting patients as they work through issues, supporting self-efficacy and self-confidence, and incorporating self-selected behavioral goal setting [14]. Involvement of the patient's family and/or caregivers in education and planning may also be helpful [14]. KDIGO acknowledges that patients benefit from repeated visits with registered dieticians, supporting them to make informed decisions about their diet, employing shared decision-making techniques, and learning from prior adjustments and their effect [14, 20].

Clinical Pearl

- Remember that choices are about trade-offs, weighing benefits and losses based on a patient's values and goals.

19.7.3 Motivational Interviewing

The successful implementation of lifestyle changes such as physical activity and dietary modification is enhanced when healthcare providers employ motivational interviewing techniques [22, 69, 70]. A strengths-based approach is of value as it reinforces a patient's abilities and successes, empowering their ongoing potential to set goals, learn, and make changes [71].

Recommendation

- Employ the five principles of motivational interviewing when engaging with patients about dietary and physical activity modifications:
  - Express empathy through reflective listening.
  - Develop discrepancy between goals/values and current behavior.
  - Avoid argument and direct confrontation.
  - Adjust to resistance, and avoid direct opposition.
  - Support self-efficacy and optimism [69].

Table 19.9 Sample of motivational interviewing phrases

"Help me understand…"
"In an ideal world, what would this look like for you?"
"What would it take to make this happen?"
"On a scale of 1–10, how motivated do you feel to make this happen?"
"What would it take to move this number up to a (fill in the blank)?"
"You used to be at a (fill in number), and now you are at a (fill in number); what made the difference?"
"So, what I hear you saying is…"
"To summarize what I understand, you would like to walk more to improve your health, *and* it's difficult to feel motivated to get outside after work"
"For you, having a regular routine and a friend to walk with have been helpful strategies for staying active"
"How would you know if/when this has become a problem for you?"

Data derived from [22, 69–71]

Table 19.9 offers a sample of motivational interviewing phrases for use during clinical appointments. A detailed overview of motivational interviewing is beyond the scope of this chapter, and the reader is encouraged to access further resources on this topic for its relevance to lifestyle management of chronic health conditions, including CKD.

19.7.4 Interprofessional Teamwork

Optimizing care for patients with CKD, particularly those at advanced stages, requires the collective expertise of an interprofessional team of healthcare providers [14, 18, 20]. At the center of the team is the patient. Wrapping directly around the patient is their family, a term which we use broadly in this chapter to describe the people who are closely involved in the patient's life as caregivers and supports.

Recommendation

- KDIGO recommends that people with progressive CKD be managed in a multidisciplinary care setting.
- Care should include CKD education and dietary counseling, in addition to counseling about other treatment options for advanced disease [14, 18, 20].

CKD healthcare team members vary depending on local resources and may include:

- **Nurse –** providing direct patient care, coordination of care and education.
- **Dietician –** providing dietary assessment, education, and nutrition management strategies.

- **Kinesiologist** – providing exercise education, fitness assessment, and supervision.
- **Physiotherapist** – providing education, rehabilitation and treatment for musculoskeletal health and mobility issues.
- **Occupational therapist** – providing rehabilitation skills, tools, and equipment to support activities of daily living and enhance daily function.
- **Pharmacist** – providing education and contributing to medication management and supply.
- **Systems navigator** – assisting patients in accessing resources in healthcare and social systems.
- **Social worker** – providing psychosocial and mental health support, education, and counseling.
- **Dialysis technician** – contributing to the safety and effectiveness of dialysis care.
- **Physician assistant** – assisting in the provision of direct medical care to patients.
- **Lab technician** – obtaining and analyzing bloodwork samples.
- **Physician** – providing clinical assessment and diagnosis, ordering clinical investigations, and managing results and treatments, providing education and support, referring to other healthcare team members.

People with CKD benefit from the involvement of physicians with varying expertise, particularly as their condition becomes more advanced. Family physicians oversee whole-person care longitudinally throughout all stages of a person's life and CKD disease trajectory. As CKD progresses toward more advanced stages, nephrology plays a key role in specialized and hospital-based management. Depending on the patient, their stage of CKD, comorbidities, and goals of care, the physician team may also include specialists in psychiatry, endocrinology, general internal medicine, cardiology, vascular surgery, radiology, transplantation surgery, and palliative care. Timely communication among all team members is essential, promoting effective collaboration of specialized aspects of patient care, as well as effective linkage between hospital and community-based care [14, 18, 20].

It is also important to acknowledge the valuable role that organizations outside of the healthcare system play in patient care and support [14, 18, 20]:

- **Peer support groups** – provide the opportunity to learn and receive support from others living with CKD and managing similar issues.
- **Community support and advocacy organizations** – provide education, support, and advocacy for issues of importance to people living with CKD.

As summarized in the CanMEDS competency framework, the work of physicians "occurs within complex systems and thus requires the development of partnerships with patients, their families and support networks, or community agencies and organizations to influence health determinants" [72].

19.7.5 Chronic Disease Self-Management (CDSM)

Although it is beyond the scope of this chapter to provide a detailed overview of CDSM, we note its importance in CKD and other chronic diseases, especially as related to lifestyle management strategies such as physical activity and nutrition [20, 73–75].

KDIGO recommends a structured self-management education program for people with diabetes mellitus and CKD and goes further to define what the key objectives of such a program should include, as follows [20]:

- Improve diabetes-related knowledge, beliefs, and skills.
- Improve self-management and self-motivation.
- Encourage adoption and maintenance of healthy lifestyles.
- Improve vascular risk factors.
- Increase engagement with medication, glucose monitoring, and complication screening programs.
- Reduce risk to prevent (or better manage) diabetes-related complications.
- Improve emotional and mental well-being, treatment satisfaction, and quality of life.

With the patient at the center of the healthcare team and bolstered by resources, education, and access to interprofessional expertise, healthcare providers can support management decisions that are consistent with patient's goals, values, and priorities. There are many tools and resources available online to assist patients in taking an active role in their CKD management, including those to guide dietary modifications and physical activity. It is the responsibility of all healthcare providers to empower and equip patients to effectively participate in CDSM [20, 73–75].

In goal setting with patients, there is also value to anticipating potential barriers and challenges, planning strategies to manage them, and identifying supports to encourage and provide accountability. It is helpful to identify motivating and enabling factors to plan for success. Table 19.10 provides examples of physical activity variables patients might consider in making plans to increase movement or exercise.

Recommendation

– Support patients in framing dietary choices as a component of chronic disease self-management over which they have control: "One of the things I have control over with regards to my health is the food choices that I make."

Table 19.10 Exploring patient preferences for physical activity

Time of day	Indoor or outdoor
Land or water	Cost or no-cost
Scheduled or spontaneous	Competitive or recreational
Solo or group	Weight bearing or non-weight bearing
Equipment or none	Weather and season dependency
Adventure or predictability	Skills-based or intuitive

KDIGO encourages the use of technology to enhance learning, including nutrition apps, social media, and online nutrient database information [20]. Refer to Table 19.4 to review various online resources to support patients in lifestyle management of their CKD.

Clinical Pearl

- Ensure that people with CKD have access to reliable resources to guide their lifestyle choices, including those available online and via mobile apps [20, 77].

Figure 19.3 illustrates the patient at the center of their own CKD management.

Recommendation

- Be attentive to the potential for unintentionally overwhelming patients with too much information at one time.
- Prioritize and provide patients with only the amount of information they feel able to manage at each visit.
- Work together to come up with small, realistic goals patients can work on in between healthcare visits.
- Reinforce small steps are the key to sustainable behavioral changes.
- Provide opportunities for questions, repetition, and follow-up [14, 20].

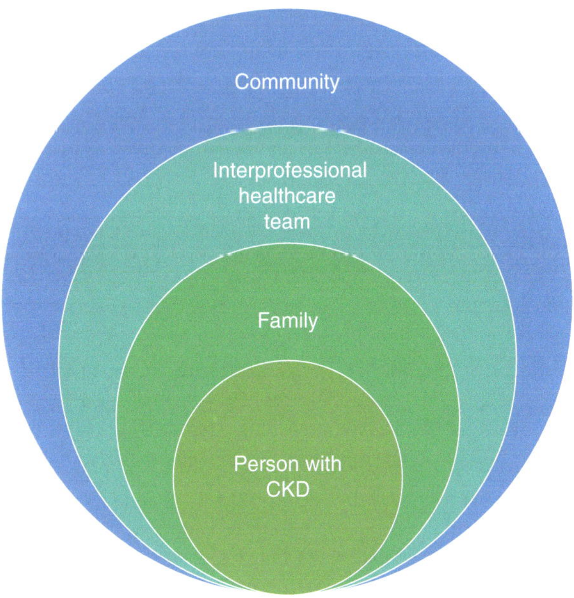

Fig. 19.3 Patient at the center of the healthcare team. (Data from [18, 65]. *"Family" denotes the people who are important to the individual and who care for and support the individual*)

19.8 Physician Advocacy

Advocacy is a key role for all physicians, as defined in the competency frameworks of the Royal College of Physicians and Surgeons of Canada (RCPSC), the College of Family Physicians of Canada (CFPC), and the Accreditation Council for Graduate Medical Education (ACGME) [72, 78, 79]. Advocacy occurs at the level of individual patients, for example, in completing forms for patients to gain access to resources through insurance or governmental programs. Advocacy also occurs at the level of the community; physicians work to streamline access to healthcare and to enhance the effectiveness of service delivery; physicians advocate for policies and planning that prioritize health equity. On an even greater scale, physicians contribute to national and international advocacy through professional organizations and charitable foundations that support individuals with CKD. This may involve scholarship, education, leadership, and fundraising initiatives.

Physicians are key influencers in the political sphere and can amplify the voice of their patients on important issues related to healthcare and healthy lifestyles. It is important to consider how the community's already-built environment promotes or discourages active living through bike lanes, green space such as parks and trails, sidewalks, and recreation facilities (both indoor and outdoor). Related to equitable access to nutrition, physicians can advocate for eradication of food deserts and distributed access to healthy food share programs and community gardens.

It is important for clinicians to identify the barriers that people with CKD face in trying to adopt healthcare recommendations. Physicians should ask patients if they are able to make ends meet each month and if security of food and/or housing is a concern. It is important to clarify if a person has health insurance and if medication costs are an issue, especially if it is noted that they are not regularly taking their medications. Similarly, clinicians should understand how people manage transportation for healthcare visits. Related to these issues, physicians play a key role in advocating for the eradication of poverty, prioritization of affordable housing, accessibility of medications and healthcare, and affordable healthy food options for all.

CanMEDS, a postgraduate training competency framework, highlights the advocate role and identifies effective physicians as those who are "accountable to society and recognize their duty to contribute to efforts to improve the health and well-being of their patients, their communities, and the broader populations they serve" [72]. The document elaborates that "improving health is not limited to mitigating illness or trauma, but also involves disease prevention, health promotion, and health protection [as well as] promoting health equity, whereby individuals and populations reach their full health potential without being disadvantaged by, for example, race, ethnicity, religion, gender, sexual orientation, age, social class, economic status, or level of education" [71].

Table 19.11 Healthcare provider resources to support lifestyle management in CKD

Organization	Web link
Canadian Society for Exercise Physiology (CSEP)	https://csepguidelines.ca/
Ontario Renal Network (ORN)	https://www.ontariorenalnetwork.ca/en/kidney-care-resources/clinical-tools
KDIGO (Kidney Disease: Improving Global Outcomes)	https://kdigo.org/guidelines/
National Kidney Foundation	https://www.kidney.org/professionals
American Kidney Fund	https://www.kidneyfund.org/training/
Kidney Foundation of Canada	https://kidney.ca
Interdisciplinary Chronic Disease Collaboration (ICDC)	http://www.ckdpathway.ca/
Kidney Supportive Care Research Group	https://www.ckmcare.com/PractitionerPathway/AtAGlance
Canadian Society of Nephrology (CSN)	https://www.csnscn.ca/_education/
Exercise is medicine (EIM)-American College of Sports Medicine (ACSM)	https://www.exerciseismedicine.org/support_page.php/health-care-providers/

Table 19.11 highlights valuable resources for healthcare providers involved in the care of patients with CKD, for continuing education, research, and advocacy initiatives.

19.9 Vignette Analyses: "Samuel and Ana: Learning and Living"

Samuel continued to receive collaborative care from his healthcare team and was actively involved in education and dialogue for self-management, including lifestyle strategies. He continued to learn ways to optimize his nutrition and to meet energy needs for his ongoing physical activity. Although he no longer played competitive soccer, he participated as a team manager and linesman during matches; between dialysis sessions he had a routine which included brisk walking, resistance training, and yoga.

Ana benefited from collaboration with members of her healthcare team to make dietary adjustments and begin supplements; as a result, her iron and vitamin D levels improved to within optimized levels. Sleep apnea was diagnosed, and she initiated treatment with a continuous positive airway pressure (CPAP) device at night, which helped to improve the quality of her sleep. Ana participated in virtual cognitive behavioral therapy (CBT) sessions, which were of benefit to managing her adjustment reaction with depressed mood. She was supported in medical modifications at work which included more frequent breaks, which she used for short periods of sitting and healthy snacks. Overall, Ana noted improved motivation and energy such that she was able to start short walks with her partner around the neighborhood most evenings after dinner.

19.10 Key Takeaways

- Physicians and healthcare providers play an important role to empower patients to engage in healthy lifestyle choices such as physical activity and balanced nutrition.
- Regular physical activity is beneficial to the physical and mental health of patients with CKD, slowing disease progression and risk of complications.
- Dietary choices are important for physical and mental health for patients with CKD, specifically related to reducing risk of cardiovascular disease and optimizing glucose, sodium, phosphorus, potassium, protein, iron, calcium, and vitamin D.
- A patient-centered approach to care that includes identifying a patient's values, priorities, goals, interests, and barriers is key to engaging patients in lifestyle management of CKD.
- Motivational interviewing, patient education, and collaborative self-management are important skills in working with patients to promote healthy lifestyle choices in CKD.
- An interprofessional team-based approach to care is key to optimally supporting patients in lifestyle management of CKD; this includes the expertise of a dietician specializing in kidney disease as patients reach more advanced stages of disease (stages 3–5).
- People with CKD and their families benefit from community connections including peer support groups, community organizations, and advocacy groups.
- Healthcare providers should provide reliable online and app-based resources to support patients with CKD in education and collaborative self-management.
- People with CKD should be encouraged to apply self-compassion in ongoing efforts toward healthy lifestyle choices, maintaining a positive future focus, and learning from challenges and setbacks.
- Physicians and healthcare providers play a key role to advocate for policies and resources that support healthy lifestyle options for all patients, including access to physical activity and financial and food security.

References

1. Chopra S, Malhotra A, Ranjan P, Vikram NK, Singh N. Lifestyle-related advice in the management of obesity: a step-wise approach. J Educ Health Promot. 2020;9:239.
2. Ockene IS, Ockene JK. Barriers to lifestyle change, and the need to develop an integrated approach to prevention. Cardiol Clin. 1996;14(1):159–69.

3. Wharton S, Lau DSW, Vallis M, Sharma AM, Biertho L, et al. Obesity in adults: a clinical practice guideline. CMAJ Aug. 2020;192(31):E875–91.
4. Statistics Canada. Tracking physical activity levels of Canadians, 2016 and 2017. Released 17 Apr 2019. Accessed 10 Apr 2021.
5. Centers for Disease Control and Prevention, National Centre for Health Statistics. Early Release of Selected Estimates based on data from the 2018 National Health Interview Survey. Accessed 10 Apr 2021.
6. Cancer Care Ontario: Insight on Cancer. News and Information on Nutrition and Cancer Prevention. Toronto: Canadian Cancer Society (Ontario Division), 2003. Accessed 10 Apr 2021.
7. Warburton DE, Charlesworth S, Ivey A, Nettlefold L, Bredin SS. A systematic review of the evidence for Canada's physical activity guidelines for adults. Int J Behav Nutr Phys Act. 2010;7:39. Published 2010 May 11.
8. Katzmarzyk PT, Powell KE, Jakicic JM, Troiano RP, Piercy K, Tennant B. 2018 PHYSICAL ACTIVITY GUIDELINES ADVISORY COMMITTEE*. Sedentary behavior and health: update from the 2018 physical activity guidelines Advisory Committee. Med Sci Sports Exerc. 2019;51(6):1227–41.
9. Preamble to the Constitution of WHO as adopted by the International Health Conference, New York, 19 June - 22 July 1946; signed on 22 July 1946 by the representatives of 61 States (Official Records of WHO, no. 2, p. 100) and entered into force on 7 April 1948.
10. Waters H, Foster F, Pieris D, Kinzie S, Zazulak J. Humanism and the Physician. In: Humanism and resilience in residency training. Hategan A, Saperson K, Harms S, Waters H, editors. Springer Nature, Switzerland; 2020.p.1–42.
11. The WHOQOL Group. The World Health Organization quality of life assessment (WHOQOL). Development and psychometric properties. Soc Sci Med. 1998;46:1569–85.
12. Centers for Disease Control and Prevention. Measuring healthy days: Population assessment of health-related quality of life. Centers for Disease Control and Prevention, Atlanta, Georgia: 2000. Accessed 10 April 2021.
13. Caspersen CJ, Powell KE, Christenson GM. Physical activity, exercise, and physical fitness: definitions and distinctions for health-related research. Public Health Rep. 1985;100(2):126–31.
14. Kidney Disease: Improving Global Outcomes (KDIGO) CKD-MBD Update Work Group. KDIGO 2017 clinical practice guideline update for the diagnosis, evaluation, prevention, and treatment of chronic kidney disease–mineral and bone disorder (CKD-MBD). Kidney Int Suppl. 2017;7:1–59.
15. Warburton D, Nicol CW, Bredin S. Health benefits of physical activity. CMAJ. Mar 2006;174(6):801–9.
16. Warburton D, Nicol CW, Bredin S. Prescribing exercise as preventive therapy. CMAJ. 2006;174(7):961–74.
17. Wilkinson TJ, Shur NF, Smith AC. "Exercise as medicine" in chronic kidney disease. Scand J Med Sci Sports. 2016;26:985–8.
18. Kidney Disease: Improving Global Outcomes (KDIGO) CKD Work Group. KDIGO 2012 Clinical Practice Guideline for the Evaluation and Management of Chronic Kidney Disease. Kidney inter., Suppl. 2013;3:1–150.
19. Ross R, Chaput JP, Giangregorio LM, Janssen I, Saunders TJ, et al. Canadian 24-hour movement guidelines for adults aged 18-64 years and adults aged 65 years or older: an integration of physical activity, sedentary behaviour, and sleep. Appl Physiol Nutr Metab. 2020; 45(10 (Suppl. 2)):S57–S102.
20. Kidney Disease: Improving Global Outcomes (KDIGO) Diabetes Work Group. KDIGO 2020 clinical practice guideline for diabetes Management in Chronic Kidney Disease. Kidney Int. 2020;98(4S):S1–S115.

21. Barcellos FC, Santos IS, Umpierre D, Bohlke M, Hallal PC. Effects of exercise in the whole spectrum of chronic kidney disease: a systematic review. Clin Kidney J. 2015;8(6):753–65.
22. Colledge E Prescribing physical activity: using a vital signs approach. Practice Based Small Group Learning Program, Foundation for Medical Practice Education. Shaw EA, editor. 2018; 26(2):1–23.
23. Jetté M, Sidney K, Blümchen G. Metabolic equivalents (METS) in exercise testing, exercise prescription, and evaluation of functional capacity. Clin Cardiol. 1990;13(8):555–65.
24. Mallamaci F, et al. Physical activity in chronic kidney disease and the EXerCise Introdo enhance trial. Nephrol Dialysis Transplant. 2020;(35):ii18–22.
25. Clarkson M, et al. Exercise interventions for improving objective physical function in patients with end-stage kidney disease on dialysis: a systematic review and meta-analysis. Am J Physiol Renal Physiol. 2019;316:F856–72.
26. Owen N, Sparling PB, Healy GN, Dunstan DW, Matthews CE. Sedentary behavior: emerging evidence for a new health risk. Mayo Clin Proc. 2010;85(12):1138–41.
27. Diaz KM, Howard VJ, Hutto B, Colabianchi N, Vena JE, et al. Patterns of sedentary behavior and mortality in U.S. middle-aged and older adults: a National Cohort Study. Ann Intern Med. 2017;167(7):465–75.
28. Rebar AL, et al. A meta-meta-analysis of the effect of physical activity on depression and anxiety in non-clinical adult populations. Health Psychol Rev. 2015;9(3):366–78.
29. Schuch F, Vancampfort D, Firth J, Rosenbaum S, Ward P, Reichert T, et al. Physical activity and sedentary behavior in people with major depressive disorder: a systematic review and meta-analysis. J Affect Disord. 2017;210:139–50. Epub 2016 Nov 29. Erratum in: J Affect Disord. 2018 Jan 1; 225:79. PMID: 28033521
30. Mammen G, Faulkner G. Physical activity and the prevention of depression: a systematic review of prospective studies. Am J Prev Med. 2013;45(5):649–57.
31. Carek PJ, Laibstain SE, Carek SM. Exercise for the treatment of depression and anxiety. Int J Psychiatry Med. 2011;41(1):15–28.
32. Dolezal BA, Neufeld EV, Boland DM, Martin JL, Cooper CB. Interrelationship between sleep and exercise: a systematic review [published correction appears in Adv Prev Med. 2017;2017: 5979510]. Adv Prev Med. 2017;2017:1364387.
33. White RL, et al. Domain-specific physical activity and mental health: a meta-analysis. Am J Prev Med. 2017;52(3):653–66.
34. Romano G, Lorenzon E, Montanaro D. Effects of exercise in renal transplant recipients. World J Transplant. 2012;2(4):46–50.
35. Bredin SSD, Gledhill N, Jamnik VK, Warburton DER. PAR-Q+ and ePARmed-X+. Canadian Family Phys. 2013;59(3):273–7.
36. Frémont P, Fortier M, Frankovich R. Exercise prescription and referral tool to facilitate brief advice to adults in primary care. Canadian Family Phys. 2014;60(12):1120–2.
37. Kondo MC, Oyekanmi KO, Gibson A, South EC, Bocarro J, Hipp JA. Nature prescriptions for health: a review of evidence and research opportunities. Int J Environ Res Public Health. 2020;17(12):4213. Published 2020 Jun 12.
38. Tillmann S, Tobin D, Avison W, et al. Mental health benefits of interactions with nature in children and teenagers: a systematic review. J Epidemiol Community Health. 2018;72:958–66.
39. Chen Y, Michalak M, Agellon LB. Importance of nutrients and nutrient metabolism on human health. Yale J Biol Med. 2018;91(2):95–103. Published 2018 Jun 28.
40. Popkin BM, D'Anci KE, Rosenberg IH. Water, hydration, and health. Nutr Rev. 2010;68(8):439–58.

41. Kidney Disease: Improving Global Outcomes (KDIGO) Anemia Work Group. KDIGO Clinical Practice Guideline for Anemia in Chronic Kidney Disease. Kidney inter., Suppl. 2012;2:279–335.
42. Głąbska D, Guzek D, Groele B, Gutkowska K. Fruit and vegetable intake and mental health in adults: a systematic review. Nutrients. 2020;12(1):115.
43. O'Neil A, Quirk SE, Housden S, Brennan SL, Williams LJ, et al. Relationship between diet and mental health in children and adolescents: a systematic review. Am J Public Health. 2014;104(10):e31–42.
44. Rabi DM, McBrien KA, Sapir-Pichhadze R. Hypertension Canada's 2020 comprehensive guidelines for the prevention, diagnosis, risk assessment, and treatment of hypertension in adults and children. Can J Cardiol. 2020;36(5):596–624.
45. Sievenpiper JL, Chan CB, Dworatzek PD, Freeze C, Williams SL. Diabetes Canada clinical practice guidelines expert Committee. Nutrition therapy. Diabetes Canada 2018 clinical practice guidelines for the prevention and Management of Diabetes in Canada. Can J Diabetes. 2018;42(Suppl 1):S1–S325.
46. Prebtani AP, Bajaj HS, Goldenberg R, Mullan Y. Diabetes Canada clinical practice guidelines expert Committee. Reducing the risk of diabetes. Diabetes Canada 2018 clinical practice guidelines for the prevention and Management of Diabetes in Canada. Can J Diabetes. 2018;42(Suppl 1):S1–S325.
47. Eckel RH, Jakicic JM, Ard JD, de Jesus JM, Houston Miller N, et al. American College of Cardiology/American Heart Association Task Force on Practice Guidelines. 2013 AHA/ACC guideline on lifestyle management to reduce cardiovascular risk: a report of the American College of Cardiology/American Heart Association Task Force on Practice Guidelines. J Am Coll Cardiol. 2014;63(25 Pt B):2960–84. Epub 2013 Nov 12. Erratum in: J Am Coll Cardiol. 2014 Jul 1;63(25 Pt B):3027–3028. PMID: 24239922.
48. Anderson TJ, Gregoire JG, Pearson GJ, Stone JA, Thanassoulis G, WArd R. 2016 Canadian cardiovascular society guidelines for the Management of Dyslipidemia for the prevention of cardiovascular disease in the adult. C J Cardio. 2016;32(11):1263–82.
49. Psaltopoulou T, Sergentanis TN, Panagiotakos DB, Sergentanis IN, Kosti R, Scarmeas N. Mediterranean diet, stroke, cognitive impairment and depression: a meta-analysis. Ann Neurol. 74(4):580–91.
50. Hardman RJ, Kennedy G, Macpherson H, Scholey AB, Pipingas A. Adherence to a Mediterranean-style diet and effects on cognition in adults: a qualitative evaluation and systematic review of longitudinal and prospective trials. Front Nutr. 2016;3:22.
51. Hansrivijit P, Oli S, Khanal R, Ghahramani N, Thongprayoon C, Cheungpasitporn W. Mediterranean diet and the risk of chronic kidney disease: a systematic review and meta-analysis. Nephrology. 2020;25:913–8.
52. Khatri M, et al. The association between a Mediterranean-style diet and kidney function in the northern Manhattan study cohort. Clin J Am Soc Nephrol. 2014;9:1868–975.
53. Beto, et al. Medical nutrition therapy in adults with chronic kidney disease: integrating evidence and consensus into practice for the generalist registered dietitian nutritionist. JADA. 2014;114(7):1077–87.
54. Leung AA, Daskalopoulou SS, Dasgupta K, et al. Hypertension Canada's 2017 guidelines for diagnosis, risk assessment, prevention, and treatment of hypertension in adults. Can J Cardiol. 2017;33(5):557–76.
55. Ikizler TA, Burrowes JD, Byham-Gray LD, et al. KDOQI nutrition in CKD guideline work group. KDOQI clinical practice guideline for nutrition in CKD: 2020 update. Am J Kidney Dis. 2020;76(3:suppl 1):S1–S107.
56. Mills KT, Stefanescu A, He J. The global epidemiology of hypertension. Nat Rev Nephrol. 2020;16:223–37.

57. Yazdi F, Morreale P, Reisin E. First course DASH, second course Mediterranean: comparing renal outcomes for two "heart-healthy" diets hypertension and obesity. (E Reisin, section editor). Curr Hypertens Rep. 2020;22:54.
58. Taghavia M, Sadeghi A, Maleki V, Nasiri M, Khodadost M, et al. Adherence to the dietary approaches to stop hypertension-style diet is inversely associated with chronic kidney disease: a systematic review and meta-analysis of prospective cohort studies. Nutr Res. 2019;72:46–56.
59. Chauveau P, Aparicio M, Bellizzi V, et al. European renal nutrition (ERN) working Group of the European Renal Association–European Dialysis Transplant Association (ERA-EDTA). Mediterranean diet as the diet of choice for patients with chronic kidney disease. Nephrol Dialysis Transpl. 2018;33(5):725–35.
60. Bach-Faig A, Berry EM, Lairon D, Reguant J, Trichopoulou A, et al. Mediterranean diet foundation expert group. Mediterranean diet pyramid today. Science and cultural updates. Public Health Nutr. 2011;14(12A):2274–84.
61. Kaidar-Person O, Person B, Szomstein S, et al. Nutritional deficiencies in morbidly obese patients: a new form of malnutrition? Obes Surg. 2008;18:870–6.
62. Kidney Disease: Improving Global Outcomes (KDIGO) Lipid Work Group. KDIGO Clinical Practice Guideline for Lipid Management in Chronic Kidney Disease. Kidney inter., Suppl. 2013;3:259–305.
63. Clegg DJ, Hill Gallant KM. Plant-based diets in CKD. CJASN Jan. 2019;14(1):141–3.
64. Kimball SM, Holick MF. Official recommendations for vitamin D through the life stages in developed countries. Eur J Clin Nutr. 2020;74:1514–8.
65. Norcross JC, Krebs PM, Prochaska JO. Stages of change. J Clin Psychol. 2011;67:143–54.
66. Zimmerman GL, Olsen CG, Bosworth MF. A 'stages of change' approach to helping patients change behavior. Am Fam Physician. 2000;61(5):1409–16. PMID: 10735346
67. Clarke S, et al. Defining elements of patient-centred care for therapeutic relationships: a literature review of common themes. Eur J Person Centred Healthcare. 2017;5(3):362–72.
68. Doran GT. There's a S.M.A.R.T. way to write Management's goals and objectives. Manag Rev. 1981;70(11):35–6.
69. Rubak S, Sandbaek A, Lauritzen T, Christensen B. Motivational interviewing: a systematic review and meta-analysis. British J General Practice J R College General Practitioners. 2005;55(513):305–12.
70. Hall K, Gibbie T, Lubman DI. Motivational interviewing techniques - facilitating behaviour change in the general practice setting. Aust Fam Physician. 2012;41(9):660–7. PMID: 22962639
71. Warburton DER, Bredin SSD. Health benefits of physical activity: a strengths-based approach. J Clin Med. 2019;8(12):2044. Published 2019 Nov 21.
72. Sherbino J, Bonnycastle D, Côté B, Flynn L, Hunter A, et al. Health advocate. In: Frank JR, Snell L, Sherbino J, editors. CanMEDS 2015 physician competency framework. Ottawa: Royal College of Physicians and Surgeons of Canada; 2015.
73. Bodenheimer T, Lorig K, Holman H, Grumbach K. Patient self-management of chronic disease in primary care. JAMA. 2002;288(19):2469–75.
74. Warsi A, Wang PS, LaValley MP, Avorn J, Solomon DH. Self-management education programs in chronic disease: a systematic review and methodological critique of the literature. Arch Intern Med. 2004;164(15):1641–9.
75. Lin M, Liu M, Hsu L, Tsai P. Effects of self-management on chronic kidney disease: a meta-analysis. Int J Nurs Stud. 2017;74:128–37.
76. Morton RL, Sellars M. From patient-Centred to Person-Centred Care for Kidney Diseases. CJASN. Apr 2019;14(40):623–5.
77. Siddique AB, Krebs M, Alvarez S, et al. Mobile apps for the Care Management of Chronic Kidney and end-Stage Renal Diseases: systematic search in app stores and evaluation. JMIR Mhealth Uhealth. 2019;7(9):e12604. Published 2019 Sep 4.

78. Ince-Cushman D. Health advocate. In: Shaw E, Oandasan I, Fowler N, editors. CanMEDS-FM 2017: a competency framework for family physicians across the continuum. Mississauga: The College of Family Physicians of Canada; 2017.
79. Kirmayer LJ, Kronick R, Rousseau C. Advocacy as key to structural competency in psychiatry. JAMA Psychiat. 2018;75(2):119–20.

20 Gender Disparity and Women's Health in Kidney Disease

Anika Lucas and Silvi Shah

20.1 Introduction

The Institute of Medicine defines gender as "self-representation as male or female, or how that person is responded to by social institutions based on the individual's gender presentation" [1, 2]. Gender therefore encompasses the social differences between men and women that are governed by culture, society, and relationships. Sex is defined as "the classification of living things, generally as male or female according to their reproductive organs and functions assigned by chromosomal complement" [1]. These distinctions between gender and sex are important when evaluating differences between men and women in the context of kidney disease. It was not until 1993 when the National Institute of Health mandated researchers to include both men and women in federally funded clinical studies through the National Institutes of Health Revitalization Act [3]. Since then, there has been an exponential increase in research studies dedicated to understanding the specific experiences of women with kidney diseases.

A. Lucas
Division of Nephrology, Department of Medicine, Duke University School of Medicine, Durham, NC, USA

S. Shah (✉)
Division of Nephrology, Kidney CARE Program, Department of Internal Medicine, University of Cincinnati College of Medicine, Cincinnati, OH, USA
e-mail: shah2sv@ucmail.uc.edu

A. Hategan et al. (eds.), *Psychonephrology*,
https://doi.org/10.1007/978-3-030-84740-1_20

20.2 Gender Disparities in Chronic Kidney Disease

Chronic kidney disease (CKD) is more prevalent among women than men in many parts of the world; for instance, the prevalence of CKD in women is double that of men in France, Thailand, Portugal, and Turkey [2, 4]. In the United States, 15% of women have CKD versus 12.8% of men [5]. Longer life expectancy in women, resulting in age-related kidney decline, may contribute to these differences. Interestingly, the Chronic Kidney Disease Epidemiology Collaboration (CKD-EPI) equation used to estimate glomerular filtration rate (GFR) assigns a lower GFR to women compared to men of the same age, race, and serum creatinine value. Measured GFR using iohexol clearance similarly demonstrates lower GFR values in women. While the CKD-EPI equation is commonly used in clinical practice, it contains measurement bias. Measured GFR is often higher than estimated GFR using the CKD-EPI equation, leading to an underestimation of kidney function in women [4]. Further epidemiological studies are needed to fully investigate accurate measurements of decreased kidney function in women and determine its actual prevalence.

Although CKD is more prevalent among women, men are at greater risk for the development of end-stage kidney disease (ESKD). In a Norwegian study evaluating the risk of kidney failure and death, the 10-year cumulative incidence of kidney failure was 0.08 (95% confidence interval [CI] 0.05–0.11) in men and 0.03 (95% CI 0.02–0.04) in women [6]. A similar trend was observed for the incidence of death in the same population. The 10-year cumulative incidence of death was 0.61 in men and 0.47 in women [6]. Similarly, the Australia and New Zealand Dialysis and Transplant Registry (ANZDATA) observed that 60% of patients with ESKD were men [2, 4].

Testosterone has been suggested as a possible contributor to decline in kidney function. Testosterone has been implicated for its pro-inflammatory effects, in contrast to estrogen which has demonstrated anti-fibrotic and anti-apoptotic characteristics. There are three different estrogen receptors in the kidney: estrogen receptor alpha, estrogen receptor beta, and G-protein-coupled receptor. Estradiol 2 decreases collagen synthesis and may increase nitric oxide synthase resulting in intraglomerular vasodilation and decreased filtration fraction [7]. Young premenopausal women, post-oophorectomy, are at increased risk for CKD. Observational studies on raloxifene and selective estrogen receptor modulators (SERM) show decreased CKD progression suggesting estrogen may be renoprotective. Selective estrogen receptor modulators or 17-ß-estradiol may reduce albuminuria, tubulointerstitial injury, and podocytopathy and improve kidney function. This suggests that sex hormones may also play an important role in kidney disease and possible progression of disease.

Estrogen and testosterone also have varying impact on the renin-angiotensin system (RAS). Estrogen decreases the synthesis of angiotensin-converting enzyme while increasing the synthesis of angiotensinogen. There is a decrease in arterial pressure via the angiotensin type 2 (AT2) and angiotensin-converting enzyme 2 (ACE2) receptors. Testosterone promotes the release of renin increasing arterial pressure. In addition to the impact of sex hormones, X-linked and Y-linked genes, chromosome mosaicism, and parental imprinting have been associated with kidney injury [5, 8]. These differences in sex hormones largely observed in animal studies may provide some explanations on how hormonal differences contribute to disparities in CKD progression between men and women.

While multiple studies demonstrate more rapid kidney disease progression in men, further evaluation for disparities in nephrology care is also needed. It is unclear if there are major differences in nephrology clinic referral rates between men and women throughout the world. We know that women are less likely to have an awareness regarding CKD, which may impact their care. Using data from NHANES, Coresh et al. observed that women with CKD had lower levels of CKD awareness [2, 9]. Additionally, there are also gender disparities in permanent dialysis access. The odds of arteriovenous fistula placement are lower in women when initiating hemodialysis compared to men. Smaller vessel size, differences in referral for vascular access procedures, and hesitancy to have surgery among women contribute to these gender disparities.

Unfortunately, racial disparities in arteriovenous fistula placement are further observed among Black women who had even lower the odds of arteriovenous fistula placement compared to men upon initiation of hemodialysis (odds ratio [OR] 0.66, 95% CI 0.62–0.69, $p < 0.0001$), while non-Black women had OR 0.70 (95% CI 0.68–0.73, $p < 0.0001$) [7]. Women are also more likely to choose conservative management of their kidney disease. Several studies have found that older women are two or three times more likely to choose conservative management of kidney disease [2, 4, 10]. More studies on how nephrology care impacts women with CKD including ESKD are needed.

20.3 Gender Disparities in Hospitalizations and Mortality in Patients with ESKD

Women receiving kidney replacement therapy are at risk for increased hospitalization and mortality. Women on hemodialysis have a 20% higher rate of all-cause hospitalization and length of stay as compared to men in the United States [4]. Women on peritoneal dialysis also have a higher risk of hospitalization, with infection-related hospitalizations accounting for 24% increased risk in women as compared to men. These risks for hospitalization are more pronounced among *younger* women receiving kidney replacement therapy compared to older women. For instance, women between the ages of 18 and 34 years had more than 50% higher risk of hospitalization than men, but women over 75 years old had only 16% higher risk of hospitalization than men of similar age. These gender differences in risks for hospitalization in patients with ESKD may be attributed to differences in hypoalbuminemia, a marker of decreased health status, nonadherence to medications, and/or other medical therapy [4].

Although women often have a survival advantage over men in the general population, this advantage is often lost with kidney replacement therapy. Younger women on dialysis under 45 years of age have shown to have a higher mortality as compared to men of the same age. Much of the higher death rate among younger women on dialysis is attributed to infection. For instance, women on peritoneal dialysis have higher rates of death due to sepsis and peritonitis. Similar results have also been observed in children, with girls having higher rates of infection-related deaths as compared to boys [11]. Data from the Dialysis Outcomes and Practice Patterns Study (DOPPS) in the United States and Japan demonstrated that urea reduction ratio, a percentage used to denote how much urea is removed with dialysis, was associated with mortality risk. Female dialysis patients with a urea reduction ratio of over 75% had a decrease in mortality risk by 15% compared to women with a urea reduction ratio of 70–75% [11]. Higher urea clearances have been associated with reduced mortality in women on dialysis. These results were supported by the Hemodialysis (HEMO) study in which women on hemodialysis also experienced reduced mortality and morbidity with intensive dialysis dose in the setting of residual kidney function [7].

20.4 Gender Differences in Kidney Transplantation

Women are more likely to be kidney transplant donors rather than recipients. Decreased numbers of male donors may be a result of comorbidities, high disease burden, and social concerns such as taking time off from work [7]. In addition, human leukocyte antigen (HLA) sensitization in multiparous women may contribute to disparities in kidney transplantation. Other barriers to transplant include referral to transplant nephrologists and placement on the waiting list. Older women may be less likely to be placed on the transplant waiting list. Women above age 55 were 29% less likely to be on the transplant list compared to women less than 45 years of age [12]. Once transplanted, there are gender differences in allograft survival. Multiple studies have observed higher or equal risk of allograft failure in women compared to men. In contrast, women age 45 years and older had reduced outcomes of allograft failure [4]. Studies on quality of life posttransplant also do not demonstrate a drastic improvement in women as they do for men.

20.5 Common Disorders and Psychosocial Concerns of Women with Kidney Disease

20.5.1 Depressive Disorders

Depressive disorder is the most common comorbid psychiatric condition among patients with ESKD on hemodialysis and has been associated with mortality and hospitalizations in patients with ESKD [3]. Patients with depressive disorder have higher rates of hospitalization than other patients without psychiatric comorbidity. Depressive disorder continues to be more prevalent in women on hemodialysis compared to men [4]. Despite these findings, patients are often untreated. Social support has been found to be a predictor of survival in patients on hemodialysis.

This is complicated by the fact that often spouses of patients may also experience depressive symptoms. Approximately 20% of spouses of patients on dialysis reported depressive symptoms in a Canadian study [13]. Women on hemodialysis additionally score higher on scales measuring anxiety as well.

Assessments on quality of life such as the health-related quality of life (HRQOL) demonstrate a lower score in women than in men. Lower scores on the HRQOL have been associated with depressive disorders [10]. Although transplant generally decreases mortality and increases quality of life, improvement in quality of life is not as commonly observed in women than men. Further studies on quality of life of women with kidney disease, including those requiring kidney replacement therapy, are needed to properly elucidate the psychosocial impact of kidney disease on patients. (For more information on psychiatric aspects in patients with CKD, see Chap. 10, Common Psychiatric Disorders in the Renal Patient.)

Clinical Pearl

- Diagnosing depressive disorder in patients with kidney disease may be challenging as symptoms of fatigue, weakness, and failure to thrive may be attributed to their underlying kidney disease and not the depressive disorder. Patients with kidney disease should be evaluated for uremia with concern for inadequate dialysis or need to initiate dialysis.

20.5.2 Sexual Dysfunction

Sexual dysfunction is common among women with kidney disease, especially those requiring kidney replacement therapy. Prevalence of sexual dysfunction is 50–80% in patients with CKD [14]. Sexual dysfunction has been associated with depressive disorder, menopause, age, diabetes mellitus, and risk for cardiovascular events. Common manifestations of sexual dysfunction in women with CKD are presented in Table 20.1 [15].

Table 20.1 Common associated factors and manifestations of sexual dysfunction in women with chronic kidney disease [15]

Associated factors	Common manifestations
Age	Atrophic vaginitis
Depressive disorder	Dyspareunia
Menopause	Decreased vaginal lubrication
Diabetes mellitus	Infertility
Risk for cardiovascular events	Early menopause
	Amenorrhea
	Loss of libido
	Difficulty with arousal or orgasm
	Hypogonadism

Hormonal abnormalities contribute to sexual dysfunction. Hyperprolactinemia is observed in women with advanced kidney disease because of decreased kidney clearance and increased prolactin production. Prolactin inhibits gonadotrophin synthesis, decreasing libido, and contributes to amenorrhea and oligomenorrhea. Decreased levels of estradiol have also been implicated in sexual dysfunction. Lower levels of estradiol cause vaginal atrophy, vaginal dryness, and dyspareunia, contributing to sexual dysfunction in women with kidney disease [10, 16]. Although hormone replacement therapy has been demonstrated to improve sexual activity in young women with advanced CKD, there is limited data on the benefits of hormone replacement therapy in postmenopausal women with advanced kidney disease [16]. Hyperparathyroidism also contributes to sexual dysfunction.

The Female Sexual Function Index (FSFI) is a 19-item questionnaire which includes the following categories: sexual desire, arousal, orgasm, satisfaction, pain, and lubrication, with a maximum score of 36. Studies utilizing the FSFI measure on women with CKD with/without ESKD demonstrate lower scores than in the general population. Scores less than 26.5 were suggestive of sexual dysfunction [15]. Dialysis modality may also impact performance on the FSFI measure, with patients on hemodialysis scoring lower. Sexual dysfunction can also impact quality of life. It has also been associated with anxiety, depression, loss of self-confidence and esteem, poor self-image, and marital issues, as well as adverse cardiovascular outcomes [10].

Treatment of sexual dysfunction involves management of underlying comorbidities and review of medications which may be associated with sexual dysfunction, such as aromatase inhibitors, antidepressants, and antipsychotics. Testosterone has also been effective in improving sexual interest in women with hypoactive sexual desire disorder [15]. Kidney transplant can improve sexual health with evidence of improvement in FSFI observed in previous studies. (For more information on sexual function aspects in patients with CKD, see Chap. 13.)

Clinical Pearl

- Many antidepressants, mood stabilizers including lithium, antipsychotics, benzodiazepines, antihypertensives, immunosuppressants, spironolactone, opioids, and glucocorticoids are associated with sexual dysfunction.

Recommendation

- In addition to a detailed medical and sexual history, the Female Sexual Function Index (FSFI), medications, and laboratory data (BUN, creatinine) should be obtained to evaluate sexual dysfunction in women with kidney disease.

20.6 Pregnancy in CKD

Pregnancy is not as common in women with CKD (including ESKD) compared to the general population. Kidney disease disrupts the hypothalamic-pituitary ovarian axis, resulting in reduction in fertility. The normal cyclical release of gonadotropin-releasing hormone does not occur, causing impaired functioning of the luteinizing hormone and follicular-stimulating hormone, leading to low estrogen levels and anovulation. Hyperprolactinemia due to overproduction and decreased kidney clearance also contributes to anovulation [17]. For example, 70% of women on dialysis either experience amenorrhea or oligomenorrhea [18]. Additionally, sexual dysfunction may limit sexual activity and become another barrier to conception for women with CKD.

Unfortunately, women with CKD including ESKD have a higher risk of adverse pregnancy outcomes than the general population. Women with CKD have fivefold increased odds of preterm birth and tenfold increased odds of preeclampsia [19]. Women with ESKD have higher rates of preeclampsia, occurring in 5–20% of pregnancies, cesarean delivery in up to 74% of pregnancies, with up to 70% of neonates requiring neonatal intensive care admission upon delivery [18].

Important adaptive physiological changes occur at 4–6 weeks gestation [20]. Systemic vasodilation occurs with an increase in plasma volume. In the kidney, vasodilation gives rise to an increase in renal plasma flow and GFR. GFR can increase up to 40–50%. Proteinuria also increases during this period due to glomerular hyperfiltration and can be as high as 300 mg/g based on 24-hour urine collection [19].

Qualitative studies that have assessed the perspectives of women with CKD regarding motherhood have shown that many women had the desire to have children and expressed sentiments of grief, guilt, and blame due to failure to conceive. Perspectives regarding motherhood varied based on country of origin. For instance, women in Brazil and Saudi Arabia defined success by marriage and motherhood, while women in the United States felt that their relationships with their partners improved because of experiencing challenges to conceive [21]. Women also expressed fear and apprehension of emotional attachment and investment to the fetus due to concerns for miscarriage, stillbirth, or genetic defects. As a result, some women were reluctant to purchase items for their unborn children. Women with kidney transplants also expressed concerns about how their babies may be impacted by exposure to immunosuppression [21].

Prenatal care of women with kidney disease requires close observation with multidisciplinary management by nephrologists, neonatologists, dieticians, social workers, nurses, as well as other specialists depending on other comorbid conditions. Low-dose aspirin should be used for the prevention of preeclampsia. Women on hemodialysis should undergo frequent and intensive hemodialysis sessions. Similarly, women on peritoneal dialysis may require increased volume and exchanges, which may be challenging with the growing fetus.

20.7 Pregnancy in Kidney Transplant

Posttransplant fertility rates increase as the function of the hypothalamic-pituitary ovarian axis is restored due to improvement in kidney function. A meta-analysis on live birth rates in kidney transplantation through 2017 demonstrated a 73% live birth rate compared to 62% in the general population [22]. Nevertheless, transplant recipients remain at risk for adverse maternal and fetal outcomes. Over 50% of pregnancies are at risk for hypertension, while up to 30% of pregnancies are at risk for preeclampsia [22]. The risk for cesarean section is higher among transplant patients compared to the general population and was observed to be at 62.6% vs. 26.9–32.7%. The risk of preterm birth can range between 43.1% and 65.4% among pregnancies in kidney transplant recipients [22]. Allograft rejection remains a concern in the immediate transplant period. Pregnant patients with allograft dysfunction, with a serum creatinine >1.3 mg/dL, hypertension, and/or proteinuria defined as >500 mg/day are at higher risk for allograft failure.

Changes to immunosuppression regimen is an important consideration prior to pregnancy. Mycophenolate mofetil can cause congenital malformations such as congenital heart defects and cleft lip and palate, as well as adverse pregnancy outcomes such as preterm birth and miscarriage [19]. Calcineurin inhibitors (e.g., tacrolimus), azathioprine, corticosteroids, and intravenous immunoglobulin can be safely used in pregnancy. In contrast, mTOR inhibitors like sirolimus and everolimus have been found to be associated with higher fetal mortality in animal studies and are contraindicated in pregnancy [19]. There are limited studies on the use of belatacept, antithymocyte globulin, basiliximab, rituximab, and alemtuzumab in pregnancy for immunosuppression, which requires further investigation [19, 22].

Clinical Pearl

- Chronic kidney disease is a risk factor for adverse maternal and fetal pregnancy outcomes.

Recommendation

- An interdisciplinary team composed of nephrologists, maternal fetal medicine physicians, and neonatologists is needed to provide effective perinatal management.

20.8 Case Vignette

A 32-year-old female sought preconception counseling. She had end-stage kidney disease due to IgA nephropathy. She received a kidney transplant from her husband 2 years previously. She had an acute rejection episode 4 months posttransplantation that was successfully treated with glucocorticoids, and kidney function had been stable subsequently. She felt well and reported no symptoms at evaluation. Vital signs included blood pressure of 114/68 mm Hg and pulse rate of 76/min. Physical examination was normal. Laboratory studies showed creatinine of 1.2 mg/dL. Her current medications were mycophenolate, tacrolimus, and prednisone. What would be the most appropriate management?

20.9 Case Vignette Analysis

Based on the patient's presentation in the vignette, mycophenolate should be switched to azathioprine. Management of immunosuppression in kidney transplant recipients is important due to the concern for teratogenic risk. Mycophenolate mofetil is a US FDA category D drug and has shown to be associated with limb and facial congenital anomalies including microtia, hypoplastic nails, shortened fifth finger, cleft lip and palate, congenital diaphragmatic hernia, and congenital heart defects. Additionally, mycophenolate mofetil increases the risk of spontaneous abortion and congenital malformation. Although data is limited with human exposure with sirolimus, sirolimus is contraindicated in pregnancy due to increased fetal mortality in animal studies. Azathioprine, low-dose corticosteroids (less than 20 mg/day in prednisone equivalents), and calcineurin inhibitors, including tacrolimus and cyclosporine, are safe to be used during pregnancy. Medications that are teratogenic should be switched or stopped at least 6 weeks before conception in kidney transplant recipients. Due to similar pharmacological class effects, it is recommended to switch mycophenolate mofetil to azathioprine and sirolimus to calcineurin inhibitors. Counseling for childbearing and risk of teratogenicity with immunosuppression should start as early as pretransplant evaluation and should be continued at every posttransplant clinic visit. Women of childbearing potential should undergo risk evaluation and mitigation strategy (REMS) and should be advised to use effective contraception while taking mycophenolate.

20.10 Postpartum Care in Patients with CKD

Careful monitoring of blood pressure should occur as women with kidney disease are at higher risk for hypertensive disorders. Additionally, medications should be evaluated to ensure they are safe if women choose to breastfeed. Ultrafiltration should also be limited in women requiring kidney replacement due to a reduction in breast milk production with aggressive fluid removal. Finally, social and emotional support should be provided to women with CKD and kidney transplant as postpartum depression is higher among women with chronic medical conditions [18, 23].

Management of women with kidney disease in the peripartum period is summarized in Table 20.2 [18, 19, 22, 24].

Clinical Pearl

- Women with CKD are at higher risk of postpartum complications.

Table 20.2 Management of women with kidney disease in the peripartum period [18, 19, 22, 24]

Prepregnancy	Pregnancy	Delivery	Postpartum
Assess underlying renal disease with stable renal function/disease and minimal proteinuria preferable prior to pregnancy	Continue to evaluate renal function and manage underlying renal disease with medications that are safe for pregnancy Common causes of acute kidney injury: Hyperemesis gravidarum Septic abortion Urinary tract infection Preeclampsia Hemolysis Elevated liver enzymes Low platelets syndrome Acute fatty liver of pregnancy Obstructive uropathy Placental abruption and placental hemorrhage	Assess renal function	Assess renal function and blood pressure
Review medications and stop teratogenic medications if pregnancy desired	Target blood pressure <150/90 mm Hg with close monitoring for preeclampsia Prescribe aspirin to decrease risk for preeclampsia	Evaluate for signs of magnesium toxicity and magnesium levels in patients with CKD who receive magnesium for prevention of eclampsia	Assess for signs of postpartum mood disorders such as depressive disorder or blues, postpartum psychosis, or posttraumatic stress disorder
Optimize blood pressure with control of additional comorbid conditions	Initiate prophylactic anticoagulation for patients with nephrotic syndrome and hypoalbuminemia and history of thrombosis (e.g., systemic lupus erythematosus with antiphospholipid antibodies) with unfractionated heparin or low molecular weight heparin Monitor for anemia	Careful evaluation of individual patient's anatomy warranted with location of a transplanted kidney and/or ureters, bladder to prevent injury during cesarean delivery	Review medications and ensure safe for breast feeding
Utilize shared decision-making to determine the best time for pregnancy	Consider if biopsy necessary with preference for first and second trimesters if warranted		Discuss plan for contraception

Recommendation

– During the postpartum period, women with CKD should be monitored for preeclampsia, acute kidney injury, thrombotic microangiopathies, venous thromboembolism, and postpartum mood disorder.

20.11 Key Takeaways

- There is a high prevalence of CKD among women as compared to men worldwide.
- Women with CKD have lower CKD awareness, inferior dialysis access placement, and decreased access to kidney transplants, as compared to men with CKD.
- Women with kidney disease have a high prevalence of depressive disorders and sexual dysfunction.
- Women with kidney disease are at increased risk of adverse maternal and fetal outcomes during pregnancy including postpartum depressive disorder.

References

1. Institute of Medicine Committee on Understanding the Biology of S. Gender D: The National Academies Collection: reports funded by National Institutes of Health. In: Wizemann TM, Pardue ML, editors. Exploring the biological contributions to human health: does sex matter? Washington, DC: National Academies Press (US); 2001. Copyright 2001 by the National Academy of Sciences. All rights reserved.; 2001.
2. Carrero JJ, Hecking M, Ulasi I, Sola L, Thomas B. Chronic kidney disease, gender, and access to care: a global perspective. Semin Nephrol. 2017;37(3):296–308.
3. Cobo G, Hecking M, Port FK, et al. Sex and gender differences in chronic kidney disease: progression to end-stage renal disease and haemodialysis. Clin Sci (Lond). 2016;130(14):1147–63.
4. Carrero JJ, Hecking M, Chesnaye NC, Jager KJ. Sex and gender disparities in the epidemiology and outcomes of chronic kidney disease. Nat Rev Nephrol. 2018;14(3):151–64.
5. Bairey Merz CN, Dember LM, Ingelfinger JR, et al. Sex and the kidneys: current understanding and research opportunities. Nat Rev Nephrol. 2019;15(12):776–83.
6. Eriksen BO, Ingebretsen OC. The progression of chronic kidney disease: a 10-year population-based study of the effects of gender and age. Kidney Int. 2006;69(2):375–82.
7. Brar A, Markell M. Impact of gender and gender disparities in patients with kidney disease. Curr Opin Nephrol Hypertens. 2019;28(2):178–82.
8. Park YJ, Kim JM. Klotho and postmenopausal hormone replacement therapy in women with chronic kidney disease. J Menopausal Med. 2018;24(2):75–80.
9. Coresh J, Byrd-Holt D, Astor BC, et al. Chronic kidney disease awareness, prevalence, and trends among U.S. adults, 1999 to 2000. J Am Soc Nephrol. 2005;16(1):180–8.
10. Guglielmi KE. Women and ESRD: modalities, survival, unique considerations. Adv Chronic Kidney Dis. 2013;20(5):411–8.
11. Vongsanim S, Davenport A. The effect of gender on survival for hemodialysis patients: why don't women live longer than men? Semin Dial. 2019;32(5):438–43.
12. Lew SQ, Patel SS. Psychosocial and quality of life issues in women with end-stage renal disease. Adv Chronic Kidney Dis. 2007;14(4):358–63.
13. Kimmel PL, Patel SS. Psychosocial issues in women with renal disease. Adv Ren Replace Ther. 2003;10(1):61–70.
14. Navaneethan SD, Vecchio M, Johnson DW, et al. Prevalence and correlates of self-reported sexual dysfunction in CKD: a meta-analysis of observational studies. Am J Kidney Dis. 2010;56(4):670–85.
15. Ali S, Dave NN. Sexual dysfunction in women with kidney disease. Adv Chronic Kidney Dis. 2020;27(6):506–15.
16. Vellanki K, Hou S. Menopause in CKD. Am J Kidney Dis. 2018;71(5):710–9.
17. Burgner A, Hladunewich MA. Women's reproductive health for the nephrologist. Am J Kidney Dis. 2019;74(5):675–81.

18. Oliverio AL, Hladunewich MA. End-stage kidney disease and dialysis in pregnancy. Adv Chronic Kidney Dis. 2020;27(6):477–85.
19. Reynolds ML, Herrera CA. Chronic kidney disease and pregnancy. Adv Chronic Kidney Dis. 2020;27(6):461–8.
20. Blom K, Odutayo A, Bramham K, Hladunewich MA. Pregnancy and glomerular disease: a systematic review of the literature with management guidelines. Clin J Am Soc Nephrol. 2017;12(11):1862–72.
21. Tong A, Jesudason S, Craig JC, Winkelmayer WC. Perspectives on pregnancy in women with chronic kidney disease: systematic review of qualitative studies. Nephrol Dial Transplant. 2015;30(4):652–61.
22. Gonzalez Suarez ML, Parker AS, Cheungpasitporn W. Pregnancy in kidney transplant recipients. Adv Chronic Kidney Dis. 2020;27(6):486–98.
23. Brown HK, Qazilbash A, Rahim N, Dennis C-L, Vigod SN. Chronic medical conditions and peripartum mental illness: a systematic review and meta-analysis. Am J Epidemiol. 2018;187(9):2060–8.
24. Pillay C, Clark K. Postpartum care of women with renal disease. Best Pract Res Clin Obstet Gynaecol. 2019;57:89–105.

Cultural Considerations When Caring for Racial and Ethnic Minority Patients with End-Stage Renal Disease

21

Emma Gregory, Tricia K.W. Woo, and Ana Hategan

21.1 The Basics of Chronic Kidney Disease and End-Stage Renal Disease

As it is also detailed elsewhere in this book, we will only briefly review chronic kidney disease (CKD) including end-stage renal disease (ESRD) here. In 2012, Kidney Disease: Improving Global Outcomes (KDIGO) updated their *Clinical Practice Guideline for the Evaluation and Management of Chronic Kidney Disease* [1]. The guideline defines CKD as "abnormalities of kidney structure or function, present for at least 3 months, with implications for health." CKD is further classified according to etiology, glomerular filtration rate (GFR), and degree of albuminuria. It is divided into five main classifications, summarized in Table 21.1 [1]. Category G5 (GFR < 15 mL/min/1.73 m^2) indicates renal failure.

In response, the Canadian Society of Nephrology suggested adding the suffix "–D" to category G5 to signify patients treated with dialysis and "–T" for those treated with renal transplantation (RTX) [2]. Dialysis and RTX are the two renal replacement therapy (RRT) options available to patients. Suffix "–ND" signifies

E. Gregory (✉)
Department of Psychiatry and Behavioural Neurosciences, Michael G. DeGroote School of Medicine, McMaster University, Hamilton, ON, Canada
e-mail: emma.gregory@medportal.ca

T. K.W. Woo
Division of Geriatric Medicine, Department of Medicine, McMaster University, Hamilton, ON, Canada
e-mail: twoo@hhsc.ca

A. Hategan
Division of Geriatric Psychiatry, Department of Psychiatry & Behavioural Neurosciences, Faculty of Health Sciences, Michael G. DeGroote School of Medicine, McMaster University, Hamilton, ON, Canada
e-mail: hategan@mcmaster.ca

A. Hategan et al. (eds.), *Psychonephrology*,
https://doi.org/10.1007/978-3-030-84740-1_21

Table 21.1 The five classifications of CKD (Adapted from KDIGO 2012) [1]

GFR category	GFR (mL/min/1.73 m^2)	Change in renal function
G1	≥ 90	Normal or high
G2	60–89	Mildly decreased
G3a	45–59	Mildly to moderately decreased
G3b	30–44	Moderately to severely decreased
G4	15–29	Severely decreased
G5	<15	Renal failure

CKD chronic kidney disease, *KDIGO* Kidney Disease: Improving Global Outcomes

patients who receive neither [2]. G5ND does not differentiate between patients for whom RRT is inaccessible, those who decline it, and those who have not yet been offered it [2]. While ESRD is not part of KDIGO's clinical nomenclature, it generally refers to patients with renal failure (defined by KDIGO) or those who require RRT to survive [3]. As one will come to see, patients with ESRD face a variety of complex medical decisions about their renal care, which may be further complicated by cultural factors.

Clinical Pearl

- CKD is "abnormalities of kidney structure or function, present for at least 3 months, with implications for health" [1].
- Patients with ESRD have renal failure (i.e., GFR < 15 mL/min/1.73 m^2) and/or rely on RRT (dialysis or renal transplantation) to survive [1, 3].

21.2 The Global Burden of CKD and ESRD

In 2017, the GBD Chronic Kidney Disease Collaboration published a systematic analysis of the estimated global burden of disease (GBD) in those with CKD [3]. At that time there were nearly 698 million cases of CKD worldwide, and the average prevalence was 9.1% (ranging from 8.5% to 9.8%) [3]. A subset of patients with CKD progress to ESRD depending on etiology, GFR, degree of albuminuria, and other important risk factors [1]. In their analysis, the Collaboration defined ESRD as patients with CKD who were treated with RRT [3]. The G5 category accounted for 0.07% of the global prevalence rate in 2017, while dialysis and RTX accounted for 0.04% and 0.01%, respectively [3].

Furthermore, CKD was associated with high morbidity in 2017, resulting in nearly 36 million disability-adjusted life years (DALYs). Patients with renal failure or on dialysis were the most affected [3]. In sum, DALYs is the number of "years of productive life lost due to disability," as well as "years of potential life lost due to premature mortality" [4]. About 2.5 million patients worldwide received RRT in 2017, and this number is expected to double by 2030 with increasing global access to RRT [3]. CKD was also associated with high mortality, ranking as the 12th leading cause of death that year (partly due to poor access to RRT) and causing over one million patient deaths [3]. Now that we have briefly reviewed CKD and ESRD as well as their global burden, we will turn our attention to the growing diversity of patients with ESRD.

Clinical Pearl

- The global prevalence of CKD was about 9% in 2017, while that of renal failure was 0.07% [3].
- CKD causes significant morbidity and mortality, in part due to limited access to RRT globally [3, 4].

21.2.1 ESRD Prevalence Among Racial/Ethnic Minority Groups

There is growing interest in the number of patients from racial/ethnic minority groups (minorities) with CKD and ESRD globally. While nearly one third of patients with CKD resided in China and India in 2017, most English-language articles focus on five countries with highly diverse populations [3]. Given the language bias inherent in our search, our references are mainly from Canada, the United States (USA), the United Kingdom (UK), Australia, and New Zealand. For example, with the increase in global migration by choice or forced, 18.5% of the US population identify as Hispanic/Latino, 13.4% as Black/African American, 6% as Asian, 1.3% as American Indian/Alaska Native, and 0.2% as Native Hawaiian/Other Pacific Islander [5]. Taken together, nearly 40% of the US population in 2019 included persons from minorities, whether they were US-born, immigrants, or other migrants.

In regard to migrants, the United Nations High Commissioner for Refugees reported 4 million asylum-seekers and 26 million refugees worldwide in 2019 [6]. Nearly 70% of these persons came from just five countries: Myanmar, South Sudan, Afghanistan, Syria, and Venezuela [6]. Asylum-seekers (i.e., persons claiming asylum but who do not yet have legal refugee status) and refugees often enter neighboring countries when displaced [6]. However, they may also arrive in Canada, the USA, the UK, the European Union (EU), Australia, and New Zealand. Moreover, unlike the initial "healthy immigrant effect" observed in new immigrants as compared to native-born citizens, these two migrant groups (asylum seekers and refugees) are at high risk of poor health for reasons related to pre-migration, migration, and post-migration conditions [7].

Clinical Pearl

- A large portion of the population in countries such as Canada, the USA, the UK, Australia, and New Zealand is comprised of racial/ethnic minority groups (minorities).
- The prevalence of CKD and ESRD is generally overrepresented among minorities, such as those in the USA, as compared to White persons [8].

Likewise, the growing diversity within countries is also reflected in CKD and ESRD patient populations. For example, the adjusted ESRD prevalence in all major minorities in the USA consistently surpassed that of White persons from 2000 to 2018 [8]. In fact, it was nearly 3.5 times as high in Black/African American persons, 2 times as high in American Indian/Alaska Native persons, and 2 times as high in Hispanic persons by 2018 (see Table 21.2) [5, 8]. While other countries may have different predominant minorities compared to the USA, ESRD is commonly over-represented among minorities. As well, while a smaller percentage of the global ESRD patient population, some will be asylum-seekers, refugees, other migrants, and new immigrants who may face significant barriers to health [9].

21.2.2 Race and Ethnicity as Social Constructs

We recognize that the terms "race" and "ethnicity," particularly the former, may be contentious among individuals. In past centuries efforts to classify humans by race included crude markers such as origin and appearance [10]. Many have since tried to define race by other "biological" markers, but historically it was done for purposes of maintaining systems of oppression (e.g., colonialism). More often now, race is understood as a social construct (i.e., there is very little that is biologically intrinsic about race) [10].

Indeed, race represents a human-made classification system that is based on various factors that people choose to assign to it. As such, there is marked heterogeneity within racial groups, and individuals may decide to self-identify as more than one race [10]. For example, the US census includes a "Mixed race" group, and it describes "Hispanic/Latino" as ethnicities because Hispanic/Latino persons can identify as any race [5]. While ethnicity is just as socially constructed as race, individuals may use it to refer to shared sociocultural and linguistic traits [11].

There continues to be conflict about the purpose of discussing race/ethnicity in medicine, but some researchers argue that they are highly relevant to health [10]. Regardless of whether individuals self-identify as a racial/ethnic group or if they are racialized or ethnicized (i.e., others ascribe race/ethnicity labels to them), it can

Table 21.2 2018 US population and adjusted ESRD prevalence among minority groups [5, 8]

Minority group	Population (%)	Adjusted ESRD prevalence (cases per million people)
Hispanic/Latino	18.5	3266.8
Black/African American	13.4	5854.8
Asian	5.9	2275.3
American Indian/Alaska Native	1.3	3163.4
Native Hawaiian/other Pacific Islander	0.2	
White	60.7	1703.5

ESRD end-stage renal disease

impact health. When race/ethnicity data is collected (recognizing the dearth of this data), it can reveal stark health disparities that may have otherwise gone unnoticed [10]. Apart from ESRD being overrepresented in minorities, we will outline a number of other concerning renal heath disparities in the next section.

Recommendation

- Be aware that commonly used terms such as "race" and "ethnicity" are understood as social constructs, meaning that they have little biological basis [10].
- However, it is still relevant to collect racial/ethnic demographic data because when analyzed against health outcomes, it may reveal health disparities [10].

21.3 Renal Health Disparities Among Racial/Ethnic Minority Groups

ESRD disproportionately affects racial/ethnic minority groups (minorities) in multiple English-speaking countries including Canada, the USA, the UK, Australia, and New Zealand. Indeed, it is one of the most understated health disparities, i.e., "health differences that adversely affect disadvantaged populations, on the basis of one or more health outcomes" [10]. In this case, renal health outcomes include risk of predisposing disorders, nephrology referral, risk of CKD progression, treatment accessibility, and risk of complications. Examples of renal health disparities among minorities are described below:

- **Risk for predisposing disorders**: Minorities are also overrepresented in prevalence rates of obesity, type 2 diabetes mellitus, and hypertension [10]. They also tend to be diagnosed with these disorders at younger ages compared to White persons [10].
- **Nephrology referral**: While timely referral to nephrology is linked with better clinical outcomes, minorities tend to experience delays in referral, if they are referred at all [10]. This puts them at risk of further CKD progression and delays in monitoring and treatment, which may partly explain why the prevalence of ESRD is higher in minorities.
- **Treatment accessibility**: Patients with ESRD rely on dialysis or RTX to survive, or else they are offered conservative care, including palliation:
  - **Dialysis**: Minorities are more likely to receive hemodialysis without arteriovenous fistulas (which provides superior vascular access), even when adjusting for age, medical comorbidities, and insurance status [11]. They are also less likely to receive peritoneal dialysis and home dialysis, which are more patient-centered than clinic–/hospital-based hemodialysis services [11, 12].
  - **Renal transplantation (RTX)**: Although RTX is considered the gold standard treatment for ESRD, minorities are less likely to be identified as candi-

dates, to be referred for evaluation, and to be waitlisted [10]. If waitlisted, they tend to wait longer than White persons and are less likely to receive RTX in the end [10]. If offered RTX, they are less likely to receive a living donor transplant kidney (LDTK) and more likely to receive one from a deceased donor. For reference, LDTK is associated with less waiting, better patient/graft survival, and increased quality of life [13].
  - **End-of-life care**: Minorities are less likely to participate in advanced care planning discussions. As such, they may be more likely to undergo invasive life-sustaining or "futile" treatments [12]. While palliation helps to improve patients' quality of life and minimize suffering, minorities are less likely to be educated about, offered, and to use these services [12].
- **Risk of complications**: Some minorities are at increased risk of complications such as infection, emergency department visits, and hospitalizations:
  - **Infection**: Black patients on peritoneal dialysis have increased risk of peritonitis compared to White patients in the USA [10].
  - **Emergency department visits**: Emergency hemodialysis is associated with greater morbidity/mortality than the recommended standard of thrice-weekly dialysis. Yet undocumented migrants in some US states, often Hispanic/Latino persons, are more likely to require emergency hemodialysis due to poor access to routine renal care [14].
  - **Hospitalizations**: In a study, dialysis was the main cause of hospitalizations for Aboriginal and Torres Strait Islander patients with ESRD in Australia [15].

Clinical Pearl

- Renal health disparities among racial/ethnic minority groups include risk of predisposing disorders, time to nephrology referral, risk of CKD progression, treatment accessibility, and risk of further complications [10–15].

Recommendation

- Reflect on your current CKD/ESRD patient population.
- Are you aware of any renal health disparities among racial/ethnic minority groups?
- Is this something that you or your workplace has considered as an area of interest or concern?

21.3.1 The Social Determinants of Renal Health Among Racial/Ethnic Minority Groups

Knowing that renal health disparities among racial/ethnic minority groups (minorities) exist, we must also consider some of the key reasons for this. Over the past decades, the understanding of health has shifted from a biological approach to the more nuanced biopsychosocial one. The latter approach recognizes that health is influenced by both individual and interlocking biological, psychological, and social factors. As such, while age, sex, genetics, lifestyle, and medical comorbidities contribute to CKD and ESRD, we must not overlook the social determinants of health [16].

The World Health Organization defines social determinants of health as the "conditions in which people are born, grow, live, work, and age," as well as the systems that construct them [17]. Studies have shown that social determinants of health may explain between 30% and 55% of health outcomes, which means that they are a substantial cause of health disparities [17]. While many clinicians are already familiar with the social determinants of health, in brief they tend to encompass historical, social, cultural, and economic factors. There is also evidence to support that social determinants of health influence renal health disparities, such as ESRD, particularly among minorities.

In 2016, Norton et al. [10] reviewed common social determinants of health for CKD among racial minorities, providing a theoretical model of how they are related. In this model, social determinants of health may affect:

- **Risk of exposure to toxins**: Low socioeconomic status (determined by education, employment, and income) may limit access to safe housing and neighborhoods, putting individuals at risk of exposure to renal toxins (e.g., lead).
- **Risk of exposure to stress**: Low socioeconomic status is associated with copious stressors that may result in chronic stress-related health outcomes (e.g., hypertension, diabetes mellitus, CKD).
- **Access to resources to sustain health**: Low socioeconomic status may limit access to nutritious foods and safe spaces for physical activity (both are factors in obesity, hypertension, and diabetes mellitus), the development of health literacy/numeracy, care affordability, and paid sick leave.
- **Access to timely, adequate healthcare**: Low socioeconomic status may limit access to health insurance, preventative care, proximity to specialized renal centers, affordable transportation, timeliness of care, and recommended treatments (e.g., renal transplantation).
- **Risk of morbidity and mortality**: Low socioeconomic status is associated with CKD prevalence, ESRD incidence, treatment nonadherence, complications (e.g., infections, emergency department visits, and hospitalizations), as well as mortality [10].

Clinical Pearl

- Research suggests that social determinants of health may account for between 30% and 55% of health outcomes [17].
- Access to social determinants of health also influences renal health disparities, including factors related to ESRD among racial/ethnic minority groups [10].

Certain sub-groups of minorities face even greater barriers in access to social determinants of health than persons who are born and raised in their home country. This includes asylum-seekers, refugees, other migrants who come through legal (e.g., temporary foreign workers in Canada or the USA) or illegal means, and immigrants. Asylum-seekers and refugees are already at risk of poor health given adverse pre-migration and migration-related exposures, including limited access to routine healthcare [7]. In addition, while each group may struggle with language proficiency on arrival, the first three are even more vulnerable if they do not have documentation or health insurance [18]. Finally, culture is another relevant factor in renal health, which we will explore in the upcoming sections.

However, it would be remiss to discuss social determinants of health without highlighting the systems of oppression that have disadvantaged minorities. For example, literature on Indigenous persons' renal health often references colonialism and its inherent violence (still ongoing in many countries), as a barrier to social determinants of health [15]. From genocides to colonization of their land and ongoing marginalization, Indigenous persons have lost access to resources to maintain health (e.g., land, work, community, culture, language, traditional knowledge). They also continue to be put at risk of poor health through other insidious means (e.g., systemic racism, intergenerational trauma, limited access to other social determinants of health) [15]. Like Indigenous persons, the social positioning of other minorities (e.g., Black, Asian, and Hispanic/Latino persons) has also been shaped by their unique experiences of colonialism.

Recommendation
- Be mindful of how social determinants of health affect your renal patients.
- If barriers are identified, consider ways that you and your interdisciplinary colleagues can support patients' health (e.g., disability applications, special diet forms).
- Patients who are asylum-seekers, refugees, other migrants, and new immigrants may need additional help navigating language proficiency, documentation, and insurance [18].

21.4 Case Vignette: "Lost in Translation"

Ms. Fernandes was a 68-year-old South-Asian widowed female who recently immigrated to Canada to be closer to her adult children and grandchildren. She was an educated woman; however, she had limited prior exposure to the healthcare system because she always felt well and thought she was fairly healthy. She had a longstanding history of type 2 diabetes mellitus and was noted by her new family physician to have moderate CKD – a new diagnosis for her. Her family physician referred her to your outpatient nephrology clinic to review non-pharmacological and pharmacological treatment recommendations. When you entered the room and introduced yourself, you realized that she did not speak English and her son and daughter-in-law were present to assist with translation. You wondered if what you were saying was being communicated accurately because her family appeared to shorten what you have said significantly. She did not appear to ask you any questions, and she seemed to defer to the wishes of her family, leaving you a bit unsure of how best to proceed. Please consider Ms. Fernandes' case as we next review culture as a determinant of renal health. We will return to her case later in this chapter for further analysis.

21.5 Culture as a Determinant of Renal Health Among Racial/ Ethnic Minority Groups

As mentioned previously, social determinants of health also include cultural factors although these can be easily missed in clinical encounters with patients. In short, culture is "the set of distinctive spiritual, material, intellectual, and emotional features" of social groups that include, "in addition to art and literature, lifestyles, ways of living together, value systems, traditions, and beliefs" [19]. Researchers have already considered how cultural factors affect renal health, especially for patients from racial/ethnic minority groups (minorities) with CKD and ESRD. Please note that while the literature references culture as pertaining to certain minorities, they are not homogenous groups and there is extensive cultural heterogeneity within them.

A number of authors over this past decade have examined cultural factors of renal health, both within and between minorities. In 2013, Crowley-Matoka examined how a variety of cultures around the world influence patients' beliefs about the kidney, as well as the etiology, significance, and treatment of renal disease [20]. In 2017, Sekkarie and Abdel-Rahman specifically assessed the cultural challenges in caring for refugees with ESRD who were from the Middle East and of Muslim faith [9]. While the examples below are by no means exhaustive, they demonstrate how cultural factors can influence a patient's beliefs about:

- **Risk factors for CKD**: For example, African American patients may describe renal disease as being "in the blood," which could be a reference to genetics and heritability, as well as the impact of predisposing disorders such as diabetes mellitus [20].
- **When to seek care**: For example, Chinese American patients may feel the need to "save face" when diagnosed. There is fear of stigma; e.g., their diagnosis may bring shame to the family, and this acts as a deterrent to seeking further medical care [21].
- **The burden of illness**: For example, African American patients may use the experiences of family/community members to influence their understanding of clinical outcomes, e.g., the belief that CKD conveys a guarded prognosis [20].
- **Medical decision-making**: For example, certain Middle Eastern cultures may value paternalism to the point that family make decisions for their loved one, including decisions around disclosure of diagnosis, prognosis, and/or treatment selection [9].
- **CKD/ESRD treatments**:
  - **Diet/medication**: For example, a Middle Eastern diet may be rich in potassium and cause hyperkalemia in patients with ESRD. As well, some Muslim patients on hemodialysis may not be able to receive pork heparin [9].

  - **Dialysis**: For example, Mexican patients may prefer to receive peritoneal dialysis because, in addition to the flexibility of care it offers, it is viewed as more "gentle" and "natural" to the body than hemodialysis [20].
  - **Organ donation**: Depending on one's spiritual beliefs, individuals may be less likely to provide kidney donations due to fear that removing an organ from the body will affect the potential donor's afterlife [20].
  - **Transplantation**: For example, African American patients may put "family first" by deciding that it is too risky for family to donate a kidney, whereas Mexican Americans may believe it is their duty to donate a kidney to their loved one [20].
- **End-of-life care**: For example, in addition to the role of family in medical decision-making, Middle Eastern families may be reluctant to accept palliative care for their loved one due to the belief that they are "abandoning" them [9].

Clinical Pearl

- Culture is often passed over as a determinant of health.
- Cultural factors may influence patient beliefs about risk factors for CKD, when to seek medical care, the burden of illness, medical decision-making, CKD and ESRD treatments, as well as end-of-life care [9, 20, 21].

21.5.1 Ethnocentrism as a Barrier to Understanding the Impact of Culture on Renal Health

Part of the reason why clinicians may overlook culture as a determinant of renal health is the fact that there is considerable ethnocentrism in medicine. Ethnocentrism is defined as the view "in which one group is the center of everything and all others are scaled and rated with reference to it" [22]. For example, medicine in Canada, the USA, the UK, Australia, and New Zealand is largely based on historically Eurocentric understandings of health. Regardless of how many cultural groups make up these countries, Eurocentric values have remained "the norm" in medicine over time. As such, common values of individualism in medicine may stand in contrast to some patients' values of collectivism (see Table 21.3 for further examples) [12, 23].

In reality, while some cultural factors may positively or negatively influence renal health, the majority likely have no particular impact on it. Yet when clinicians meet patients whose cultural contexts of health are different from the norm, how they respond also has the potential to affect patient care. For example, some clinicians may have little curiosity about patients' cultural contexts and never ask, others may ask but be unsure of how to respond in meaningful ways, and others may have implicit biases toward other cultures. At its most benign, this may represent a missed opportunity for patient-centered care, but at its worst, a negative response could potentially marginalize and disadvantage a patient clinically [15].

Table 21.3 Examples of individualistic vs. collectivistic values in medicine [12, 23]

	Individualistic values	Collectivistic values
Knowledge	Evidence-based	Traditional knowledges
Risk factors	Individual factors (e.g., lifestyle)	Communal factors (e.g., social determinants)
Disclosure	Full disclosure for diagnosis and prognosis	Withhold "bad" news from loved ones
Decision-making	Autonomy Patient is provided choices in healthcare Patient is the most important decision-maker	Paternalism Acquiesce with clinicians or other traditional providers Family/community are key decision-makers
End of life	Biomedical approach Avoidance of suffering Advanced care planning Withdrawal of "futile" care	Spiritual approach Avoidance of death Emphasis on the living Life-prolonging care

Culture matters to renal health and clinicians should consider inquiring about it with ESRD patients, including, but not limited to, those from minorities and those who are new to a country. If cultural factors are neglected, there may be delays in diagnosis and treatment, treatment may be less appropriate, and there may be treatment nonadherence and complications [9]. Ultimately, there may be a disconnect between patients and clinicians, causing mistrust in the healthcare system and resulting in poor patient satisfaction and renal care outcomes [9]. In effort to combat this, we will next review strategies to help clinicians, organizations, and health systems gain comfort in assessing and addressing cultural factors in ESRD care.

Recommendation

- Be aware of the danger of ethnocentrism in medicine.
- Remember that while some cultural factors influence renal care, not all do, so we must be careful not to make assumptions about patients of different cultures.
- However, if we never consider cultural factors, it can cause rifts between patients and clinicians and mistrust in health systems and result in suboptimal renal care [9].

21.6 Establishing Cultural and Linguistic Competency in Renal Care

Given that racial/ethnic minority groups (minorities) are overrepresented in poor renal outcomes, including ESRD, and that inequitable access to social determinants of health and neglect of cultural factors in health are some of the reasons for this, there needs to be meaningful change. Clinicians must especially consider the needs of minority patients who are specifically asylum-seekers, refugees, migrants, or new immigrants and are in precarious positions in regard to health [7]. Cultural and linguistic factors may be all the more important to their health, versus minority patients who are born and raised in the country and/or have acculturated over time [9].

Assessing and addressing cultural factors in ESRD care is one of the ways we can continue working toward renal health equity both within countries and globally [24]. Cultural and linguistic competency has gained traction to respond to demographic changes and to reduce health disparities among minorities [24]. These competencies support "health services that are respectful of and responsive to the health beliefs, practices and needs of diverse patients" [24]. By recognizing and responding to patients' cultural and language needs in renal care settings, clinicians, organizations, and health systems can improve minorities' health. For those particularly interested in developing these competencies, we will review recommendations for how this can be done at individual, organizational, and systemic levels.

Clinical Pearl

- Culturally and linguistically competent care is one of the ways that we can advance renal health equity for racial/ethnic minority groups [24].
- This is especially relevant for patients with ESRD who face a number of complex decisions about their care and whose values and preferences may vary.

21.6.1 Clinician, Know Thyself: Individual-Level Strategies

The literature recommends building cultural self-awareness, conducting culturally competent assessments, and being open to negotiating ESRD care with patients at this level. First, clinicians should be mindful that their own cultural and linguistic backgrounds may result in implicit biases toward patients of other cultures [25]. These types of bias are not always benign as they may affect clinicians' beliefs, attitudes, and behavior toward patients and their clinical care [25]. Interestingly, Harvard University created the Implicit Association Test (IAT) as a means for individuals to assess implicit biases [26]. The IAT can measure an individual's bias toward race, among other factors such as age, gender, sexuality, and disability. Biases are not uncommon, and there is opportunity to challenge them through exposure to diverse patients so as to gain insight into and respect for differences.

Second, conducting culturally competent assessments can help clinicians develop skills in cross-cultural communication, psychoeducation, and negotiation. Important areas to ask patients about, especially if they are newcomers to a country, include their explanatory model of renal health as well as psychosocial and acculturation factors [25, 27]. Clinicians may also find that some questions about explanatory models and psychosocial factors are applicable to all patients. Table 21.4 has examples of questions that clinicians may choose to incorporate into patient assessments to assess cultural and linguistic needs [25, 27]. Being open to learning about their needs, listening effectively to patients, providing psychoeducation when there are

Table 21.4 Questions to consider in a culturally competent clinical assessment [25, 27]

Explanatory models of health	Psychosocial and acculturation factors
Explanation of illness: What do you call this illness? What do you think caused it? What does it do to your body?	Psychosocial coping: How do you normally cope with stress? How are you personally coping now? How are your loved ones coping?
Burden of illness: How severe do you think it is? How does it affect your life? What do you fear most about it? What do you think will happen?	Migration: What is your country of origin? Where were you before coming here? What made you decide to come here? What were some of the difficulties?
Truth-telling: Do you prefer that I tell you all the information that I have about your illness now?	Family Are your loved ones here with you? If not, are they safe elsewhere? Do you speak with them?
Decision-making: Who advises you or makes decisions about your health? Should I talk to anyone else besides you about your health?	Community: What is your cultural background? Do you prefer to be with people from the same background as you?
Treatment: Who do you seek treatment from? Have you tried any other treatments? What kind of treatment do you think would help you now?	Language: What is your first language? Do you speak any other languages? What language do you speak at home? How well can you read, speak, or understand the main language(s) here? Do you prefer to use interpreters in your appointments?
Goals of care: What are your goals of care? What is most important for you in life?	Documentation/health insurance: Do you have access to documentation? Do you have access to health insurance? Do you know what you are covered for and how to access care?

differences, and negotiating care is essential. It is one step toward translating knowledge into patient-centered care so that patients receive appropriate ESRD care for their needs and clinical outcomes are optimized.

21.6.2 Case Vignette Analysis: "Lost in Translation"

Now that you have learned about culture as a determinant of renal care and the importance of delivering culturally and linguistically competent care, how would you approach the conversation with Ms. Fernandes and her family? While there is not one correct answer, a good place to start is to reflect on your own cultural and linguistic background and any implicit biases you may have toward patients of other cultures that could interfere with this encounter. Being mindful of these factors, consider also asking questions such as those in Table 21.4 to assess areas such as migration, family, language, and explanatory models of health. Doing so may help determine specific cultural and linguistic needs that she may have. One clear issue was the fact that her family was translating on her behalf, which was less than ideal so, if possible, you can access on-demand professional translators via phone or video to ensure that all information is communicated. If her needs cannot be accommodated in the initial appointment, it may be necessary to plan for a close follow-up and in the meantime to find out what resources your organization and local health system offer that can help support her. It is important to understand that her needs may change, so reassessing areas such as decision-making, treatment, and goals of care may be necessary – especially if she advances to severe CKD or ESRD later in life.

21.6.3 Through the Looking Glass: Organizational-Level Strategies

In order to adapt clinical ESRD care to patients' cultural contexts of health, cultural and linguistic competency should be reflected in an organization's policies and practices. Remember that clinicians are also part of an overarching medical culture, which may be predominantly Eurocentric depending on where they are based [25]. As such there is still a need to identify and challenge implicit beliefs in the workplace among all clinical and nonclinical staff. It is often suggested to form a working group with adequate funding that comprises key stakeholders, including patient and cultural community members [15]. The group will be responsible for assessing cultural and linguistic competency in the workplace, as well as developing, implementing, and evaluating any relevant interventions.

It is necessary for organizations to conduct a local needs assessment around key areas of cultural and linguistic competency that may affect ESRD care. It may cover areas such as workplace recruitment, staff beliefs/attitudes, communication, patient resources, health programming, clinical outcomes, and research. If the working group does not have the means to develop their own assessment tool, there are resources available to help guide these types of assessments. For example, Georgetown University's National Center for Cultural Competence has a range of free assessment checklists [28]. Assessment findings will focus on the working group's actionable goals, measurable objectives, and priority interventions (see Table 21.5 for examples in renal care) [9, 15, 21, 29].

An exemplar of organizational-level interventions in ESRD care is Northwestern University's Hispanic Kidney Transplant Program (HKTP) which was founded in 2006 in the USA [29]. In response to disparities in access to transplantation for Hispanic/Latino patients, Gordon et al. used a quality improvement lens to design, implement, and evaluate the HKTP [29]. Their program identified and rectified patient/donor, clinician, workplace, and system factors responsible for low rates of live donor kidney transplantation. Their interventions were extensive and incorporated cultural and linguistic congruence between staff and patients, culturally targeted psychoeducation, community engagement, and patient advocacy among others. In the end, they achieved a 74% increase in the number of Hispanic/Latino

Table 21.5 Examples of culturally and linguistically competent interventions in renal care [9, 15, 21, 29]

Area of interest	Culturally competent intervention
Recruitment	Increase recruitment of culturally and linguistically diverse staff [15]
Education (staff)	Mandate, or at least offer, cultural competency training for staff [15] Offer training for working effectively with interpreters/cultural brokers
Assessment	Train clinicians in how to conduct culturally competent assessments Offer the use of interpreters/cultural brokers in patient care encounters [9] Involve family, community members, and/or spiritual leaders in care at the patient's preference [9]
Education (patients)	Develop psychoeducational materials in appropriate languages and formats for patients [21] that also address cultural concerns (if needed) [27] Provide education to other people involved in the patient's care and medical decision-making (e.g., family) [21]
Treatment	Be willing to appropriately negotiate treatment and tailor it to cultural preferences if possible [9]
Supports	Offer patient navigation [15] and peer support [21] from individuals of the same cultural background
Research	Include relevant cultural groups in all stages of qualitative and quantitative research (if produced by the workplace) [15]

patients receiving live donor kidney transplantation, thereby drastically decreasing the discrepancy between these patients and non-Hispanic White patients [29].

21.6.4 Challenging Eurocentrism in Medicine: Systemic-Level Strategies

Some countries have not only identified cultural and linguistic competency in healthcare as a priority but have established specific standards to support clinicians and workplaces. For example, the US Department of Health and Human Services created the Office of Minority Health (OMH) with the goal of achieving health equity for racial/ethnic minority groups [30]. They developed the *National Standards for Culturally and Linguistically Appropriate Services in Health and Health Care*. The standards cover three main areas: "governance, leadership, and workforce," "communication and language assistance," and "engagement, continuous improvement and accountability" [30]. An example of an organization that has incorporated the standards into daily ESRD care includes the HKTP through Northwestern University (mentioned previously) [29]. The OMH further offers a detailed implementation guide, e-learning programs targeted to a variety of health professionals, and many other online educational resources.

Standards such as these make it clear that it is not enough to pursue equality in ESRD care because health inequities demonstrate that healthcare is not "one size fits all." We often talk about cultural humility as something that individual clinicians should develop over their careers; however, this also needs to be applied at the systemic level. It implores all involved in upholding healthcare systems, based largely on Eurocentric values, to engage in an active and lifelong process of critical reflection [27]. It challenges us to acknowledge shameful historical legacies against racial/ethnic minority groups that are reflected in today's disparities and to work toward reducing ongoing power imbalances [15]. In doing so, it encourages us to be open to ESRD patients' cultural contexts of health, to empower patients as partners in care, and to be genuinely ready, willing, and able to adapt renal care planning, programming, and monitoring as needed [15].

Recommendation

- We should identify and challenge implicit beliefs about other cultures at all levels of healthcare [25].
- Individually, you can work toward building cultural self-awareness, conducting culturally competent assessments, and negotiating ESRD care with patients [27].
- In the workplace, consider forming working groups that focus on developing culturally and linguistically appropriate services for patients [15, 30].
- At the systems level, we can acknowledge histories of oppression against racial/ethnic minority groups and work to minimize any power imbalances that still exist and contribute to renal health disparities [15].

21.7 Key Takeaways

- The demographics of ESRD patient populations are shifting along racial/ethnic lines as global migration increases.
- There are significant renal health disparities among racial/ethnic minority groups (minorities) which include:
  - Risk of predisposing disorders
  - Time to nephrology referral
  - Risk of CKD progression
  - CKD (including ESRD) prevalence
  - Treatment accessibility
  - Risk of complications
- Access to social determinants of health influences renal health disparities, including the rates of ESRD among minorities.
- Minority patients who are asylum-seekers, refugees, other migrants, and new immigrants may face even greater barriers in access to social determinants of health.
- Culture is an overlooked determinant of renal health; it may influence beliefs about the kidney as well as the etiology, significance, and treatment of renal disease.
- If overlooked, it may cause rifts between patients and clinicians and mistrust in the healthcare system, resulting in suboptimal renal care.

- Assessing and addressing cultural factors in ESRD care is one of the ways we can advance renal health equity globally.
- Clinicians can develop cultural self-awareness, skills in conducting culturally competent assessments, and the ability to negotiate renal care.
- Workplaces can design, implement, and evaluate culturally and linguistically appropriate services based on local needs assessments.
- Finally, health systems can promote cultural humility so as to acknowledge unjust legacies against minorities and to reduce ongoing power imbalances.

References

1. Kidney Disease: Improving Global Outcomes (KDIGO) CKD Work Group. KDIGO 2012 clinical practice guideline for the evaluation and management of Chronic Kidney Disease. Kidney Int Suppl. 2013;3(1):1–150. https://kdigo.org/wp-content/uploads/2017/02/KDIGO_2012_CKD_GL.pdf.
2. Akbari A, Clase CM, Acott P, Battistella M, Bello A, Feltmate P, et al. Canadian Society of Nephrology commentary on the KDIGO clinical practice guideline for CKD evaluation and management. Am J Kidney Dis. 2015;65(2):177–205.
3. GBD Chronic Kidney Disease Collaboration. Global, regional, and national burden of chronic kidney disease, 1990–2017: a systematic analysis for the Global Burden of Disease Study 2017. 2020;395(10225):709–33.
4. World Health Organization (WHO). DALYs/YLDs definition [Internet]. Geneva: WHO; 2021 [cited 2021 Jan 24]. https://www.who.int/mental_health/management/depression/daly/en/.
5. United States Census Bureau. QuickFacts [Internet]. Suitland: United States Census Bureau; 2019. [cited 2021 Jan 24]. https://www.census.gov/quickfacts/fact/table/US/PST045219.
6. United Nations High Commissioner for Refugees (UNHCR). Figures at a glance [Internet]. Geneva: UNHCR, The UN Refugee Agency; 2020 [cited 2021 Feb 2]. https://www.unhcr.org/figures-at-a-glance.html.
7. Pottie K, Greenaway C, Feightner J, Welch V, Swinkels H, Rashid M, et al. Evidence-based clinical guidelines for immigrants and refugees. Can Med Assoc J. 2011;183(12):E824–925.
8. United States Renal Data System (USRDS) ESRD Database. Incidence, prevalence, patient characteristics, and treatment modalities [Internet]. Bethesda: USRDS; 2020 [cited 2021 Jan 24]. https://adr.usrds.org/2020/end-stage-renal-disease/1-incidence-prevalence-patient-characteristics-and-treatment-modalities.
9. Sekkarie MA, Abdel-Rahman EM. Cultural challenges in the care of refugees with End-Stage Renal Disease: what Western nephrologists should know. Nephron. 2017;137(2):85–90.
10. Norton JM, Moxey Mims MM, Eggers PW, Narva AS, Star RA, Kimmel PL, et al. Social determinants of racial disparities in CKD. J Am Soc Nephrol. 2016;27(9):2576–95.
11. Norris KC, Williams SF, Rhee CM, Nicholas SB, Kovesdy CP, Kalantar-Zadeh K, et al. Hemodialysis disparities in African Americans: the deeply integrated concept of race in the social fabric of our society. Semin Dial. 2017;30(3):213–23.
12. Harding K, Mersha TB, Webb FJ, Vassalotti JA, Nicholas SB. Current state and future trends to optimize the care of African Americans with End-Stage Renal Disease. Am J Nephrol. 2017;46(2):156–64.
13. Gordon EJ, Lee J, Kang RH, Caicedo JC, Holl JL, Ladner DP, Shumate MD. A complex culturally targeted intervention to reduce Hispanic disparities in living kidney donor transplantation: an effectiveness-implementation hybrid study protocol. BMC Health Serv Res. 2018;18(1):368.
14. Desai N, Lora CM, Lash JP, Ricardo AC. CKD and ESRD in US Hispanics. Am J Kidney Dis. 2019;73(1):102–11.

15. Schwartzkopff KM, Kelly J, Potter C. Review of kidney health among Aboriginal and Torres Strait Islander people. Aust Indig Health Bull. 2020;20(4):1–40. http://healthbulletin.org.au/wp-content/uploads/2020/10/AIH_Review-of-kidney_Post-Publication-peer-reviewed-011220-WEB.pdf.
16. Crews DC, Bello AK, Saadi G. Burden, access, and disparities in kidney disease. Nephron. 2019;141(4):219–26.
17. World Health Organization (WHO). Social determinants of health [Internet]. Geneva: WHO; 2021 [cited 2021 Jan 31]. https://www.who.int/health-topics/social-determinants-of-health#tab=tab_1.
18. Dawson AZ, Garacci E, Ozieh M, Walker RJ, Egede LE. The relationship between immigration status and Chronic Kidney Disease risk factors in immigrants and US-born adults. J Immigr Minor Health. 2020;22(6):1200–7.
19. United Nations Educational, Scientific and Cultural Organization (UNESCO). UNESCO universal declaration on cultural diversity [Internet]. Paris: UNESCO; 2001 [cited 2021 Feb 1]. http://portal.unesco.org/en/ev.php-URL_ID=13179&URL_DO=DO_TOPIC&URL_SECTION=201.html.
20. Crowley-Matoka M. Anthropological issues in renal care. Kidney Int Suppl. 2013;3(2):219–22.
21. Luk M. Cross-cultural considerations: the Asian perspective [Internet]. Vancouver: BC Renal. 2016 [cited 2021 Feb 3]. http://www.bcrenal.ca/resource-gallery/Documents/1.%20M.%20Luk%20-%20Cross%20Cultural%20Considerations.pdf.
22. Sumner WG. Folkways: a study of the sociological importance of usages, manners, customs, mores, and morals. Boston: Ginn and Company; 1907. 692 p.
23. Harris HA. Cultural considerations in decision-making and goals of care discussions [Internet]. Stanford: Stanford Geriatric Education Center; 2015 [cited 2021 Feb 1]. https://sgec.stanford.edu/content/dam/sm/sgec/documents/conferences/Nephrology_Jan_9/Harris%20Heather_Cultural%20Considerations%20in%20Decision-Making%20and%20Goals%20of%20Care%20Discussions.pdf.
24. Office of Minority Health (OMH), US Department of Health and Human Services. Culturally and linguistically appropriate services (CLAS) [Internet]. Rockville: OMH; 2021 [cited 2021 Feb 4]. https://thinkculturalhealth.hhs.gov/clas/what-is-clas.
25. Kodjo C. Cultural competence in clinician communication. Pediatr Rev. 2009;30(2):57–64.
26. Project Implicit. Project Implicit [Internet]. Boston: Project Implicit, Inc.; 2011 [cited 2021 Feb 4]. https://www.projectimplicit.net/.
27. Vo D, Mayhew M. Cultural competence for child and youth health professionals. Ottawa: Canadian Paediatric Society. 2018 [cited 2021 Feb 4]. https://www.kidsnewtocanada.ca/culture/competence.
28. Georgetown University Center for Cultural Competence. Self-assessments [Internet]. Washington, DC: Georgetown University National Center for Child and Human Development; 2021 [cited 2021 Feb 4]. https://nccc.georgetown.edu/assessments/index.php.
29. Gordon EJ, Romo E, Amórtegui D, Rodas A, Anderson N, Uriarte J, et al. Implementing culturally competent transplant care and implications for reducing health disparities: a prospective qualitative study. Health Expect. 2020;23(6):1450–65.
30. Office of Minority Health (OMH), US Department of Health and Human Services. National culturally and linguistically appropriate services standards [Internet]. Rockville: OMH; 2021 [cited 2021 Feb 4]. https://thinkculturalhealth.hhs.gov/clas/standards.

22 Occupation-Related Stress Affecting Physicians Caring for Patients with Renal Disease

Emma Gregory, Tara Riddell, and Ana Hategan

22.1 The Basics of Burnout

Given the uptake in interest in physician wellness over the past decade, most residents, fellows, and other physicians have likely heard about burnout before now. However, each individual may have their own understanding and experience of burnout. For example, one may think of it as chronic stress, or as significant emotional distress, or even as becoming too sick to function daily at work. Before discussing the current issue of burnout in nephrology, it is helpful to define what is meant by burnout, including means of measuring it.

22.1.1 Defining Burnout

The term burnout was first established in the literature by German-born American psychologist Herbert Freudenberger. In 1974, he published an article titled "Staff burn-out" that described burnout, its risk factors, and its prevention [1]. Burnout has

E. Gregory (✉)
Department of Psychiatry and Behavioural Neurosciences, Michael G. DeGroote School of Medicine, McMaster University, Hamilton, ON, Canada
e-mail: emma.gregory@medportal.ca

T. Riddell
Department of Psychiatry and Behavioural Neurosciences, McMaster University, Hamilton, ON, Canada
e-mail: tara.riddell@medportal.ca

A. Hategan
Division of Geriatric Psychiatry, Department of Psychiatry & Behavioural Neurosciences, Faculty of Health Sciences, Michael G. DeGroote School of Medicine, McMaster University, Hamilton, ON, Canada
e-mail: hategan@mcmaster.ca

A. Hategan et al. (eds.), *Psychonephrology*,
https://doi.org/10.1007/978-3-030-84740-1_22

been widely discussed in the literature over the past decades, but the main concept has stayed the same. While it is not included as a psychiatric disorder in the *Diagnostic and Statistical Manual, 5th Edition*, it is clinically defined elsewhere.

The *International Classification of Diseases, 11th Revision*, describes burnout as a syndrome resulting from chronic occupational stress which includes the following [2]:

1) Emotional exhaustion: feeling that one's emotional reserve is depleted.
2) Depersonalization: a cynical, negative, or detached response to one's work.
3) Low personal accomplishment: feeling less effective or accomplished at one's work.

In other words, burnout is akin to saying, "I have nothing left to give," "I just don't care anymore," or "I'm not even helping." Perhaps these are thoughts that one has had before or has even voiced to others at work.

22.1.2 Measuring Burnout

Having a shared definition of burnout is important, but knowing how to measure it is also useful as one can track existing workplace patterns and changes over time. It can be measured by a variety of methods, but a well-known instrument in the literature is the Maslach Burnout Inventory (MBI). The MBI was developed by psychologists Maslach and Jackson in 1981 to assess an individual's experience of burnout. The MBI has been long-recognized as a highly reliable and validated instrument, and it continues to be the gold standard of measuring burnout [3].

There are different versions of the MBI for various professions, including the Human Services Survey for Medical Personnel (MBI-HSS (MP)). It consists of 22 items divided into 3 domains that measure emotional exhaustion (9 items), depersonalization (5 items), and personal accomplishment (8 items). An example item is the statement, "I feel emotionally drained from my work" [3]. Individuals can select from "never, a few times a year or less, once a month or less, a few times a month, once a week, a few times a week, or daily" as options [3]. Rather than having one overall cutoff score that signifies burnout or not, it is now recognized as a continuum. Individuals can have low, moderate, or high levels of each domain.

Clinical Pearl

- Brief burnout screens are available if the full MBI is not accessible to physicians. A 1–2-item screen may include:
  1) "I feel burned out from my work" (emotional exhaustion).
  2) "I have become more callous toward people since I took this job" (depersonalization).
- Not only do these items correlate strongly with each respective burnout domain in trainees and physicians who completed the full MBI, but they performed well across a variety of predictive models for negative burnout outcomes, e.g., suicidality [4].

Recommendation

- Familiarize yourself with the signs and symptoms of burnout in yourself and colleagues.
- Be aware that burnout is a syndrome caused by chronic work stress that includes emotional exhaustion, depersonalization, and reduced personal accomplishment.
- Be able to measure it using tools such as the MBI, which will help identify individual physicians at high risk of burnout, as well as any concerning patterns of burnout in the workplace.

22.2 Burnout in the Medical Profession

Burnout has become an "occupational hazard" for physicians and this is the case regardless of one's specialty. For example, in 2018, the Canadian Medical Association conducted a national health survey of physicians, including residents, and found that 30% of respondents reported high levels of burnout. This included measuring the main domains of burnout with participants reporting especially high levels of emotional exhaustion as well as burnout as a syndrome [5]. The rate of burnout in physicians generally continues to increase even though physicians actually entered the medical profession with an advantage regarding levels of psychological stress, as further explained in the next section.

22.2.1 A Leg Up on a Difficult Climb

Students entering medical school often have a leg up and begin their careers with lower levels of psychological distress than their nonmedical peers. In 2014, Brazeau et al. [6] compared rates of burnout and depression among matriculating medical students with age-matched college graduates. Matriculating medical students reported lower rates of burnout (27% vs. 37%) and depressive symptoms (26% vs. 42%), as well as higher scores of quality of life compared to controls [6]. Yet this trend reverses later in a medical career, and so there is something about the medical profession itself that impacts physician wellness.

Indeed, physicians go on to experience high rates of burnout across their careers. Dyrbye et al. [7] also compared burnout and other forms of psychological distress among medical students, residents and fellows, and graduate physicians up to 5 years into practice with other-employed age-matched controls. Regardless of career stage, all groups were more likely to experience burnout compared to controls, but medical students, residents, and fellows reported higher rates of burnout and depressive symptoms [7].

Though the abovementioned study explored burnout only as far as the first 5 years into practice, physicians remain at high risk of burnout throughout their entire career. Prior to the aforementioned study, Dyrbye et al. [8] compared burnout among staff physicians at different career stages. They found that physicians were at highest risk of burnout in middle career (11 to 19 years of practice post-residency/fellowship), then early career (up to 10 years), and, finally, in late career (21+ years) [8]. Table 22.1 is a summary of Dyrbye et al.'s overall findings [7, 8].

Clinical Pearl

- While medical students begin their careers with lower rates of burnout and distress than their nonmedical peers, this trend reverses quickly [6, 7].
- Medical students, residents, fellows, and other physicians continue to be at high risk of burnout through their careers, particularly during medical training and in middle career [7, 8].

22.3 Case Vignette: "A Slow Burn"

Samantha was a nephrologist who was 10 years into practice post-fellowship and worked as an associate professor at a major teaching hospital in a variety of roles. She often oversaw a nephrology fellow, a general internal medicine resident, and at least one medical student. Clinically she spent her mornings in an outpatient general nephrology clinic, noon at "lunch and learn" sessions, and afternoons rounding on inpatients and supervising consults. In addition, she either initiated her own research or worked with fellows to complete their projects, as well as contributing to the academic curriculum. When she finished her fellowship training, she had looked forward to a rewarding career in nephrology, but her joy and interest dwindled as her roles and responsibilities increased. By the end of the day, she felt like she was "crawling home" to her partner, children, and pets, trying to gear herself up for whatever was waiting when she walked in the door. She sometimes reviewed lab results and other clinical documentation in the evening, ensuring that nothing was missed, and practically fell into bed, hoping that tomorrow would be better.

Yet Samantha woke up feeling more exhausted each day and nothing changed because she was steadfast in her work, taking on more of it rather than reflecting on what it did to her. She worked a busy call shift with her team one weekend, dealing with several complications involving her inpatients and reviewing multiple ER and ward consults. She found herself criticizing her fellow for taking more time to round

Table 22.1 Burnout across the medical career (Data derived from [7, 8])

Stage of career	Rate of burnout (%)
Medical school	56
Residency/fellowship	60
Very early career (< 5 years post completion of specialty training)	51
Early career (0–10 years)	50
Middle career (11–20 years)	54
Late career (21+ years)	40

and do consults than she would have: "What's with him? Doesn't he know how to be efficient by now? He's practically staff." Later she could barely hear about another ER patient with chronic renal disease who presented after not seeing their nephrologist for years and not adhering to treatment. "Why don't they just listen? Don't they take their life seriously? Why do we even bother?" She left her call shift utterly dejected and wondered if she could even keep going at this rate. Keep Samantha in mind as we review occupation-related stress in nephrology, and we will return to her case later in this chapter.

22.4 Burnout in the Nephrology Workforce

When burnout is discussed in the literature, it is often done in relation to physicians working in areas such as family medicine, general internal medicine, emergency medicine, or intensive care medicine. Beyond general internal medicine, there are specialties such as nephrology that may be overlooked despite burnout still being a critical issue. Fortunately, there have been several surveys in recent years that have prioritized this issue in North American nephrology fellows and practicing nephrologists. While nephrologists may not have the absolute highest rates of burnout in medicine, burnout remains ever-present and cannot be minimized or dismissed.

22.4.1 A Concerning Trend in Nephrology

In 2016, the American Society of Nephrology released the results of a national US survey that included nephrologists aged 55 years and older with a response rate of 20%. Despite 94% of respondents being in a good or better overall health, approximately 52% of respondents reported less work satisfaction than 5 years ago, 79% worked over 40 hours weekly, 38% reported increased patient care hours, and 60% would consider switching to part-time work [9]. While the authors did not measure burnout directly, these types of responses may indirectly reflect domains such as emotional exhaustion and reduced personal accomplishment.

In 2020, Medscape published the results of another national US survey that included nephrologists of all ages. In this case, the prevalence of burnout among nephrologists was 49%, which is higher than the average for all physicians (41%). Beyond this, only 23% reported being very or extremely happy at work, which was lower than the average for all physicians (27%) [10]. There appears to be a discrepancy between the 2016 and 2020 survey results, with respondents for the former generally reporting positive well-being and those in the latter reporting burnout. This may in part be due to career stage as it has already been established that physicians in early and middle career tend to be at the highest risk of burnout.

Concerned with the lack of data on medical trainees' burnout experiences, Agrawal et al. [11] released the results of a national US survey of nephrology fellows in 2020. They had a 42.9% response rate and used a 2-item screen to assess for key domains of burnout including emotional exhaustion and depersonalization. In the first study of burnout in nephrology fellows ever, 28% reported the former and 14% reported the latter, with the overall prevalence of burnout being 30% [11]. As one will see later, this may be one of the reasons why there is less interest among medical students and general internal medicine residents in pursuing nephrology.

Clinical Pearl

- As is the case for many physicians, burnout is an ongoing issue for the nephrology workforce.
- While not often highlighted in the literature, nephrology fellows and practicing nephrologists continue to report high rates of burnout up to 30% and 49%, respectively [10, 11].

22.5 Contributing Factors to Burnout in Nephrology

While a degree of stress comes with any profession, the risk of burnout for physicians is significantly higher than for the general population employed in other careers. This suggests that there is something about the medical profession itself that affects physician wellness and causes them to feel burned out at such high rates. In fact, there is a multitude of contributing factors to burnout in medicine that reach across individual, organizational, and systemic levels. While nephrology fellows and other physicians are also impacted by these general factors (see Table 22.2), they also face distinctive ones that exacerbate their risk [10–16].

22.5.1 Individual Risk Factors

Often in medical culture, the responsibility for maintaining wellness falls to the individual, and so psychological distress may be internalized as a personal weakness. On the one hand, there are certain demographic criteria that put physicians at increased risk of burnout, such as being of the female gender [12] and being younger (age < 55 years) [15]. In Medscape's 2020 national US survey, female physicians reported higher rates of burnout than their male colleagues across generations [12].

Table 22.2 Known factors in physician burnout [10–16]

Individual	Organization	Systems
Age	Excessive bureaucratic tasks	Culture of medicine
Gender	Long work hours	Regulatory pressures
Personality traits	Computerization of practice	Lack of autonomy
Unhelping coping styles	Insufficient compensation, reimbursement	Lack of control
	Lack of respect from colleagues	Lack of flexibility
		Lack of resources
		Moral distress

Moreover, the American Society of Nephrology reported that the age distribution in their specialty makes it one of the "youngest" medical specialties [9].

Physicians may also possess certain personality traits such as perfectionism, which likely helped propel them into medicine, but also puts them at risk of burnout [13]. As well, some individuals may engage in unhelpful coping mechanisms such as neglecting basic needs, socially withdrawing, or turning to substances for relief/escape. Medscape reported that 42% of nephrologists reportedly coped with burnout by isolating themselves, as well as by binge eating and drinking alcohol (22% in each area) [10]. On the other hand, most factors affecting physician wellness go far beyond the individual, and this is where one's focus should be attuned.

22.5.2 Organizational Risk Factors

At this level, which includes one's practice and larger institution, there are several risk factors that physicians continue to identify across different specialties. In Medscape's 2020 US national survey of nephrologists [10], their answers mirrored those of a much larger sample of over 15,000 physicians in 29 specialties [12]. When asked to identify what contributes to burnout, the top five answers included excessive bureaucratic tasks, long work hours, lack of respect from colleagues, increasing computerization of practice, and insufficient compensation/reimbursement [10]. Issues such as increased workload, changing practices, and remuneration are reflected in the literature time and again, and yet there are even higher-level factors that exist too.

Additionally, the 2020 national survey results of US nephrology fellows showed that a disruptive work environment was also strongly associated with burnout [11]. Disruptive behavior is understood as that which violates societal norms of respectful and appropriate behavior and results in a perceived threat to others. It tends to be experienced by clinicians in more acute settings, and those survey authors recognized that fellows often consult in acute medical and surgical units. As it was not the focus of their survey, the authors could not tease apart whether fellows were victims or witnesses of this behavior or if this behavior stemmed from patient or colleague interactions (or both). Given the number of international medical graduates (IMG) in nephrology fellowships too, the authors wondered whether some IMG fellows were also subject to racializing experiences [11]. If that were the case, racialization (i.e., the process of social construction of race) could also be considered another type of disruptive behavior.

22.5.3 The Impact of Moral Distress

Nephrologists routinely manage complex patients in a variety of settings across a spectrum of acuity ranging from emergent to chronic care. Pawlowicz and Nowicki published the results of a national Polish survey of nephrology fellows and practicing nephrologists in 2020, and, expectedly, the results mirrored the US experience

[14]. They also queried whether those working in dialysis care may be at greater risk of burnout compared to colleagues working in settings such as inpatient care. Indeed, they found that those working in dialysis care reported higher rates of reduced personal accomplishment than their colleagues working in other settings [14].

When discussing why nephrology fellows and practicing nephrologists in dialysis care may experience more burnout, they described a host of factors. Patients are often chronic, have medical comorbidities, have low adherence to diet and fluid recommendations, and may subsequently have poorer prognoses [14]. Physicians may also experience difficult patient interactions, including serious illness or end-of-life discussions, they may provide futile care to some very ill patients, or they may be forced to treat undocumented patients with emergent-only dialysis [17]. With the increase in migration globally, the moral distress inherent in working with possibly undocumented patients in many countries is an emerging concern [18].

While nephrology fellows and practicing nephrologists are not the only clinicians exposed to suffering, trauma, and death, moral distress is recognized as a unique factor in burnout. Moral injury or distress is a term borrowed from military personnel that has been more recently applied to clinicians. It occurs when clinicians cannot act according to their ethical beliefs because of constraints imposed upon them in the work culture and environment [18]. When considering the organizational and systemic factors in burnout mentioned above and below in nephrology, it is reasonable to understand how it develops and how insidious it can be. If moral distress is left unsaid and unmanaged, it too can result in burnout and other forms of serious psychological distress.

22.5.4 Systemic Risk Factors

In terms of health systems, which vary according to country, nephrologists describe additional factors that contribute to burnout. Regulatory pressures and "protocol-driven environments" are frustrating as they result in a perceived lack of physician control, autonomy, and flexibility [15]. Added to this is a lack of time and material resources that make physicians feel like another "cog in the wheel" [10]. Overriding the above is the culture of medicine that they are exposed to from the start of training and which continues to shape how they live and work.

The culture of medicine is part of the hidden curriculum that physicians know and abide by, but do not often openly discuss or critique. The medical profession tends to reward those who are most willing to push themselves beyond what is expected of other professionals. Work often requires some strife and sacrifice that physicians are expected to tolerate, if not overcome. If they cannot, then they face feelings of fear, shame, and stigma. Particularly when they experience psychological distress, it may be framed as an internal failure rather than the result of being worn down by external factors [16].

This culture becomes a barrier to physicians identifying burnout in themselves and their colleagues, intervening early, and optimizing outcomes. In Medscape's

2020 national US survey of nephrologists, 75% of respondents stated that they have not previously sought help despite experiencing burnout and/or depressed mood and they do not intend to seek help in the future either [10]. Physicians often think that their symptoms are not severe enough to warrant help, that they can manage alone, or that they are, ironically, too busy. A further subset may not want to risk disclosure and its perceived consequences in the workplace [12]. In any case, they are left vulnerable by the system they work in and become conditioned to suffer alone and in silence through their careers.

Clinical Pearl

- Moral distress results when there is a discrepancy between what clinicians think is right to do and what they can actually do. If it is a pattern, burnout can ensue.
- Patient, practice, and system factors, i.e., things often beyond an individual's control, can affect the degree of moral distress that nephrology fellows and practicing nephrologists face.

Recommendation

- Recognize that the factors which have the largest impact on physician burnout are those at the *organizational* and *systemic* levels, not the *individual* level.
- In particular, the culture of medicine encourages physicians to push themselves to the extreme, to sacrifice what makes them well, and to do so alone and without question.

22.6 Case Vignette Analysis: "A Slow Burn"

Based on Samantha's case described previously in the vignette and the information we have since reviewed, it is likely that she was experiencing burnout for several reasons. While not explicitly stated, she appeared to be a high-achieving individual who eagerly took on multiple roles and responsibilities early in her career as a nephrologist. Yet the same joy and excitement with work faded as she transitioned to middle career and tried her best to juggle clinical, teaching, and scholarly roles at a busy academic center. While we did not delve into the particularities of her work as a nephrologist, one can expect that the system in which she worked did not prioritize her well-being, so neither did she. Instead, she experienced a slow burn. While the signs and symptoms may not have been clear to her or her colleagues early on, they eventually became undeniable at work.

The triad of emotional exhaustion, depersonalization, and reduced self-efficacy was evident as she wearily trudged through another day of the same work with no reprieve. Her situation may not have been unique, but that is problematic. She joined the ranks of many physicians before and alongside her who were similarly left vulnerable. However, burnout is not the be-all, end-all of her experience. In fact, it is associated with several other harms that she was also at risk for and may have endured too. Perhaps how she felt when she finished her shift provided a moment to pause and reflect on the bigger picture of burnout and what she genuinely needed to recover and reengage. Yet as one will see, burnout is not an individual problem requiring an individual solution. Rather, it is a systemic issue with far-reaching consequences that requires a shared response.

22.7 The Consequences of Burnout in Nephrology

Although physicians may prefer to think otherwise, given the culture of medicine, they are human and do experience emotional responses that affect their life and work. They are empathic, they often form long-term relationships with patients and colleagues, and they witness daily suffering – and this is in addition to the above factors for burnout. While some researchers may consider burnout to be the main outcome of interest, it is also associated with a range of individual, patient care, and health systems consequences (see Table 22.3) [9, 12, 17, 19–21]. Therefore, burnout matters not only because of how it touches individual physicians, but because of how it subsumes others in equally troubling ways.

22.7.1 Individual Effects

At this level, physicians who experience burnout also suffer psychological distress that further puts them at risk of depression, suicidality, and substance use. Medscape's 2020 national US survey results of physicians found that 16.3% of respondents reported depression ranging from "colloquial" to "clinical." Indeed, the rate of major depressive disorder is higher in physicians compared to the general population [12]. Moreover, 22.3% reported previous suicidal ideation with no suicide attempts, while 1.7% reported past attempts. It is also disconcerting that 39% of respondents reported suicidality that they did not disclose to others, and up to 400

Table 22.3 Adverse outcomes associated with physician burnout [9, 12, 17, 19–21]

Individual	Patient care	Health systems
Depressive disorders	Medical errors	Low interest in training
Suicidality	Safety incidents	Unfilled fellowship positions
Post-traumatic stress disorder	Professional misconduct	Fellow dropout from training
Substance use disorders	Low patient satisfaction	Low work satisfaction
	Reduced quality of patient care	Turnover and part-time work
		Difficulty maintaining the nephrology workforce

physicians die by suicide annually [12]. Finally, studies have shown that rates of substance use disorders are similar for physicians as for the general population (e.g., 10–15%), but alcohol misuse is especially problematic [19]. Alcohol use disorder is highly prevalent in physicians, and it is further associated with burnout, depression, suicidal ideation, and recent medical errors [19].

22.7.2 Patient Care Effects

The impact of physician burnout extends beyond the confines of an individual's "personal" life to their day-to-day work. In terms of practice, physicians who are burned out tend to have decreased work satisfaction and productivity in clinical, scholarly, and teaching work [20]. Again, this not only means that burnout affects physicians' patients but also their colleagues who they may work with in any of their various roles. Some studies also show that burnout is linked to increased rates of referrals to other specialists and increases in resource utilization [20], which further strains the system.

Argentero et al. [21] released the results of an Italian study in 2008 that explored the relationship between burnout in dialysis care nurses and nephrologists and patient satisfaction. Burnout was assessed via the Maslach Burnout Inventory, and patient satisfaction was based on completeness of medical information, their relationship with staff, staff performance, and organization of the service. There was a negative correlation between staff reports of emotional exhaustion and patient satisfaction, no correlation for depersonalization, and a positive correlation between high personal accomplishment and patient satisfaction [21].

Not only do burned out physicians risk low patient satisfaction, but there is increased risk of medical errors, safety compromise incidents, and malpractice claims [20]. Burnout is associated with reduced quality of care and puts the very patients who physicians are trying to treat at possible risk of harm. However, these negative patient care outcomes do not occur in a vacuum, and they often cause significant distress for physicians confronted by them. Physicians named in a patient complaint may experience a cascade of responses ranging from poor sleep to anxiety, depression, and suicidal ideation [22].

22.7.3 Health Systems Effects

More recently there has been specific interest in how burnout affects the sustainability of the nephrology workforce in caring for renal patients. Several articles have noted the declining interest of medical students and general internal medicine residents in nephrology, which is also related to organizational-level factors in burnout [17]. Not only is there decreased entry into nephrology training, meaning unfilled fellowship positions, but there are also fellows who do not complete training. Even for fully qualified nephrologists, survey results demonstrate an interest in changing practices, moving to part-time hours, or even retiring earlier [9]. This also taxes the system as a conservative estimated cost of turnover per physician per year is already between 5000 and 10,000 USD [20]. With depleted numbers in training and in the workforce, one worries about how nephrologists will continue to meet the growing needs of renal patients worldwide.

Clinical Pearl

- Physicians' work can have profound emotional impacts, leading to a range of outcomes, some of which can be devastating, e.g., suicide.
- These outcomes matter not only because of how they deeply affect individuals, but because of how they also impact patient care and health systems.

Recommendation

- If conducting a wellness survey in the workplace, consider screening for other markers of psychological distress related to burnout such as anxiety, depression, suicidality, and personal, social, or occupational impairment.
- Further, when examining issues in patient satisfaction, team morale, or work processes and sustainability, consider the health and wellness of the workforce and whether key factors such as burnout are being missed.

22.8 Facilitating Physician Wellness in Nephrology

Before considering the evidence base for specific interventions, it is important to discuss what is meant by physician wellness. Having a better understanding of this will help direct one's efforts toward relevant targets and strategies for shifting physicians along the wellness continuum. From there, one can consider individual, organizational, and systemic changes to optimize wellness, including how to possibly address moral distress in nephrology. Above all, pursuing these endeavors requires a change in the culture of medicine to one that genuinely supports and promotes wellness.

22.8.1 Redefining Physician Wellness

Physician wellness is a common term in the literature, and yet it is less common for stakeholders to consider what it actually entails. For example, Brady et al. [23] published a systematic review in 2018 that analyzed over 75 articles on physician wellness in which only 14% of them defined wellness. Even when this information was provided, descriptions varied, but they often recognized that one's quality of life is of paramount importance. When wellness was measured, tools used varied again, but they tended toward measuring negative outcomes such as burnout and depression rather than wellness itself [23]. As such, impaired well-being becomes conflated with distress and disorder. Thus, rather than interventions designed to target wellness, they are designed to prevent illness [23]. Even if physicians are *not ill*, it does not necessarily mean that they are *well*. There are many other strategies that can be used to optimize their sense of wellness.

If we consider physician wellness as more than the absence of illness, then we can focus on enhancing positive well-being, quality of life, and helping them reach full potential [23]. "We" is used intentionally, as physician wellness is not just the *individual's* responsibility, but rather it should be conceptualized as a shared responsibility among *all key stakeholders*. To this point, the Stanford WellMD Professional Fulfillment Model is a widely accepted model that illustrates the idea of collective responsibility. It identifies three main areas to promote physician wellness, including the areas of personal resilience, efficiency of practice, and culture of wellness [24]. In doing so it acknowledges that wellness reaches beyond the individual to incorporate organizational and systemic changes (see Table 22.4) [14, 16–18, 20, 25, 26]. While it further suggests that organizations and systems should be mainly responsible for changes in the latter two [24], each still has a role in encouraging and supporting individual resilience efforts.

22.8.2 Boosting Physician Resilience

When one speaks of individual interventions to address burnout, often one hears the critique that physicians just need to be more resilient. Resilience is another term with various definitions, but it is generally considered as "qualities that enable a person to adapt well and even thrive in the face of adversity" [27]. While physicians may be led to think otherwise, there is evidence that physicians maintain high levels of resilience throughout their careers. West et al. [27] published the results of a national US survey of physicians in 2020 that compared the level of resilience between physicians and the general population. They found that resilience was higher among physicians, but even those with high scores still reported burnout [27], indicating that resilience alone does not guarantee wellness.

While resilience is likely one small part of the wellness picture, there are still some strategies that are effective in boosting resilience. Interventions such as gratitude (i.e., partaking in positive psychology exercises such as keeping a gratitude journal or writing a gratitude letter), mindfulness (i.e., maintaining a present

Table 22.4 Interventions to enhance physician wellness [14, 16–18, 20, 25, 26]

Personal resilience	Efficiency of practice	Culture of wellness
Self-care	Decrease workload	Educate leaders and staff
Gratitude	Increase efficiency	Challenge implicit beliefs
Self-compassion	Enhance teamwork	Prioritize staff wellness
Mindfulness		Peer support groups
Narrative medicine		Access to formal supports

moment awareness of thoughts, feelings, bodily sensations, and surrounding environment through a variety of practices to help reduce stress), narrative medicine (i.e., utilizing people's narratives in clinical practice as a way to promote healing), and self-compassion (i.e., extending compassion to one's self when perceived inadequacy, failure, or suffering) may lessen distress, help process difficult emotions, and foster well-being [17, 18, 20]. While not specific to nephrology, a variety of organizations targeting medical students, resident physicians, fellows, and other physicians have developed resilience programs. See Table 22.5 for a summary of these wellness initiatives. While they are not the endpoint for physician wellness, they engage in a harm reduction approach to wellness. Beyond this, we need to continue to advocate for more effective interventions that address work culture and environment.

Table 22.5 Selected physician wellness resources

Selected wellness resources	Description
McMaster University "Resilience in the Era of Sustainable Physicians: An International Training Endeavour" (RESPITE) https://respite.machealth.ca/	Online resident modules designed by a multisite, international team, to help residents understand personal resilience and how to address it, and other strategies to mitigate risk of burnout
Resident Doctors of Canada "Resiliency Curriculum" https://residentdoctors.ca/areas-of-focus/resiliency/	Interactive resident and leadership modules facilitated by resiliency peer trainers, as well as booster modules in development to supplement core training
Stanford Medicine "WellMD Center" https://wellmd.stanford.edu/center1.html	Information on physician health and wellness, including strategies for personal resilience, efficiency of practice, and culture of wellness
Canadian Medical Association "Physician Wellness Hub" https://www.cma.ca/physician-wellness-hub	Online hub of original CMA content and other trusted tools and resources for medical trainees and physicians to support their health and wellness
American Medical Association "STEPS Forward" https://edhub.ama-assn.org/steps-forward	Online modules on how to engage leadership, understand physician burnout and how to address it, and develop a culture of wellness
International Conference on Physician Health 2021 "A vision for humanity in medicine" https://www.bma.org.uk/events/international-conference-on-physician-health-2021	An international online conference in collaboration with the British, American, and Canadian Medical Associations that aims to support physician health with key knowledge and interventions
Your local clinic or hospital website	Check online for workplace wellness committees, assessments, initiatives, and other helpful resources

22.8.3 Driving Efficiency of Practice

While individual interventions are not enough to promote physician wellness, there is promise in pursuing higher-level solutions. At minimum, there should be training in wellness for key stakeholders within the organization, specific workplace interventions offered, and a referral system to formal supports. Panagioti et al. [25] published a meta-analysis of controlled interventions in 2017 which determined that organizational interventions were associated with higher treatment effects for physician burnout compared to individual ones [25]. The authors suggested that individual interventions would likely have been more effective had organizations and systems supported their work [25], again recognizing that physician wellness is a shared responsibility. As for interventions, organization efforts involved reduced workload and increased workflow as well as teamwork and peer support.

Nephrologists also acknowledge these areas as key recommendations when considering how to optimize nephrology fellows and other physicians' wellness. For example, Rosner and Berns [26] considered how nephrologists can re-establish joy, meaning, and engagement in their work. They advocated for having standardized work processes, pre-visit planning/testing, using interdisciplinary teams and physician extenders to share the work, as well as scribes and better EMR tools to manage documentation. While not exactly peer support, they also advocated for virtual and in-person communities of practice in nephrology where physicians can share best practices, establish research networks, and create other network opportunities [26]. While no one is expecting organizations to put all these interventions in place at once, each contributes to positive changes in physician wellness.

22.8.4 Alleviating Moral Distress

In identifying moral distress as a unique contributor to burnout in nephrology, while there is no evidence supporting one intervention over another, there are ways we can help. Ducharlet et al. [18], who presented international cases of moral distress in nephrology, discussed the importance of first acknowledging moral distress and using the term in practice. They also advocate for providing evidence and support in difficult care decisions and encouraging leadership to be active role models in this work. More specifically, they suggest the equivalent of complex case rounds; team debriefs after distressing patient events; training in ethics, advocacy, and advanced communication skills; and, of course, access to formal psychological supports [18].

While Ducharlet et al. [18] did not consider formal peer support in their article, others have discussed its use and benefit in nephrology for similar purposes. Roberts stated that facilitated small groups may provide opportunities to discuss distressing cases as well as to manage difficult emotions, build connectedness, and reduce burnout [17]. For example, Balint groups are structured groups that help physicians explore and process difficult patient-physician relationships. Given their popularity, Pawlowicz and Nowicki also suggested these groups for Polish nephrologists experiencing burnout [14]. It becomes clear that alleviating moral distress often requires organizational and systemic changes rather than falling to individual physicians alone.

22.8.5 Fostering a Culture of Wellness

At the systemic level, it is recommended to align the culture of medicine, a main contributor to physician burnout, with that of a culture of wellness. Joan Anzia is a US psychiatrist who has presented on this topic and identified several implicit beliefs that sustain the culture of medicine. For example, physicians are expected to sacrifice basic needs, have endless reserves of energy, strive for perfection in work, and manage alone when they are struggling [16]. In stark contrast, a culture of wellness challenges these beliefs and prioritizes physician wellness. Moreover, the system's policies, practices, and procedures reflect such values [16]. We hope that physicians can fulfill their basic needs so they can function optimally, that they recognize their limitations and show self-compassion, and that they remain connected and seek help when needed.

Cultural change is worthwhile because these interventions have some of the greatest impacts on physician wellness while also reducing psychological distress. Change can be difficult and so the literature offers some advice for enacting systemic change in medicine [28]. First, it is important to recruit key stakeholders who can act as wellness champions, develop relevant initiatives, and be involved in their implementation. Next, it may be helpful to conduct a local needs assessment to explore the unique factors, challenges, and barriers to physician wellness in one's setting. Since physicians' needs vary and their degree of wellness influences others, there should also be at least several initiatives to target major domains of wellness. Finally, it is advised to use a quality improvement approach as wellness is a dynamic process that requires ongoing evaluation and optimization [28].

Clinical Pearl

- Physicians are a highly resilient group when compared to the general population.
- While resilience may help mediate distress in medicine, it is not enough on its own to maintain wellness or prevent psychological harms.
- Instead, organizational and systemic interventions have been shown to be the most effective for these purposes [25] and should be the focus of our efforts.

Recommendation

- We need to start challenging our implicit beliefs about what it means to be a physician today.
- In doing so, we take steps at the systemic level to shift the culture of medicine toward a culture of wellness that prioritizes our health and wellness.
- Once there is commitment at this level from relevant stakeholders, we can use a targeted approach to designing, implementing, and evaluating wellness initiatives.

22.9 Key Takeaways

- While not specific to nephrology alone, occupation-related stress is an ongoing concern for nephrology fellows and other physicians caring for renal patients.
- Burnout is a syndrome caused by chronic work stress that encompasses a triad of:
  - Emotional exhaustion
  - Depersonalization
  - Reduced sense of personal accomplishment
- Measuring it with tools such as the Maslach Burnout Inventory will help identify individual physicians at high risk of burnout, as well as any concerning patterns of burnout in the workplace.
- There is a multitude of contributing factors to burnout in medicine that reach across individual, organizational, and systemic levels.
- While nephrology fellows and other physicians are also impacted by these general factors, experiences such as moral distress may be more unique.
- Burnout matters not only because of how it affects individuals, but how it also goes on to affect patient care and health systems.
- To optimize wellness, we need to maintain a broader definition of wellness beyond the absence of illness, as there is always opportunity to improve.
- While individual resilience can help mediate distress, it is only a temporizing measure, and it is not enough on its own to maintain wellness.
- We should focus on organizational and systemic change as this is where interventions in efficiency of practice and culture of wellness have the most impact
- To enact systematic change, it is helpful to engage key stakeholders, conduct a local needs assessment, trial a range of interventions, and use a quality improvement model.

References

1. Freudenberger HJ. Staff burn-out. J Soc Issues. 1974;30(1):159–65.
2. ICD-11 for Mortality and Morbidity Statistics [Internet]. World Health Organization; updated 2020 Sep. QD85 Burnout; [cited 2020 Dec 28]; [about 1 screen]. https://icd.who.int/browse11/l-m/en#/http://id.who.int/icd/entity/129180281.
3. Maslach C, Jackson SE. MBI: Human Services Survey for Medical Personnel [Internet]. Menlo Park, CA: Mind Garden: Tools for Positive Transformation; 2019 [cited 2020 Dec 28]. https://www.mindgarden.com/315-mbi-human-services-survey-medical-personnel#horizontalTab4.
4. West CP, Dyrbye LN, Satele DV, Sloan JA, Shanafelt TD. Concurrent validity of single-item measures of emotional exhaustion and depersonalization in burnout assessment. J Gen Intern Med. 2012;27(11):1445–52.
5. Canadian Medical Association. CMA national physician health survey: a national snapshot [Internet]. Canada: Canadian Medical Association; 2018 Oct [cited 2020 Dec 28]. 31 p. https://www.cma.ca/sites/default/files/2018-11/nph-survey-e.pdf.
6. Brazeau CM, Shanafelt T, Durning SJ, Massie FS, Eacker A, Moutier C, et al. Distress among matriculating medical students relative to the general population. Acad Med. 2014;89(11):1520–5.

7. Dyrbye LN, West CP, Satele D, Boone S, Tan L, Sloan J, et al. Burnout among U.S. medical students, residents, and early career physicians relative to the general U.S. population. Acad Med. 2014;89(3):443–51.
8. Dyrbye LN, Varkey P, Boone SL, Satele DV, Sloan JA, Shanafelt TD. Physician satisfaction and burnout at different career stages. Mayo Clin Proc. 2013;88(12):1358–67.
9. Salsberg E, Quigley L, Mehfoud N, Masselink L, Collins A. The US adult nephrology workforce 2016: developments and trends [Internet]. Washington, DC: George Washington University Health Workforce Institute, prepared for the American Society of Nephrology; 2016 [cited 2020 Dec 29]. 28 p. https://www.asn-online.org/education/training/workforce/Nephrology_Workforce_Study_Report_2016.pdf.
10. Martin KL. Medscape nephrologist lifestyle, happiness, & burnout report 2020 [Internet]. Medscape; 2020 Feb [cited 2020 Dec 29]. 23 p. https://www.medscape.com/slideshow/2020-lifestyle-nephrologist-6012499#1.
11. Agrawal V, Platinga L, Abdel-Kader K, Pivert K, Provenzano A, Soman S, et al. Burnout and emotional well-being among nephrology fellows: a national online survey. J Am Soc Nephrol. 2020;31(4):675–85.
12. Kane L. Medscape national physician burnout & suicide report 2020: the generational divide [Internet]. Medscape; 2020 Jan [cited 2020 Dec 29]. 29 p. https://www.medscape.com/slideshow/2020-lifestyle-burnout-6012460#1.
13. Giroux C. 5: Personal coping styles and resilience. 2018 [cited 2020 Dec 29]. In: Resilience in the Era of Sustainable Physicians: An International Training Endeavour [Internet]. Hamilton, ON: McMaster University. 2018 – [about 1 screen]. https://respite.machealth.ca/know_5.html.
14. Pawłowicz E, Nowicki M. Burnout syndrome among nephrologists – a burning issue – results of the countrywide survey by the Polish Society of Nephrology. BMC Nephrol. 2020;21(1):177.
15. Williams AW. Addressing physician burnout: nephrologists, how safe are we? Clin J Am Soc Nephrol. 2018;13(2):325–7.
16. Anzia J. Physician wellness. Session presented at: Women in Medicine Symposium at Northwestern University Feinberg School of Medicine; 2018 Oct 25; Chicago, IL.
17. Roberts JK. Burnout in nephrology: implications on recruitment and the workforce. Clin J Am Soc Nephrol. 2018;13(2):328–30.
18. Ducharlet K, Philip J, Gock H, Brown M, Gelfand SL, Josland EA, et al. Moral Distress in nephrology: perceived barriers to ethical clinical care. Am J Kidney Dis. 2020;76(2):248–54.
19. Oreskovich MR, Shanafelt T, Dyrbye LN, Tan L, Sotile W, Satele D, et al. The prevalence of substance use disorders in American physicians. Am J Addict. 2015;24(1):30–8.
20. West CP, Dyrbye LN, Shanafelt TD. Physician burnout: contributors, consequences and solutions. J Intern Med. 2018;283(6):516–29.
21. Argentero P, Dell'Olivo B, Santa Ferretti M. Staff burnout and patient satisfaction with the quality of dialysis care. Am J Kidney Dis. 2008;51(1):80–92.
22. Bourne T, Wynants L, Peters M, Van Audenhove C, Timmerman D, Van Calster B, et al. The impact of complaints procedures on the welfare, health and clinical practise of 7926 doctors in the UK: a cross-sectional survey. BMJ Open. 2015;5(1):e006687.
23. Brady KJS, Trockel MT, Khan CT, Raj KS, Murphy ML, Bohman B, et al. What do we mean by physician wellness? A systematic review of its definition and measurement. Acad Psychiatr. 2017;42(1):94–108.
24. Stanford Medicine Well MD Center [Internet]. Stanford, CA: Stanford Medicine; c2016. 2017 WellMD Model Domain Definitions; 2017 [cited 2020 Dec 31]; [about 1 screen]; https://wellmd.stanford.edu/content/dam/sm/wellmd/documents/2017-WellMD-Domain-Definitions-FINAL.pdf.
25. Panagioti M, Panagopoulou E, Bower P, Lewith G, Kontopantelis E, Chew-Graham C, et al. Controlled interventions to reduce burnout in physicians: a systematic review and meta-analysis. JAMA Intern Med. 2017;177(2):195–205.
26. Rosner MH, Berns JS. Transforming nephrology. Clin J Am Soc Nephrol. 2018;13(2):331–4.

27. West CP, Dyrbye LN, Sinsky C, Trockel M, Tutty M, Nedelec L, et al. Resilience and burnout among physicians and the general US working population. JAMA Netw Open. 2020;3(7):e209385.
28. Linzer M, Guzman-Corrales L, Poplau S. Physician burnout: improve physician satisfaction and patient outcomes. 2015 Jun [cited 2021 Jan 3]. In: AMA STEPS Forward [Internet]. Chicago, IL: American Medical Association. 2015 – [about 1 screen]. https://edhub.ama-assn.org/steps-forward/module/2702509.

Modernizing Continuing Professional Development Using Social Media

23

Natasha Snelgrove, Matthew A. Sparks, Javeed Sukhera, Joel M. Topf, and Teresa M. Chan

23.1 Introduction

In the domain of psychonephrology, readers may be wondering why there is a chapter written by an interdisciplinary team about the use of social media for continuing professional development. It is our hope that by the end of this chapter, it will be clear that social media has a great potential of helping to foster and grow a community of diverse individuals interested in the intersection of psychiatry/psychology and nephrology in patients with renal disease.

N. Snelgrove
Department of Psychiatry and Behavioural Neurosciences, McMaster University, Hamilton, ON, Canada
e-mail: natasha.snelgrove@medportal.ca

M. A. Sparks
Division of Nephrology, Department of Medicine, Duke University, Durham, NC, USA

Renal Section, Durham Veterans Affairs Health Care System, Durham, NC, USA
e-mail: matthew.sparks@duke.edu

J. Sukhera
Division of Child and Adolescent Psychiatry, Department of Psychiatry, Schulich School of Medicine, Western University, London, ON, Canada
e-mail: jsukhera@uwo.ca

J. M. Topf
Department of Internal Medicine, Oakland University, Detroit, MI, USA
e-mail: jtopf@scsp.net

T. M. Chan (✉)
Division of Education & Innovation/Division of Emergency Medicine, Department of Medicine & Office of Continuing Development, Faculty of Health Sciences, McMaster University, Hamilton, ON, Canada
e-mail: teresa.chan@medportal.ca

A. Hategan et al. (eds.), *Psychonephrology*,
https://doi.org/10.1007/978-3-030-84740-1_23

We must acknowledge that staying current in a field where multiple disciplines may intersect can be particularly difficult. When we train and interact almost exclusively within our academic silos, it can be difficult to bring those of different disciplines together. Social media has provided us with a mechanism to break down the traditional silos of academia and bring together many scholars and practitioners in a truly interdisciplinary fashion.

23.1.1 What Is SoMe?

Social media (SoMe) has now become an inextricable modality used for facilitating communication globally. Clinicians, researchers, and members of the public all communicate within this space and use it to connect with each other [1–4]. Although many healthcare practitioners have often used these modalities for communication and connection with friends and families for decades, it is only in the 2010–2020s that many healthcare and medical professionals began harnessing its power for continuing professional development and scholarly discourse [1, 5].

Social media is defined as any technology-mediated communication platforms that allow individuals to distribute and curate content in digital communities [1, 6, 7]. There are dozens of platforms that currently exist, and many have emerged and disappeared throughout the decades since these platforms first gained popularity. One of the advantages of social media is its ability to connect individuals and allow for ample opportunities to create a virtual "interstitial space" that allows idea exchange and forming a sense of community [6].

Social media platforms come in two major forms: (1) open platforms (e.g., Twitter, Facebook, Instagram LinkedIn, Instagram, TikTok, Reddit, podcasts, blogs) or (2) closed platforms (e.g., WhatsApp, Slack, Microsoft Teams). Though various platforms typify open or closed forms, they often have features that cross this dichotomy (e.g., direct messaging on Twitter and stories on WhatsApp). There are ample reasons why groups would pick one or the other strategy – but often, open platforms will allow for more emergent communities to develop, while close platforms will lend themselves more to a targeted audience [8]. Furthermore, as communities mature, hybrid models often develop using both open and closed communication channels [9]. Even the classic discussion modality of an email listserv or online webforum could be seen as an early form of social media [9]. Today's social media platforms, however, allow individuals to go beyond selected closed groups where they can connect – and in this particular emergent community of psychonephrology – openly accessible communities of practice may be the way that we can engage in key exchanges of ideas across disciplines [10].

23.1.2 Networked Learning

In continuing professional development, one of the great challenges is the lack of clear guidance for our continued exposure to new ideas as we train. Whereas the bulk of the literature suggests that continuing professional development should be a singular and lonely burden for each individual practitioner to engage in by themselves [11], the reality is that we rarely learn exclusively on our own. Rhizomatic learning [12] has been described as a nonhierarchical learning approach that hinges on the development and usage of personal learning networks [13].

As individuals begin to engage in online communities, they establish a variety of relationships or connections. These connections can be thought of as a spoke on a wheel. When conceptualizing this, it is important to note that the robustness of the community develops by having more connections that communicate frequently. It is also important to note that these connections (spokes) should be bidirectional. This allows for more collaboration and a sense of community to develop. Hierarchy should be avoided whenever possible. However, it is important for leadership to consider strategies to continually reinforce communication and groupthink and ultimately build a community.

Recommendation

- Social media (SoMe) should be considered as a mechanism that all practicing professionals use to stay connected with others interested in similar domains (such as psychonephrology).

Clinical Pearl

- SoMe can be a powerful mechanism for staying up-to-date and connected with an interdisciplinary field such as psychonephrology.

23.2 Case Vignette

A 35-year-old South-Asian female Assistant Professor of Psychiatry presented to her Chair's office with a query. She had found it difficult to find a local community of practice within the department. She was interested in the domain of psychonephrology and felt rather disconnected since there were very few opportunities to engage in discussions and scholarly activities on this topic. Everyone in her department already seemed to have an academic niche, and she had only recently started to carve out an interest in this area, but wanted to find mentors and collaborators. She had reached out to the Division of Nephrology within the Department of Medicine at her institution, but she had received very little meaningful response. She was invited to present a guest rounds in the coming months, but she was unsure of how she could make a compelling case for collaboration in her upcoming talk. She wished she could pick the brain of nephrologists but did not know where to turn. As her Chair, what would you have advised? A case analysis is also presented at the end.

23.3 Problems and Barriers to Using Social Media for Continuing Professional Development

Despite the benefits that social media can provide to physicians collaborating across disciplines, barriers and challenges arise in the use of this medium. Firstly, getting started in setting up your digital identity can be a challenge and can take time and effort. Secondly, two major barriers of the medium itself can dissuade physicians from joining and engaging on social media professionally – professionalism and privacy concerns.

23.3.1 Digital Identity Formation and Personal Bandwidth

Many physicians begin to use social media as a way to meet an educational need [14]. During the process of setting up and using social media, a digital identity is formed. Often physicians wish for more boundaries between personal and professional use, but challenges can arise when one decides how much personal information or insights ought to be shared. Navigating this space requires care and thought. In addition, as you first start to use social media to connect with others in your field, finding and seeking out appropriate sources of information, people to connect with, and mentors can take time. Often this upfront investment can be time-consuming or seem arduous. This chapter includes tips and tricks for overcoming these issues in the next section.

As a start, one should ask themselves about their reasons for using social media. Is it just to meet educational needs? Stay up-to-date on the latest advances? Are you hoping to connect with others in your field? Do you have an advocacy position to advance? Do you want to provide public information for the greater good? This ethos may evolve over time, but having a good sense of why you are using SoMe to begin with can set you up to create a persona and identity that will meet your definition of success and conform to your personal bandwidth needs.

23.3.2 Professionalism

Concerns around professionalism on social media are as old as the medium itself. However, this is not unique to social media and the same principles that govern day-to-day life should be used. This concern is intimately tied to concerns around formation of digital identity. Digital professionalism for health professionals is a concept that emphasizes that social media use has the potential to blur the lines between personal and professional identities [15]. There is also a gap between what is taught in regard to digital professionalism and what is perceived by medical students [16]. Despite increased teaching, reported incidents of unprofessional posts including violations of patient confidentiality are still quite common. For example, 60% of US medical schools have reported incidents where medical students make posts considered unprofessional with 13% of schools reporting violations of patient confidentiality [16, 17].

As a professional, you can decide why you are using social media, what types of things you feel comfortable sharing, and how these fit with professional society and/or employer recommendations. It is important to remember that giving general advice on a topic, networking with colleagues, and sharing research are generally encouraged, but giving specific patient advice is not. Gray areas remain around sharing personal opinions on politicized issues, so you may want to consider staying away from these types of conversations until you feel confident in your own digital identity.

Another important aspect to social media use is that the platform may lack nuance, depth, or the opportunity for misinterpretation of well-intended commentary. An example of this is humor, which can be easily misinterpreted and sometimes with devastating consequences [18]. Should you engage in discourse with other professionals and sense that misinterpretation has occurred, we advise you to seek an opportunity to apologize and connect directly or privately with the other party. When in doubt, you can delete offending tweets and seek repair.

23.3.3 Privacy

Many physicians also worry about privacy in the social media setting [5]. If you wish to be on an open platform, such as Twitter, your ability to engage with other like-minded professionals will be much higher with lower privacy settings. This will allow others to see what you share, follow you, and build your community of practice. However, this is balanced with concerns around who can see what you share. Patients may be online and may contact you. As you form your digital identity, you may share information or perspectives that you wish you had not – and although you can delete a posting, if it has been seen or shared, it may never truly disappear.

Understanding privacy legislation and having a philosophy of social media use can be helpful in avoiding privacy slips. Most social media recommendations authored by physician organization advise that identifying patient information never be disclosed. Be mindful of what this may be for a particular patient, especially if you work in a small field. For specific patient advice, take the discussion offline – to the phone or in person. Sometimes, despite your best efforts, "trolls" may follow you and harass you on social media. This can be particularly common in psychiatry where anti-psychiatry groups may critique and criticize efforts. Social media platforms have a variety of ways you can respond, such as by increasing privacy settings, muting, or blocking users. Note that the behavior and definitions of these various defensive actions will vary from platform to platform.

Clinical Pearl

- There are many considerations that one should consider before entering into social media for learning. Key considerations to weigh are: (a) personal bandwidth, (b) professional and personal identity (and portrayal of this identity), and (c) privacy concerns.

Recommendation

- Weigh each of these aforementioned considerations (personal bandwidth, professional and personal identity, and privacy concerns) carefully, and make a strategic plan for yourself when you begin engaging in SoMe for learning.
- Start off slow and use high security settings initially.

23.4 A "How To" Guide for Harnessing the Power of SoMe for Continuing Professional Development

Writing this about 1 year into the coronavirus infectious disease 2019 (COVID-19) pandemic, it is clear that Twitter should be your primary social media platform for medical education and professional development. To understand why this is, it is useful to look at the core features of Twitter compared with the other social media platforms. See the list below for some details:

- **Open.** For people trying to start their engagement in social media, an open platform is essential. In symmetric systems like Facebook, both parties need to agree to engage in order to interact. This is the process of friend requests. This controls interaction but slows the process of onboarding. Twitter (with its default privacy settings), like Instagram, allows people to follow the content of any creator.
- **Flexible.** Twitter is usually described as a social network that allows people to broadcast short strings of text, limited to 280 characters, but this underplays its flexibility. Each tweet is a container for a variety of contents including text, images, animations, and most importantly links. Links are essential for substantive medical education. Links provide the opportunity to cite original literature, a staple of modern medical education. They allow deeper immersion in an argument, allowing the social media to be a teaser to draw in curious learners. Instagram does not allow links in the content (only a single link in the account owner's biography) [19].
- **Networked.** Metcalfe's law states the value of a network is proportional to the square of the number of connected users of the system. Twitter has a large foundation of medical educators, clinicians, and scientists already using it, so the value of the Twitter medical education network is very large. Twitter allows even very specific subjects within medicine, like nephrology and psychonephrology, to build communities of practice. At the time of writing this chapter, other platforms have yet to build up the human capital to surpass Twitter. Few have been able to do that and this will likely mean that Twitter will endure as an effective social media platform. Reddit is a social network that has the critical features of a medical social media platform but lacks the size to have sufficient network effect. By following others on these platforms, you can begin to create a personal learning network to support your own development.

Clinical Pearl
- SoMe is an undeniable part of our lives, and there are many advantages to using it for Continuing Professional Development. It will allow you an open, flexible, and networked way to engage in your personal learning.

Recommendation
- Select a SoMe platform, and then start finding and following other psychologists, psychiatrists, and nephrologists to start your own personal learning network.

23.4.1 Getting Started on Twitter

The first step is to set up your professional account with a login name and description that reflects your role and goals on social media. Typically, most professionals will use their names and highlight their qualifications in their profile description. Make sure to add a picture to your bio. A complete bio makes it easier for others to find and engage with you so you can start engaging in the free open-access medical education (#FOAMed) community. If you are hesitant to engage on social media, start an account, and start to look around, there is no obligation to contribute; consuming social media is a natural first step in engagement [4].

One of the challenges to Twitter is the onboarding process. When one opens a Twitter account, it is empty, and it only becomes meaningful as one follows people. This is a "catch-22", as one wants to follow people who post relevant and interesting tweets, but one cannot see those tweets unless one already follows them. Twitter tries to ease this by suggesting people to follow based on some questions while establishing the account. However, there are two additional ways to see tweets from people one does not follow: retweets and hashtags.

A retweet is when a person posts another user's content to their feed. Suppose one follows a college friend and the friend retweets a post about the immune system by @EdYong209. Even if the user does not follow @EdYong209, they will see this tweet because they follow their college friend.

Similarly, hashtags allow you to break from the timeline of people they follow and see tweets tagged with a particular hashtag regardless of the author. Hashtags develop around sporting and entertainment events but can be particularly granular.

One of the most important nephrology hashtags is #KidneyWk which denotes American Society of Nephrology's annual meeting. Following that hashtag during the annual meeting will reveal tweets about good sessions, bad speakers, tasty places to eat, and interesting posters. Users can then decide to follow people from that stream. Other important hashtags to follow in nephrology include:

- #NephJC. NephJC is a twice a month journal club that meets on Twitter. A discussion of the importance of NephJC to the nephrology twitter community is examined later in this chapter [20, 21].
- #NephMadness. Every March the *American Journal of Kidney Diseases* and the National Kidney Foundation have sponsored NephMadness. NephMadness is a collaborative educational game where participants discuss and debate the merits of 32 nephrology concepts that compete to advance through a single elimination bracket. A deeper exploration of #NephMadness can be found later in this chapter [22–24].
- #AskRenal. One of the frustrations with getting started on Twitter is that it is easy to follow people in nephrology and hear their opinions and observations but when one wants to share one's own opinion, if they have no followers, the tweet is like a tree falling in the forest without anyone around to hear it. #AskRenal allows people to access a significant portion of the nephrology Twitter community so their tree does not fall unnoticed. People with questions that they want the nephrology community to answer just need to tweet the question and add the hashtag #AskRenal. A software program continuously scans Twitter for any new tweets with this hashtag and then retweets the original tweet from a dedicated account called @AskRenal. @AskRenal has over 5000 followers so this retweet reaches a broad swath of the nephrology community on Twitter.

Hashtags that are useful in psychiatry are:

- #PsychTwitter. This is a hashtag that connects those who are interested in psychiatry across Twitter. Similar to the larger hashtag #MedTwitter, which is a broader interdisciplinary hashtag for all who identify as physicians, this hashtag can be applied to most psychiatry or psychology tweets that are for other practitioners within the field.

Clinical Pearl

– Hashtags can help you to locate groups of messages that are tagged. Think of them as MeSH terms for SoMe. You can search for messages (and accounts) that associate themselves with hashtags to help you find other like-minded individuals.

Recommendation

– Use Twitter hashtags to discover new groups of individuals or topics. For instance, try joining tweet chats like #NephJC to see how they operate, and learn more about nephrology. Consider using #AskRenal to ask nephrologists for advice.

One of the reasons that nephrology is developing a robust social media infrastructure is a formal nephrology social media training program called the Nephrology Social Media Collective (NSMC). The NSMC, established in 2015, is a means to ensure a consistent entry of new voices into the nephrology social media space [19]. It is a 1-year program of remote learning that trains people in many aspects of social media education and presentation. The program is defined by four rotations focusing on various types of social media:

1. Blogs and Tweetorials
2. Nephrology journal clubs and Twitter-based discussions
3. Digital communications focusing on visual abstracts
4. Podcasts and audio communication

Faculty mentors are included in each pod to help provide mentorship and feedback throughout the year. In addition, monthly lecture series are incorporated into the curriculum, and daily communication is achieved through Slack [9, 25]. The internship trains 28 interns a year. Graduates have gone on to leadership roles throughout nephrology including academia, private practice, and industry [9, 19].

23.5 Building and Sustaining Cross-Disciplinary Virtual Communities of Practice

An increasing number of health professionals are moving from faculty development activities that take place on an individual level to informal collective learning exemplified by the idea of a community of practice (CoP) [6, 26]. A CoP refers to a group of individuals that shares both concern and interest for something they do and wish to improve it through interacting with one another (CoP is a term coined by Lave and Wenger). When applied to a virtual setting, virtual CoPs (VCoPs) involve individuals coming together through technology in a virtual space. In business, VCoPs have been shown to be effective in improving knowledge sharing, thus reducing professional and structural isolation [27].

Building and maintaining a VCoP can be challenging when groups are diverse. For example, different specialties may have different interests and professional identities. Although VCoPs can improve knowledge sharing and foster connection, virtual communities may also reflect inter-group biases and group-based behavior that limit knowledge sharing [26].

Despite these challenges, there is evidence that VCoPs can improve and enhance interprofessional collaboration and education. In a 2018 review, McLoughlin et al. found that VCoPs can offer an informal method of development and can decrease isolation [28]. However, success was limited by issues such as privacy, trust, encouragement, technological infrastructure, and technological ability [28]. These challenges can be overcome by using easily accessible tools that allow for real-time communication [22, 23]. VCoPs should also consider safety and create low-risk environments to reduce barriers within and between professions. Ultimately, VCoPs have value for individuals who are working in isolation to come together in ways that would not be possible due to geographical barriers.

23.5.1 Bringing Disciplines Together

Bringing psychiatry and nephrology together through a VCoP may seem like an unusual or eclectic idea. Yet, there are several examples of how different disciplines have come together virtually over mutual and shared interest that we may draw inspiration from.

The first is an example from the field of pediatric pain research. Led by clinical psychologist, Dr. Christine Chambers, #itdoesnthavetohurt is a science-media partnership that brings evidence-based information about children's pain directly to parents [29]. In her journey, Dr. Chambers found that numerous eHealth tools for pain assessment and management are developed, yet have a reduced impact because they are rarely made available to end users [30]. She and her team targeted their digital strategy directly at caregivers, whom they empowered with knowledge on best practices for managing pediatric pain.

After the initial work to build a community of practice that includes patients and health professionals, a community of practice with diverse disciplines has grown and spread [31]. The group contains strong interprofessional and interregional communication. The network comes together on a shared focus and passion for improving pediatric pain management. It is built around a democratized approach to knowledge translation led by Dr. Chambers' initial work.

In the field of psychonephrology, VCoPs could be helpful with helping those who are new to the field to engage in distance-based mentorship. In smaller fields or in fields where providers may lack local support, digital mentorship (e.g., via Twitter) can be useful to help others find their footing [32].

Clinical Pearl

- Virtual Communities of Practice (VCoPs) can be highly influential for supporting cross-disciplinary practice. There is an opportunity for psychonephrology-interested individuals to bring psychiatry, psychology, and nephrology together via SoMe.

23.5.2 Creating an Online Rally Point

While much of social media consists of random interactions, it became evident that some order is needed to establish a robust CoP. For nephrology, the creation of a bimonthly Twitter-based journal club [20, 33], called NephJC (nephrology journal club), was instrumental in serving this purpose. Founded in 2014, the goal of NephJC is to discuss high-impact research that drives the field forward. What started as a scholarly series of discussions of research advances on Twitter became an important activity that resulted in continual growth of the nephrology social media community. The presence of a regularly occurring meeting place on Twitter helped to introduce like-minded people and strengthen connections and served as a de facto social media equivalent of an in-person grand rounds conference series. Moreover, NephJC has become an activity that nephrologists look forward to participating in every 2 weeks, not only to further their education but to chat with collaborators, colleagues, and friends.

NephJC provided the necessary ingredient to enable nephrologists to meet regularly in social space [34]. However, it was evident that people still craved the big once a year meeting. This calling was filled by NephMadness [22–24, 35]. NephMadness, founded in 2013, is a yearly education-based game that pits nephrology concepts against each other in a single elimination tournament throughout the month of March modeled after the annual US collegiate basketball tournament. While learning nephrology concepts is fundamental to the activity, it became clear that community building was just as important. Each year over 1000 participants submit entries into NephMadness, and 1500 individual Twitter accounts use the #NephMadness hashtag. Importantly, fellowship programs, practices, and academic groups throw NephMadness parties and share photos across social media. Participation is global with participants in over 30 countries and over 50% of NephMadness users located outside of the USA. NephMadness continues to serve as a yearly opportunity for nephrologists to discuss and debate important topics in the field. It is also an opportunity to continue to grow one's network, reinforce existing connections, and serve as a positive community builder.

Clinical Pearl

- Creating an online rallying point for groups can be important. The creation and maintenance of the #NephMadness hashtag and annual event has become a cultural phenomenon and acts as a rallying point for the community.

23.5.3 Sustainability and Structures

The key to maintaining a robust online community is multiple successive waves of increasing enthusiasm and structure. For the larger open-access movement within medical education, referred to popularly as the *Free Open Access Medical education* movement (FOAM or by the hashtag #FOAMed), there have been four waves of citizens that have been described to each hold a key role toward both establishing and sustaining it [36]. The first wave is the founders, those who bravely charged ahead and decided to become active in creating online education without regard to reward structures or academic merit. Next came the enthusiasts, those who were inspired by the founders and took up the similar mantle. These individuals tended to be very enthusiastic about the movement, improving and bringing great energy and contributions in their own right. The third wave of participants for the FOAM movement were the structuralists, those who sought to bring the disruptive nature of the movement back into the academy – formalizing structures (editorial boards, organizational structures), creating new avenues for academic merit or reward, and teaching others to be critical of the movement for its own sake. The last movement is the entry of more and more participants – those who now have access and ability to engage within the movement because of increasing availability of mentors or programs for training [9, 37, 38].

Clinical Pearl

- Sustainability is, and likely always will be, a key challenge for emerging academic practices like this. Learning from other online education movements (such as the Free Open Access Medical education movement) can help newly established VCoPs to best anticipate potential roadblocks.

23.6 The Future

Social media has changed the world so drastically in the past few decades that it is certain that it will slowly have influence on the tried-and-true academic structures. As we have described previously, it can be seen as a disruptive force for individual careers, essentially upending traditional academic trajectories of scholars [39]. It is also challenging traditional models of continuing professional development, shifting us from an individualistic approach to learning within our careers to a more networked possibility. Most interesting may be that the disruptive nature of social media is now in a phase of formalization and structuralization [36]. Free and open-access movements such as FOAM are starting to organize and take on structure [36]. Social media groups are emerging organizations [38, 40].

Social media now has such a great power and influence, that many practitioners are seeing that it is in need of shape and formalization. And whereas this has been met with some resistance [36], increasingly the once-disruptive social media groups are increasingly taking on familiar formalized structures such as governance models, codes of conduct, and formal mergers or collaborations, suggesting that disruption is now facing increasing institutionalization.

What does the future of continuing professional development for the psychonephrology community look like? Only time will tell. But perhaps with some of the precedents and lessons learned from nephrology, a new community of practice may be formed and sustained to give rise to a new exciting way to engage in continuing professional development.

Recommendation

- While social media platforms will come and go, it can be beneficial for members of the community to connect via digital means. We recommend that members of the #Psychonephrology community consider either forming their own virtual community of practice or integrating with nephrology and psychiatry communities online.

23.7 Case Vignette Analysis

Referring to the case vignette outlined in Sect. 23.2, here are some suggestions that the authors present in line with the previous discussions. Based on this Assistant Professor's problem, one of the approaches she could take would be to engage in various virtual communities of practice to find like-minded individuals who are also interested in this topic. In preparation for her upcoming talk to her local nephrologists, she posted a question to several hashtags (#AskRenal and #PsychTwitter) and found an interdisciplinary cadre of individuals who all provided her relevant and useful opinions for her talk. Several members of this community welcomed her and began to digitally mentor her in developing her academic niche. One nephrologist from another country even reached out to say that she would be thrilled to host her as a digital grand rounds speaker on the same topic if she would like. She also contemplated applying to one of the many digital social media fellowships she has discovered, as she was hoping to develop an academic niche in this area as well.

23.8 Key Takeaways

- Social media (SoMe) is a must-use technology for continuing professional development.
- Virtual communities of practice (VCoPs) established through social media can be a powerful tool to connect individuals who may be geographically distant and yet share common interests.
- To sustain a VCoP, members must be mindful to create sustainable structures and systems. Looking to successes within other fields and seeking mentorship from other established SoMe educators may be prudent when embarking in this mission.

References

1. Chan TM, Dzara K, Dimeo SP, Bhalerao A, Maggio LA. Social media in knowledge translation and education for physicians and trainees: a scoping review. Perspect Med Educ. 2020;9(1):20–30.
2. Choo EK, Ranney ML, Chan TM, Trueger NS, Walsh AE, Tegtmeyer K, et al. Twitter as a tool for communication and knowledge exchange in academic medicine: a guide for skeptics and novices. Med Teach. 2015;37(5):411–6.
3. Chan T, Seth Trueger N, Roland D, Thoma B. Evidence-based medicine in the era of social media: scholarly engagement through participation and online interaction. Can J Emerg Med. 2018;20(1):3–8.
4. Jaffe RC, O'Glasser AY, Brooks M, Chapman M, Breu AC, Wray CM. Your @Attending Will #Tweet You Now: Using Twitter in Medical Education. Acad Med [Internet]. 2020 Apr 21 [cited 2020 Apr 28];Publish Ahead of Print. Available from: https://journals.lww.com/academicmedicine/Citation/9000/Your__Attending_Will__Tweet_You_Now__Using_Twitter.97237.aspx.

5. Lu D, Ruan B, Lee M, Yilmaz Y, Chan TM. Good practices in harnessing social media for scholarly discourse, knowledge translation, and education. Perspect Med Educ [Internet]. 2020 Aug 20 [cited 2020 Sep 7]; Available from: https://doi.org/10.1007/s40037-020-00613-0.
6. Yarris LM, Chan TM, Gottlieb M, Juve AM. Finding your people in the digital age: virtual communities of practice to promote education scholarship. J Grad Med Educ 2019;11(1):1–5.
7. Hafeez K, Hafeez K, Alghatas F, Alghatas F. Knowledge Management in a Virtual Community of practice using discourse analysis. Electron J Knowl Manag. 2007;5(1):29–41.
8. Chan TM, Gottlieb M, Sherbino J, Cooney R, Boysen-Osborn M, Swaminathan A, et al. The ALiEM faculty incubator: a novel online approach to faculty development in education scholarship. Acad Med. 2018;93(10):1497–502.
9. Ramakrishnan M, Sparks MA, Farouk SS. Training the public physician: the nephrology social media collective internship. Semin Nephrol. 2020;40(3):320–7.
10. McAloon CJ, Makin SDJ, Warriner DR, Norrington KDFM, Francis R, McGinnigle E, et al. How Twitter can enrich professional development. BMJ. 2016;352:i1327.
11. Allen LM, Palermo C, Armstrong E, Hay M. Categorising the broad impacts of continuing professional development: a scoping review. Med Educ. 2019;53(11):1087–99.
12. Cabrera D. FOAM and the Rhizome: an interconnected, non-hierarchical approach to MedEd [Internet]. ICE Blog. 2015 [cited 2020 Dec 23]. Available from: https://icenetblog.royalcollege.ca/2015/01/27/foam-and-the-rhizome-an-interconnected-non-hierarchical-approach-to-meded/.
13. fkankel. Personal Learning Networks: A hack to maintain competence [Internet]. ICE Blog. 2015 [cited 2020 Dec 23]. Available from: https://icenetblog.royalcollege.ca/2015/10/02/personal-learning-networks-a-hack-to-maintain-competence/.
14. Ruan B, Yilmaz Y, Lu D, Lee M, Chan TM. Defining the digital self: a qualitative study to explore the digital component of professional identity in the health professions. J Med Internet Res. 2020;22(9):e21416.
15. Ellaway RH, Coral J, Topps D, Topps M. Exploring digital professionalism. Med Teach. 2015;37(9):844–9.
16. Mostaghimi A, Olszewski AE, Bell SK, Roberts DH, Crotty BH. Erosion of digital professionalism during medical students' Core clinical clerkships. JMIR Med Educ. 2017;3(1):e6879.
17. Chretien KC, Greysen SR, Chretien JP, Kind T. Online posting of unprofessional content by medical students. JAMA. 2009;302(12):1309–15.
18. Ronson J. How one stupid Tweet Blew Up Justine Sacco's Life. The New York Times [Internet]. 2015 Feb 12 [cited 2021 Feb 6]; Available from: https://www.nytimes.com/2015/02/15/magazine/how-one-stupid-tweet-ruined-justine-saccos-life.html.
19. O'Glasser AY, Jaffe RC, Brooks M. To tweet or not to tweet, that is the question. Semin Nephrol. 2020;40(3):249–63.
20. Chan TM, Thoma B, Radecki R, Topf J, Woo HH, Kao LS, et al. Ten steps for setting up an online journal club. J Contin Educ Heal Prof. 2015;35(2):148–54.
21. Stoneman S, Hiremath S. Twitter-based journal clubs: bringing critical appraisal to the social table. Semin Nephrol. 2020;40(3):264–72.
22. Sparks MA, Lerma EV, Kupin W, Phelan PJ, Jhaveri KD, Topf J. NephMadness 2015: nephrology as a cornerstone of medicine. Am J Kidney Dis. 2015;65(3):375–7.
23. Sparks MA, Topf JM. NephMadness after 5 years: a recap and game plan for the future. Am J Kidney Dis. 2018;71(3):299–301.
24. NephMadness: Lessons from Seven Years on the Leading Edge of Social Media Medical Education [Internet]. Eur Med J. 2019 [cited 2020 Dec 23]. Available from: https://www.emjreviews.com/nephrology/article/nephmadness-lessons-from-seven-years-on-the-leading-edge-of-social-media-medical-education/.
25. Shah S, Topf J. Mentorship in the digital age: nephrology social media collective internship. Clin J Am Soc Nephrol. 2019;14(2):294–6.
26. Rolls K, Hansen M, Jackson D, Elliott D. How health care professionals use social media to create virtual communities: an integrative review. J Med Internet Res. 2016;18(6):e166.

27. Barnett S, Jones SC, Bennett S, Iverson D, Bonney A. General practice training and virtual communities of practice – a review of the literature. BMC Fam Pract. 2012;13(1):87.
28. McLoughlin C, Patel KD, O'Callaghan T, Reeves S. The use of virtual communities of practice to improve interprofessional collaboration and education: findings from an integrated review. J Interprof Care. 2018;32(2):136–42.
29. Chambers CT. From evidence to influence: dissemination and implementation of scientific knowledge for improved pain research and management. Pain. 2018;159(Suppl 1):S56–64.
30. Higgins KS, Tutelman PR, Chambers CT, Witteman HO, Barwick M, Corkum P, et al. Availability of researcher-led eHealth tools for pain assessment and management: barriers, facilitators, costs, and design. Pain Rep. 2018;3:e686.
31. Chambers CT, Dol J, Parker JA, Caes L, Birnie KA, Taddio A, et al. Implementation effectiveness of a parent-directed YouTube video ("it Doesn't have to hurt") on evidence-based strategies to manage needle pain: descriptive survey study. JMIR Pediatr Parent. 2020;3(1):e13552.
32. Landry A, Lewiss R. Is good mentorship found on Twitter? We think so. Eur J Emerg Med [Internet]. 2020 Dec 14 [cited 2020 Dec 23];Publish Ahead of Print. Available from: https://journals.lww.com/euro-emergencymed/Citation/9000/Is_good_mentorship_found_on_Twitter__We_think_so.99063.aspx.
33. Topf JM, Sparks MA, Phelan PJ, Shah N, Lerma EV, Graham-Brown MPM, et al. The evolution of the journal Club: from Osler to Twitter. Am J Kidney Dis. 2017;69(6):827–36.
34. Colbert GB, Topf J, Jhaveri KD, Oates T, Rheault MN, Shah S, et al. The social media revolution in nephrology education. Kidney Int Rep. 2018;3(3):519–29.
35. AJKDblog. #NephMadness 2018: Let the Games Begin! [Internet]. AJKD Blog. 2018 [cited 2020 May 27]. Available from: https://ajkdblog.org/2018/03/09/nephmadness-2018-let-the-games-begin/
36. Chan TM, Stehman C, Gottlieb M, Thoma B. A short history of free open access medical education. The past, present, and future. ATS Sch. 2020;1(2):ats-scholar.2020-0014PS.
37. Dave NN, Sparks MA, Farouk SS. An introduction and guide to becoming a social media savvy nephrologist. Nephrol Dial Transplant [Internet]. 2020 May 8 [cited 2020 Dec 23],(gfaa067). Available from: https://doi.org/10.1093/ndt/gfaa067.
38. Ting DK, Thoma B, Luckett-Gatopoulos S, Thomas A, Syed S, Bravo M, et al. CanadiEM: accessing a virtual community of practice to create a Canadian National Medical Education Institution. AEM Educ Train. 2019;3(1):86–91.
39. Chan TM, Stukus D, Leppink J, Duque L, Bigham BL, Mehta N, et al. Social media and the 21st-century scholar: how you can harness social media to amplify your career. J Am Coll Radiol. 2017:1–7.
40. McMaster Education Research, Innovation & Theory. Academic Life in Emergency Medicine | Dr. Michelle Lin | MERIT Rounds [Internet]. 2020 [cited 2020 Dec 23]. Available from: https://www.youtube.com/watch?v=NHp63LSo4c4&feature=youtu.be.

24 Psychonephrology of the Future: A Global Psychiatry and Nephrology Inter-specialty Curriculum for Training the Next Generation of Specialists

James A. Bourgeois, Ana Hategan, and Amanjot Sidhu

24.1 Introduction

We are in the throes of two convergent vectors regarding delivery of clinical services. The first is best thought of as *increasing specialty and subspecialty differentiation*, wherein the knowledge base, clinical literature, and technical aspects of care delivery proceed along ever narrower, focused lines [1, 2]. Nephrology evolved as a subspecialty of internal medicine, and transplant nephrology is an even more specialized area within nephrology, a "sub-subspecialty" of nephrology. In psychiatry, there is a directly analogous evolution from the specialty of psychiatry to the subspecialty of consultation-liaison psychiatry and to the "subspecialty" of psychonephrology and/or transplant consultation-liaison psychiatry.

In parallel with the focal vector leading to subspecialty and sub-subspecialty differentiation (which are areas of differentiation "within" a medical specialty), there is the unmistakable (and welcomed) trend toward *greater inclusion of other medical specialties and other clinical professions* in the multispecialty and multidisciplinary

J. A. Bourgeois (✉)
Department of Psychiatry, Baylor Scott & White Health, Central Texas Division, Department of Medical Education, College of Medicine, Texas A&M University Health Science Center, Temple, TX, USA
e-mail: james.bourgeois@bswhealth.org

A. Hategan
Division of Geriatric Psychiatry, Department of Psychiatry & Behavioural Neurosciences, Faculty of Health Sciences, Michael G. DeGroote School of Medicine, McMaster University, Hamilton, ON, Canada
e-mail: hategan@mcmaster.ca

A. Sidhu
Division of Geriatric Medicine, Department of Medicine, Faculty of Health Sciences, McMaster University, Hamilton, ON, Canada
e-mail: Sidhua4@mcmaster.ca

A. Hategan et al. (eds.), *Psychonephrology*,
https://doi.org/10.1007/978-3-030-84740-1_24

areas of patients. Regarding nephrology, there is the need for regular collaboration with physician assistants, nurse practitioners, clinical pharmacists, registered dieticians, urologists, transplant surgeons, infectious disease physicians, and immunologists. Relating to psychiatry, there is increasing interaction with psychiatric physician assistants, nurse practitioners, psychologists, and social workers.

Accepting the axiom that kidney disease inherently is associated with a great deal of psychiatric comorbidity (e.g., the risk of major depressive disorder is estimated at up to 50% in chronic renal failure), management of comorbid psychiatric illness is expected to improve patient symptom burden, increase compliance with medical regimens, and improve clinical outcomes [3, 4]. Indeed, as in many chronic illness states, psychiatric intervention for comorbid psychiatric illness may tangibly improve patient function and clinical outcomes, even if the natural history of the underlying kidney disease is progressive and likely to require major clinical interventions [5]. As such, having regular, available, and engaged psychiatric consultants should be considered part of any system that offers comprehensive care for chronic kidney disease. This need is all the more obvious when patients require hemodialysis or consideration of kidney transplantation to improve the clinical course.

In some cases, the use of multidisciplinary teams is driven by cost considerations. For example, standardized clinical management of many patients can be safely delivered by well-supported physician assistants and nurse practitioners. Psychosocial assessment for transplant candidacy and psychotherapy interventions to assist patients in dealing with chronic illness can be cost-effectively delivered by psychologists and social workers. The system approach of having physicians to be responsible for only the most complex clinical responsibility in their discipline is referred to "working at the top of one's license." Given the worldwide imperative to provide efficiently delivered care in all healthcare systems, the use of multidisciplinary teams in a carefully crafted system is imperative. Moreover, integration of behavioral health and general medicine services is another imperative, because this care model has been shown to improve patient outcomes, reduce healthcare utilization, and reduce stigma associated with mental health illnesses and interventions [6, 7]. (For more information on integrated care of the patient with kidney disease, see Chap. 9, Consultation-Liaison Psychiatry and Collaborative Care Models of the Patient with Renal Disease).

24.2 Future Developments in Psychonephrology

Taking the current state as the starting point, clinical leaders are challenged to anticipate future trends in care delivery and provide didactic and experiential models to achieve them in as seamless a way as possible.

24.2.1 Educational Milestones

Similar to other collaborative subspecialty education programs such as geriatric nephrology, educational milestones should be differentiated and catered toward the subspecialty to avoid redundancy and thereby offer a novel educational experience. For example, transplant recipients in many centers undergo psychiatric evaluation prior to the transplant surgery, as well as postoperative psychiatric follow-up. A key milestone offered to nephrology trainees would be additional training in psychosocial assessments. In psychiatry, understanding the transplant procedure and complexity around posttransplant care, including the use of multiple antirejection medications, would be a key milestone. Tables 24.1 and 24.2 identify key milestones that would be achieved by each subspecialty through a psychonephrology-based curriculum.

24.2.2 Educational Models

Educational model innovations for both multispecialty and multidisciplinary care of kidney patients with psychiatric comorbidity can take several forms. From mandating a designated amount of time toward psychonephrology training to incorporating the curriculum didactically, psychonephrology is already present in some academic institutions. Most psychonephrology experience for psychiatry trainees occurs in the context of the standard consultation-liaison (CL) psychiatry rotation. This rotation could be required or offered to other specialties (e.g., internal medicine, surgery, nephrology) as elective rotations. In addition to the CL psychiatry rotation, rotations in renal pharmacology, palliative care, geriatric nephrology, transplant medicine, and outpatient based multi-care kidney clinics would offer additional training and cover the key milestones outlined in Tables 24.1 and 24.2.

Table 24.1 Key milestones for nephrology trainees

Area	Milestones
Transplant medicine	Training in pre-op evaluation of kidney transplant candidates by performing psychosocial assessments for transplant qualification Training in post-op assessments to help patients adapt to life as a transplant recipient
Psychopharmacology	Understanding the role of psychotropic medications and their importance while balancing renal function and other comorbid conditions
Chronic kidney disease	Screening for and identifying depressive disorders with development of a preliminary management plan Perform psychiatric examination including suicide risk assessment
Chronic kidney disease including end-stage kidney disease	Performing psychological and cognitive assessments and recognizing the neurocognitive ramifications of kidney disease Approach to goals of care and decisional capacity determinations around dialysis modality and end-of-life care Recognizing substance use disorders

Table 24.2 Key milestones for psychiatry trainees

Area	Milestones
Pathophysiology	Understanding the aging kidney and the physiological and pathological implications
Transplant medicine	Understanding kidney transplant medicine from procedure to complexity of care required posttransplant and the effects of antirejection medications
Psychopharmacology	Identifying renal toxicity of psychotropic medications Identifying the psychiatric side effects of immunomodulators
Chronic kidney disease including end-stage kidney disease	Identifying unmet psychiatric needs in this population Understanding role of diet and exercise in kidney disease

Within the clinical operations of nephrology teams, clinical "bedside" teaching rounds could model multispecialty and multidisciplinary care delivery. Rehabilitation rounds could incorporate dialysis discussion and its relevance and/or barrier to rehabilitation. These multispecialty team rounds could include nephrology, psychiatry, transplant surgery, social work, health psychology, clinical pharmacy, and others.

Furthermore, specific applied clinical rotations with nephrology patients with comorbid psychiatric illness could be developed as components in training programs for multidisciplinary fields. Psychology graduate students and postgraduate trainees could receive experience in health psychology approaches to chronically ill renal patients, perform psychosocial assessments for transplant qualification, and assist patients in postoperative adaptation to life as a transplant recipient including medication and other clinical compliance. Pharmacy students could gain experience in therapeutic drug monitoring, renal adjustment of drug doses, and ascertainment of drug-drug interactions for kidney patients on complex regimens.

Currently, psychiatric care is embedded in the multi-care kidney clinic (a specialized multidisciplinary care model for patients with advancing chronic kidney disease), and this model, whether offered in-person or virtually/by telemedicine, facilitates the management of mild to moderate psychiatric comorbidity (psychiatric illness that is not of sufficient acuity to require psychiatric clinic referral) within the nephrology care model. By offering access to psychiatric care in this clinic model, nephrologists and trainees can further understand certain psychosocial implications, use of psychotropic agents, while uncovering other relevant issues that may have not been discussed in a general follow-up visit. For example, issues such as substance use disorder may arise during the psychiatric interview and warrant referral to an addiction psychiatry specialist. A patient with a history of a prolonged period of substance abstinence and stability requires further psychiatric intervention to then qualify for a kidney transplant, and thus the collaborative relationship between psychiatry and nephrology facilitates the delivery of patient-centered care.

Patients with bipolar disorder on lithium therapy who develop renal insufficiency need psychotropic medication protocols to be switched to alternative psychopharmacology regimens with ongoing therapeutic drug monitoring. By offering formal training in psychonephrology in a multi-care kidney clinic setting or the CL psychiatry rotation, these matters are better recognized and managed, often avoiding potential catastrophic complications.

24.3 Future Directions and Fostering Collaboration

With the rapid advancement in the use of virtual care and digital technology in patient management, collaboration among subspecialties can be facilitated with greater convenience and efficiency. Telemedicine sessions with (distantly located) nephrology and consultation-liaison psychiatry with local clinical laboratory and primary care physician management will become increasingly normative. Use of patient-friendly apps could further assist in gathering data regarding psychiatric symptom burden, as well as track data required for transplant work-up. The combination of using apps, electronic medical charting, as well as other digital platforms creates greater opportunity to manage psychiatric issues "collectively and effectively."

Paralleling the rapid evolution of evidence-based psychiatric care, psychiatric symptom assessment tools (both in-person and virtually) will be used increasingly routinely. These include but are not limited to the Montreal Cognitive Assessment (MoCA), Patient Health Questionnaire (PHQ-9), Hamilton Depression Rating Scale (Ham-D), and Generalized Anxiety Disorder (GAD-7). Within psychonephrology, specifically, further development of objective and numerical assessments of medication compliance, delirium screening tools, standardized protocols for informed consent, and psychiatric assessment of transplant candidacy would be encouraged.

Other areas of likely clinical evolution pertinent to the integrated practice of psychonephrology include artificial intelligence (AI) applications and high-level data management applications. These may include "big data sourcing" for clinical research and protocol development, coordination of transplant candidacy across transplant centers, monitoring of substance use/drug screening, and facilitated interface among services in nephrology, psychiatry, other mental health clinicians, primary care clinicians, and social work. This may prove to be especially helpful where kidney transplant centers have a wide geographic catchment area that requires centralized data management.

24.4 Key Takeaways

- Over the last decade, there has been a push toward the integration of behavioral health and general medicine services, as it has been shown to improve patient outcomes, reduce healthcare utilization, and reduce stigma associated with mental health care.
- By offering formal training in psychonephrology, the collaborative care model would be strengthened and therefore adopted in other subspecialties.

- Fellows in both psychiatry and nephrology would have increased competence in the prevention, evaluation, and management of psychiatric aspects of nephrology, including kidney transplant, disorders of the aging kidney, renal and psychopharmacology, and decisional capacity around life-prolonging technologies and end-of-life care.
- By introducing a formal psychonephrology curriculum, the next generation of nephrologists and psychiatrists would be better prepared to offer care that is more comprehensive and holistic.

References

1. Bourgeois JA, Hategan A, Eppel AB. Psychiatry of the future – 2030 and beyond. Journal of Psychiatry Reform. Vol 8 #6, July 27, 2020. ISSN 2371-4301. https://journalofpsychiatryreform.com/2020/07/27/psychiatry-of-the-future-2030-and-beyond/. Accessed 17 Apr 2021.
2. Dalen JE, Ryan KJ, Alpert JS. More sub-subs are coming! Am J Med. 2019;132(2):132–3.
3. Simoes E, Silva AC, Miranda AS, Rocha NP, Teixeira AL. Neuropsychiatric disorders in chronic kidney disease. Front Pharmacol. 2019;10:932.
4. Kimmel PL, Fwu CW, Abbott KC, et al. Psychiatric illness and mortality in hospitalized ESKD dialysis patients. Clin J Am Soc Nephrol. 2019;14(9):1363–71.
5. Sharaf El Din UA, Salem MM, Abdulazim DO. Stop chronic kidney disease progression: time is approaching. World J Nephrol. 2016;5(3):258–73.
6. APA, APM. Dissemination of integrated care within adult primary care settings: The collaborative care model. American Psychiatric Association, Academy of Psychosomatic Medicine; 2016. https://www.psychiatry.org/psychiatrists/practice/professional-interests/integrated-care/learn. Accessed 17 Apr 2021.
7. Huang H, Forstein M, Joseph R. Developing a collaborative care training program in a psychiatry residency. Psychosomatics. 2017;58(3):245–9.

Index

A. Hategan et al. (eds.), *Psychonephrology*,
https://doi.org/10.1007/978-3-030-84740-1

T

GPSR Compliance

The European Union's (EU) General Product Safety Regulation (GPSR) is a set of rules that requires consumer products to be safe and our obligations to ensure this.

If you have any concerns about our products, you can contact us on ProductSafety@springernature.com

In case Publisher is established outside the EU, the EU authorized representative is:

Springer Nature Customer Service Center GmbH
Europaplatz 3
69115 Heidelberg, Germany

Batch number: 10777424

Printed by Printforce, the Netherlands